AF759461

Anorectal Disorders - From Diagnosis to Treatment

Edited by Alberto Vannelli

Published in London, United Kingdom

Anorectal Disorders - From Diagnosis to Treatment
http://dx.doi.org/10.5772/intechopen.111137
Edited by Alberto Vannelli

Contributors
Ajit Naniksingh Kukreja, Andrea Pierre Luzzi, Antonio d'Alessandro, Anup Chalise, Bhupesh Dewan, Bishnu P. Kandel, Branko Branković, Béatrice Vinson-Bonnet, Chris Gillespie, Dimitrios Christoforidis, Erin Santos, Goran Stanojević, Guilherme Macedo, Isabel Garrido, Jeffrey Van Eps, Jerry Xiao, Jiawei Zhao, Jinshi Huang, João Afonso, Juaquito M. Jorge, Li-Hua Fang, Marianne Cusick, Michael Eisenberg, Mihai-Teodor Georgescu, Milica Nestorović, Nana-Yaw Bonsu, Nathalie Mantilla, Nikola Milutinović, Rosa Coelho, Salahedin Delshad, Satyadeep Bhattacharya, Shweta Kondekar, Siddheshwar Shinde, Sotirios-Georgios Popeskou, Tommaso Cipolat Mis, Valeria Basso, Weihong Guo, Woihwan Kim, Yanan Zhang, Yu Xiong

© The Editor(s) and the Author(s) 2024

The rights of the editor(s) and the author(s) have been asserted in accordance with the Copyright, Designs and Patents Act 1988. All rights to the book as a whole are reserved by INTECHOPEN LIMITED. The book as a whole (compilation) cannot be reproduced, distributed or used for commercial or non-commercial purposes without INTECHOPEN LIMITED's written permission. Enquiries concerning the use of the book should be directed to INTECHOPEN LIMITED rights and permissions department (permissions@intechopen.com).

Violations are liable to prosecution under the governing Copyright Law.

Individual chapters of this publication are distributed under the terms of the Creative Commons Attribution 3.0 Unported License which permits commercial use, distribution and reproduction of the individual chapters, provided the original author(s) and source publication are appropriately acknowledged. If so indicated, certain images may not be included under the Creative Commons license. In such cases users will need to obtain permission from the license holder to reproduce the material. More details and guidelines concerning content reuse and adaptation can be found at http://www.intechopen.com/copyright-policy.html.

Notice

Statements and opinions expressed in the chapters are these of the individual contributors and not necessarily those of the editors or publisher. No responsibility is accepted for the accuracy of information contained in the published chapters. The publisher assumes no responsibility for any damage or injury to persons or property arising out of the use of any materials, instructions, methods or ideas contained in the book.

First published in London, United Kingdom, 2024 by IntechOpen
IntechOpen is the global imprint of INTECHOPEN LIMITED, registered in England and Wales, registration number: 11086078, 167-169 Great Portland Street, London, W1W 5PF, United Kingdom

British Library Cataloguing-in-Publication Data
A catalogue record for this book is available from the British Library

Additional hard and PDF copies can be obtained from orders@intechopen.com

Anorectal Disorders - From Diagnosis to Treatment
Edited by Alberto Vannelli
p. cm.
Print ISBN 978-1-83769-956-8
Online ISBN 978-1-83769-955-1
eBook (PDF) ISBN 978-1-83769-957-5

We are IntechOpen, the world's leading publisher of Open Access books

Built by scientists, for scientists

7,100+
Open access books available

188,000+
International authors and editors

205M+
Downloads

156
Countries delivered to

Our authors are among the
Top 1%
most cited scientists

12.2%
Contributors from top 500 universities

WEB OF SCIENCE™

Selection of our books indexed in the Book Citation Index in Web of Science™ Core Collection (BKCI)

Interested in publishing with us?
Contact book.department@intechopen.com

Numbers displayed above are based on latest data collected.
For more information visit www.intechopen.com

For EU product safety concerns:
IN TECH d.o.o., Prolaz Marije Krucifikse Kozulić 3, 51000 Rijeka, Croatia, info@intechopen.com or visit our website at intechopen.com.

Meet the editor

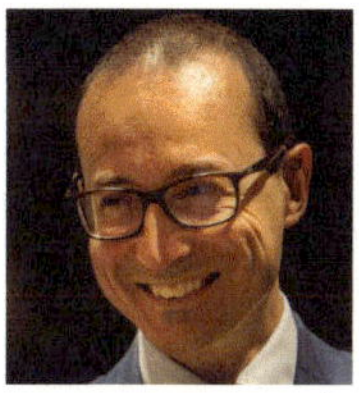

Dr. Vannelli completed medical school, postgraduate research and general surgical training in Milan, Italy before training in colorectal surgery at the National Cancer Institute. Currently, he is the Director of General Surgery at Valduce Hospital, Como, Italy. Dr. Vannelli is focused on advanced minimally invasive techniques, including multidisciplinary management of patients with colorectal cancers. Furthermore, his division is a referral center for colorectal disease and is well known for sphincter-saving procedures for rectal cancer and inflammatory bowel disease (IBD). In 2012, Dr. Vannelli founded Erone Onlus to assist cancer patients and their families. He collaborates with the School of Specialization in General Surgery at the Emergency Department of the University of Milan.

Contents

Preface

Benign anorectal disorders carry significant morbidity and place financial burden on the healthcare system. Benign anorectal disorders of structure and function are common in clinical practice. When a patient comes to your office with anorectal complaints, chances are that they have progressed to the point of extreme discomfort.

For any problem, performing a complete history and physical examination is mandatory. Information on bleeding, pain, discharge, swelling, changes in bowel habits, pruritus, prolapse, fever, incontinence, prior sexual contacts, and dyspareunia is valuable. Digital rectal and bimanual examinations are mandatory. Also important are sphincter tone, presence of gross blood, and presence or absence of hemorrhoids. Endoscopy (ano and proctoscopy) is among the possible diagnostic tests. Understanding anorectal anatomy is key to evaluating patients with benign anorectal disease. The anorectal area is the terminal portion of the lower gastrointestinal tract. It is a part of the pelvic district that includes urogenital organs and muscular, ligamentous, and connective tissue structures. As a functional unit, the anorectal area maintains fecal continence by acting as both a reservoir and an expulsion unit for feces.

The rectum has both intraperitoneal and extraperitoneal segments. The rectum begins at the confluence of the taeniae coli at the rectosigmoid junction. We commonly define the rectum as the last 12 cm above the anal verge. The anal canal is roughly 4 cm in length and extends from the anal verge to the proximal level of the levator-external anal sphincter complex. The sphincter mechanisms and the dentate line are of great importance when addressing the anal canal surgically.

The dentate line (pectinate line) is approximately 2 cm from the anal verge and is a place of transition from columnar epithelium (endoderm) to squamous epithelium (ectoderm). Between these layers is a transitional area called the cloacogenic zone. The dentate line is a line that divides the upper two-thirds and lower third of the anal canal. Developmentally, this line represents the hindgut proctodeum junction, an important landmark because of differences in innervation, blood supply, and lymphatic drainage of the anal canal; several distinctions and pathologies can be made based upon the location of a structure relative to this line. The anal glands, of which there are typically four to eight, empty into the anal canal at the base of the anal columns. These extend through the full thickness of the mucosa and submucosa and even into the muscularis externa. They are branched, straight tubular glands with ducts lined with stratified columnar epithelium, and their function is mucus secretion.

Moreover, during the physical examination temperature, body habitus, the abdomen, and the perineum need special attention.

This book summarizes the preferred approach to the evaluation and management of defecation disorders, proctalgia syndromes, hemorrhoids, anal fissures, and fecal incontinence in adults and children. Each section contains key concepts, recommendations, and summaries of the available evidence. Written by highly experienced physicians, the book provides detailed notes on optimal management of these disorders including pre- and post-operative management. Chapters cover the entire range of benign and malignant disorders, including hemorrhoids, fissures, fistula-in-ano, anorectal injuries, anal incontinence, rectal prolapse, pelvic floor disorders, and anal cancer.

Alberto Vannelli
Director of General Surgery,
Valduce Hospital,
Como, Italy

Section 1

Anal Cancer

Chapter 1

Anal Cancer Screening: Unveiling Its Importance

Isabel Garrido, João Afonso, Rosa Coelho and Guilherme Macedo

Abstract

Anal dysplasia, a precancerous condition of the anal canal, is increasingly recognized as a significant health concern, particularly among individuals with high-risk factors such as patients living with human immunodeficiency virus, men who have sex with men, a history of anogenital cancer, and immunosuppression. Screening for anal dysplasia has emerged as a critical measure for early detection and treatment, in order to prevent progression to invasive AC. This chapter provides an overview of anal dysplasia screening modalities, including anal cytology and high-resolution anoscopy, while discussing their benefits and limitations. The significance of risk stratification and prevention measures is also emphasized. The potential benefits of anal dysplasia screening in reducing the burden of anal cancer and improving patient outcomes are highlighted, along with the need for further research and comprehensive screening programs to optimize early detection and management of anal dysplasia.

Keywords: screening, anal dysplasia, anal cancer, anal cytology, high-resolution anoscopy, HPV, HIV, MSM, anus

1. Introduction

The anal cancer (AC) incidence has been rising in most of the developed countries, particularly in high-risk populations such as men who have sex with men (MSM), immunocompromised individuals, and patients infected with human papillomavirus (HPV) [1, 2]. Currently, the incidence of squamous cell carcinoma of the anus (SCCA) among MSM infected with human immunodeficiency virus (HIV) has surpassed the incidence of cervical cancer in women. Moreover, in contrast to other HIV-related neoplasia, the incidence of SCCA in patients living with HIV has been rising even after the advent of antiretroviral drugs, probably due to a longer life expectancy and an increase in the incidence of sexually transmitted infections (ISTs) [3, 4].

AC prevention works in two distinct phases. Primary prevention focuses on reducing the incidence of malignant and premalignant lesions, and secondary prevention focuses on the early diagnosis and treatment of those lesions [5].

Primary prevention can be accomplished through HPV vaccination. This should occur before HPV infection, at a targeted age of 11-12 years old, before sexual initiation. Adequate vaccination policies can prevent high-risk genotype infection, leading to a decrease of mucosal infection and reducing the carcinogenic cascade that is initiated by HPV infection [5].

Secondary prevention occurs through AC screening. Screening plays a major role in the early detection and prevention of AC and allows the timely diagnosis of precancerous lesions and early AC, thus enabling prompt intervention and treatment [5].

The first screening test, usually done through anal cytology, allows for the identification of high-risk patients. According to those results, patients with abnormal cytology are proposed to do a high-resolution anoscopy (HRA), which is the gold standard for the diagnosis and management of high-grade squamous intraepithelial lesions (HSIL) [6, 7].

This step-up approach allows for balanced resource management, limiting the number of patients that are submitted to a costly and time-consuming intervention and allowing for the monitoring of a higher number of patients.

The impact of AC screening was clearly demonstrated by the ANal Cancer/HSIL Outcomes Research (ANCHOR) trial, where patients living with HIV with anal HSIL were randomly assigned to receive treatment or active monitoring with HRA every 6 months. The primary endpoint was to evaluate the SCCA progression, and the study had to be terminated early due to a clear increase in SCCA in the monitoring group [5]. However, there is still some lack of information and guidelines on how to perform those screening programs.

Through this chapter, we intend to provide a practice-oriented and up-to-date review of the importance of AC screening with a brief description of the current guidelines published by several societies about AC screening programs. It reinforces who is most at risk and how screening should be performed. Finally, we describe the various treatment options for anal dysplasia, from topical therapies to surgical options.

2. Epidemiology of AC

AC is a relatively rare neoplasia with a worldwide incidence of 50,865 new cases per year, according to GLOBOCAN 2020. However, its incidence is rising worldwide, and it is estimated that in the USA alone, the number of new cases per year doubled from 2001 to 2015. This can be partially justified by STIs, including HPV infection, and the longer overall survival of people living with HIV [8].

The incidence of SCCA is not homogenously distributed throughout the population. There are some groups of individuals presenting with a higher risk of developing AC. HIV-infected patients, MSM, women with HPV-related gynecologic lesions, or solid-organ transplant recipients present a much higher incidence of SCCA and so represent a particularly important subset of individuals when referring to AC screening [9].

The highest risk group has been consistently demonstrated in different studies to be the group of patients that combined HIV infection and MSM, showing a synergistic effect between these two risk factors [9].

Before the HIV epidemic, it was estimated that the rate of AC MSM was as high as 37 cases per 100,000 individuals [10]. This incidence was comparable to the rate of cervical cancer in women before the introduction of cervical Papanicolaou smear screening. In HIV-positive MSM, the incidence of AC has been estimated to be roughly double that of HIV-negative MSM [11].

Moreover, compared to other cancers commonly found in HIV-positive individuals, such as Kaposi sarcoma and non-Hodgkin lymphoma, the occurrence of AC has not decreased with the advancement of potent antiretroviral therapy. As a matter of fact, a study demonstrated that the incidence of AC in males aged 40 to 64 years more than quadrupled from the pre-HIV era to the present era, despite the availability of effective antiretroviral therapy. Rates rose especially dramatically for San Francisco men ages 40 to 64, from 3.7 cases per 100,000 in 1973-1978 to 8.6 cases per 100,000 in 1984-1990 and 20.6 cases per 100,000 in 1996-1999 [12].

Other immunosuppressive conditions such as solid-organ transplant recipients or some patients with autoimmune diseases may have a similar effect, mainly due to a higher HPV replication [9].

Less is known about the epidemiology and natural history of SCCA in patients with inflammatory bowel disease. A systematic review that included 11 studies from 1940 to 2005 revealed that the incidence of SCCA was 0.02 per 1000 patient-years in patients with Crohn's disease and 0.009 per 1000 patient-years in patients with ulcerative colitis, similar to that of the general population [13]. The majority of the cases were diagnosed in the context of long-standing Crohn's disease (>10 years) and underlying chronic perianal disease. Indeed, patients with chronic perianal Crohn's disease may be at increased risk of developing SCCA [14]. However, studies are scarce and have conflicting results [15].

3. Current guideline recommendations for AC screening

The level of evidence on the different guidelines addressing this issue is generally low, with some of the statements resulting from expert opinions without clear data supporting them. However, some general rules are common to the different organizations that issued guidelines on the topic.

The low prevalence of AC in the general population is low and so, no organization recommends a global screening program outside the scope of high-risk populations.

Therefore, the screening programs are restricted to high-risk groups such as people living with AIDS (PLW), MSM, and women with genital HPV-related lesions. There is not enough evidence to include immunocompromised patients without other risk factors in the screening program, so no organization recommends routine screening of those patients.

Most guidelines do not specify the screening starting age, except the guidelines issued by the New York State Department of Health AIDS Institute (NYSDHAI) on March 2020 that stated that screening should start annually at 35 years old in every HIV-positive patient and before that, only in the presence of anal signs or symptoms [16]. In **Table 1**, the authors resumed the latest and most important guidelines about AC screening.

Also, the screening method varies between societies (**Table 1**), but most state that visual inspection and digital anorectal examination (DARE) should be done yearly, and cytology should also be performed in centers with HRA availability.

In case of abnormal pathological results, patients should undergo HRA and biopsy if possible, and visible lesions should be managed accordingly.

Society	Title	Year	Patient populations	Screening methodology	Age
American Society of Colon & Rectal Surgeons (ASCRS) [17]	"Anal Squamous Cell Cancers"	2018	High-risk population: PLWH; Genital HPV-related disorders; MSM	Anal cytology: Considered in high-risk patients with or without HPV testing	Not defined
American Society of Transplantation Infectious Diseases Community of Practice (ASTIDCP) [18]	"Human papillomavirus infection in solid-organ transplant recipients: Guidelines from the American Society of Transplantation Infectious Diseases Community of Practice"	2019	Solid-organ transplant recipients if there is a history of receptive anal intercourse or cervical dysplasia.	Anal cytology: • If normal repeat for 1-3 years • If abnormal, perform HRA	Not defined
AIDS Study Group (GeSIDA) of the Spanish Society of Infectious Diseases and Clinical Microbiology [19]	"Executive summary of the GeSIDA consensus document on control and monitoring of HIV-infected patients"	2019	PLWH; PLWH + risk factors: MSM Genital HPV-related disorders; Genital warts	Anal symptoms inquiry; Anal examination and digital anorectal examination (DARE) in every PLWH; Anal cytology in high-risk patients HRA if abnormal cytology	NA
HIV Medicine Association of the Infectious Diseases Society of America (HIVMA/IDSA) [20]	"Primary Care Guidance for Persons With Human Immunodeficiency Virus: 2020 Update by the HIV Medicine Association of the Infectious Diseases Society of America"	2020	PLWH; PLWH + risk factors: Receptive anal intercourse Abnormal Pap test Genital wards	Cytology in high-risk patients HRA if abnormal cytology	NA
New York State Department of Health AIDS Institute. (NYSDHAI) [16]	"Screening for Anal Dysplasia and Cancer in Adults With HIV"	2020	PLWH	AC screening in every patient - > Decision on cytology, patient based; HRA if abnormal cytology	≥35 years old

AC—anal cancer; HPV—human papillomavirus; HIV—human immunodeficiency virus; HPV—human papillomavirus; HIV—human immunodeficiency virus; NA—Not applicable; PLWH—People living with HIV.

Table 1.
Guidelines recommendations regarding AC screening.

4. Who is most at risk?

Many risk factors for anal squamous intraepithelial lesions and AC are described, such as sexual behavior, HIV, and iatrogenic immunosuppression. **Table 2** provides an overview of the patient populations that are most vulnerable to developing AC.

The screening benefit and risk ratio for detecting anal HSIL has not been established for any of the groups listed in this table. However, recently the ANCHOR trial,

Risk factor	Risk or IR of developing AC
People living with HIV (PLWHIV) [21]	IR (cases per 100,000 person-years) MSMLWH IR: 85 (82-89) MLWH (non-MSM) IR: 32 (30-35) Females: 22 (19-24)
Men who have sex with men [21]	IR (cases per 100,000 person-years) MSM without HIV IR: 19 (10-36)
Women with a history of cervical, vulvar, or vaginal SIL (also termed intraepithelial neoplasia) or cancer [21]	IR (cases per 100,000 person-years) Cervical cancer IR: 9 (8-12) Cervical precancerous lesions: 6 (5-7) Vaginal cancer IR: 10 (3-30) Vaginal precancerous lesions: 19 (9-43) Vulvar cancer IR: 48 (38-61) Vulvar precancerous lesions: 42 (33-52)
Individuals with a history of anogenital warts (AW) [22]	Risk of AC: Previous history of AW: 17 of 383 (4.4%) vs. Without AW: 17 of 6132 (0.3%) (P < .001)
Iatrogenic immunosuppression	
Solid-organ transplant recipients [21]	IR (cases per 100,000 person-years) IR: 13 (12-15) By ten years posttransplant: IR: 24.5 (males) and 49.6 (for females)
Other immunocompromised individuals without HIV infection (long-term oral corticosteroids) [21]	IR (cases per 100,000 person-years) SLE: was 10 (95% CI 5-19) UC IR: 6 (95% CI 3-11) CD IR: 3 (95% CI 2-4)
Smoking [23]	RR 1.9 for 20 pack-years RR 5.2 for 50 pack-years
Age [24]	The incidence of AC increases by 2.7% per year, with pronounced increases in age groups 50 years and older
Gender [25]	AC incidence in women vs. men: 2.52 versus 1.26 per 100,000 people

CD—Crohn's disease; HIV—human immunodeficiency virus; IR—incidence rates; MSMLWH—Male sex male who are living with HIV; MLWH—males living with HIV; RR—relative risk; SLE—systemic lupus erythematosus; SIL—squamous intraepithelial lesions; UC—ulcerative colitis.

Table 2.
Risk factors and the estimated risk or IR of developing AC according to each group.

as previously described, strongly supports the importance of screening and early identification of HSIL in high-risk individuals [5].

4.1 People living with HIV (PLWHIV)

It is not clear whether HIV infection itself has a direct effect on the development of AC or if this is mediated through HPV infection. However, the incidence of dysplastic lesions and AC is higher in males living with HIV (MLWH), particularly MSM who are living with HIV. It has also been demonstrated that PLWHIV has a higher risk of progression from low-grade squamous intraepithelial lesions (LSIL) to HSIL and AC [9]. It is also important to emphasize that the incidence of HPV infection and HPV-associated preinvasive and invasive malignancy is higher in PLWH, regardless of sexual practice [26]. Moreover, a meta-analysis that included a total of 53 studies showed that the prevalence of both high-risk anal HPV subtypes and AC was significantly higher among MSMLWH as compared with MSM without HIV [3].

4.2 MSM

There have been multiple studies showing a high prevalence of anal HSIL in MSM, both with and without HIV. In fact, MSM are considered at increased risk of developing AC compared with males who do not have sex with men. Moreover, the number of sexual partners and a history of anal-receptive intercourse are associated with anal SIL in this population [18].

4.3 HPV-related gynecological diseases

Women with HPV-related gynecological precancerous lesions or cancer are those in which HPV plays a significant role in the pathophysiology. This group includes cervical cancer, which is nearly entirely dependent on HPV infection, and vaginal and vulvar cancer, which are related to HPV infection in about 78 and 24.9% of cases, respectively, along with the corresponding precancerous lesions [21]. Women with a history of HPV-related disease have a significantly increased risk of anal intraepithelial neoplasia (AIN) and AC. Survivors of vulvar cancer have the highest risk of developing AC, followed by vaginal survivors and cervical cancer survivors. In light of this information, it is evident that patients who have received treatment for HPV-related diseases should be closely monitored to prevent the occurrence of another HPV-related illness [27].

4.4 HPV infection

The most commonly diagnosed sexually transmitted infection in the USA is HPV infection, and there is a close link between HPV infections, particularly patients infected with high oncogenic strains, such as HPV 16 and 18, and the development of genital and AC. Epidemiologic studies link more than 90% of squamous cell carcinoma cases to HPV infection, and their presence is higher in patients with concomitant HIV infection [9]. Therefore, it is not surprising that there is a strong correlation between the presence of anal squamous intraepithelial lesions and the prevalence of anal HPV infection. Studies have shown that as the severity of anal SIL increase, the prevalence of HPV also increases. Specifically, HPV type 16 is strongly associated with high-grade SIL and invasive AC [28].

However, it is important to highlight that HPV infection is necessary but insufficient for the development of squamous intraepithelial lesions, including HSIL. Moreover, not all cases of anal HPV infection, including those with high-risk (hr)-HPV types, result in anal squamous intraepithelial lesions [29]. Therefore, a full understanding of the factors that dictate the development of HSIL in the presence of hr-HPV infection remains elusive.

4.5 Genital warts

A longitudinal cohort study of 6515 PLWHIV concluded that a previous history of anogenital warts is associated with a higher risk of developing AC. After adjusting for covariates, the odds of developing AC were 12.79 (95% CI, 6.19-26.45; $P < .001$) times higher in individuals with a history of anogenital warts compared with individuals without a history of anogenital warts [22]. Moreover, it seems that the presence of perianal warts is a suitable risk marker for anal HPV 16 detection and anal dysplasia [30].

4.6 Iatrogenic immunosuppression

- **Solid-organ transplant recipients:** Other causes of chronic immunosuppression, such as solid-organ transplantation, also may be associated with the development of high-grade SIL and invasive AC. For example, among renal transplant recipients, the risk of anogenital cancer has been associated with persistent HPV infection [31, 32].

- **Other immunocompromised individuals without HIV infection**: Autoimmune diseases such as inflammatory bowel disease and systemic lupus erythematosus seem to be a risk factor for AC, probably due to chronic glucocorticoid therapy [21].

4.7 Smoking

It increases the risk of developing AC. In fact, several case–control studies demonstrated a statistically significant risk of AC in smokers, especially current smokers [33]. In one series, cigarette smoking was associated with a significantly increased risk of AC. Moreover, cigarette smoking is highly associated with cervical neoplasia and is thought to act as a cocarcinogen for anogenital squamous cell carcinoma [34].

4.8 Gender

AC incidence is the highest in women compared to men and is rising more rapidly in women compared to men (28.6 versus 13.5%, respectively), considering data from England between 2013 and 2017 [25]. Moreover, females are more likely to present late with advanced cancers, taking into consideration data from the Surveillance, Epidemiology and End Results Program (SEER) demonstrated that women are more likely to present with advanced staging, receive radiotherapy, and die of AC [35].

5. Screening techniques: from anal cytology to HRA

Anal HSIL is typically a not palpable lesion; therefore, it is unlikely to be diagnosed or suspected on routine DARE. The AC screening programs have relied on cytology as the initial screening examination. In the presence of an abnormal cytology result (e.g., LSIL, atypical squamous cells of undetermined significance (ASCUS) or HSIL), the anal canal and perianal area should be observed with HRA in order to identify areas of potential HSIL that should be confirmed by biopsy. These precancerous lesions could be properly treated to prevent AC.

It is crucial to note that screening should only be offered to at-risk populations if there is local expertise in interpreting screening results and if there is a referral system in place for HRA with biopsy, as well as access to ablative treatments and follow-up care.

5.1 Anal cytology

This procedure involves the insertion of a swab in the anal canal (without direct visualization), allowing the collection of epithelial cells from the lower rectum, squamocolumnar transformation zone, and anal canal. It is typically done using a moistened polyester fiber swab (**Figure 1**), which is preferred over a cotton swab because it releases the collected cells more easily and has a plastic shaft that does not break during the procedure. In fact, it is not advisable to use cotton swabs with marked or wooden sticks because they may fracture.

After insertion of the swab, the cloth is removed with sideways force, employing a rotating movement to obtain samples from all sides of the anal canal, and then, the material is transferred to a liquid transport medium (ethanol or processed using a liquid cytology technique) to be analyzed.

To obtain the maximum number of cells and preserve their original appearance, anal cytology sampling should be conducted before DARE or anoscopy.

The cytological changes are reported using the Bethesda nomenclature, as negative for squamous intraepithelial lesions (NILM), atypical squamous cells of undetermined significance (ASCUS), low-grade SIL (LSIL), atypical squamous cells cannot exclude high-grade SIL (ASC-H), and high-grade SIL (HSIL) [36].

Although clinician-collected samples are the standard practice, self-collected anal cytology may be an option to increase patient compliance and reduce the cost of screening. However, a study performed to compare these two procedures concluded that the sensitivity of cytology to detect AIN is higher for clinician-collected versus self-collected specimens [37].

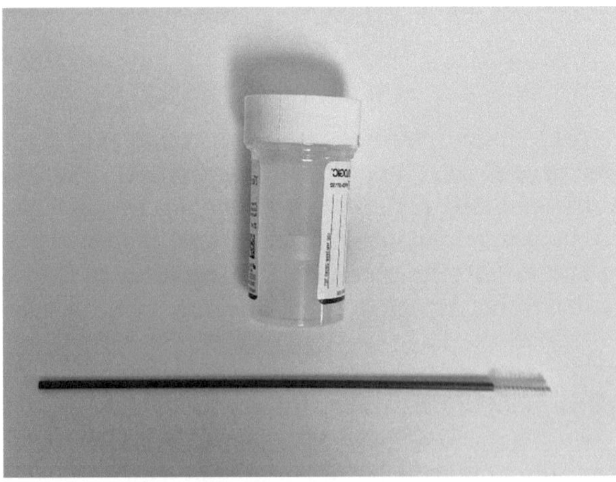

Figure 1.
Polyester fiber swab and transport medium.

A recent systematic review and meta-analysis that included a total of 18 studies described the performance of anal cytology (any abnormality as a threshold) to detect HSIL, in PLWH, with a sensitivity of 82% and specificity of 45% [38]. The positive predictive value was 36%, and the negative predictive value was 87%. These results align with previous studies that consider any cytologic abnormality, including ASCUS, as a referral threshold for HRA [38]. However, limited resources prevent HRA from being performed on all at-risk individuals. Therefore, cytology helps to prioritize those who would benefit most from HRA, starting with individuals with HSIL and then those with LSIL.

5.2 High-resolution anoscopy

It should be performed after an abnormal anal cytology screening test to visualize the anal and perianal regions using a colposcope (**Figure 2**). Compared with cervical colposcopy, HRA presents several additional challenges such as uneven topography, obscuring of lesions due to hemorrhoids, folds or presence of stools, or lesions being located at the base of folds and anal glands. Therefore, a long learning curve is typically required before becoming fully competent in this technique [39].

HRA is usually performed without previous bowel preparation in the left lateral position (fetal position); however, other positions are acceptable as well. After the insertion of an anoscope, a systematic inspection of the squamocolumnar junction, the anal canal, and the perianal skin with no staining should be performed.

Figure 3 illustrates that the anal canal is divided into distal/proximal regions: distal rectum, squamocolumnar junction, dentate line, mid-canal, distal canal, and anal verge. The perianal skin should also be visualized by gentle retraction of the buttocks and is considered the area that extends 5 cm laterally from the anal margin [40].

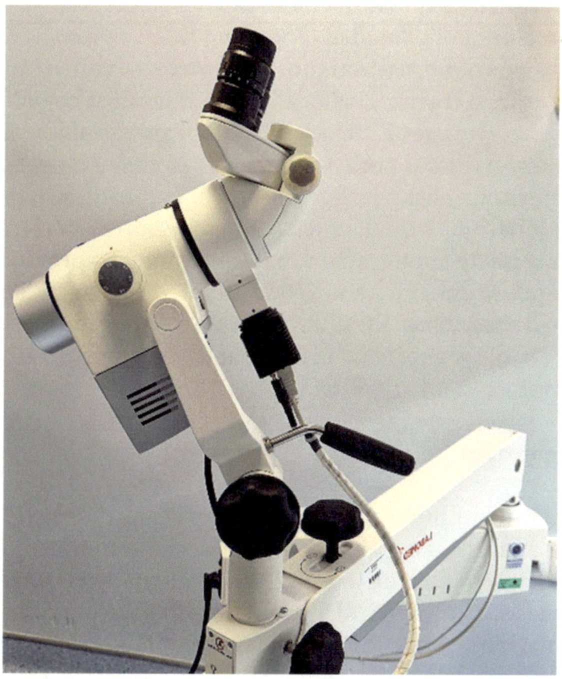

Figure 2.
Colposcope: High-resolution mobile microscope.

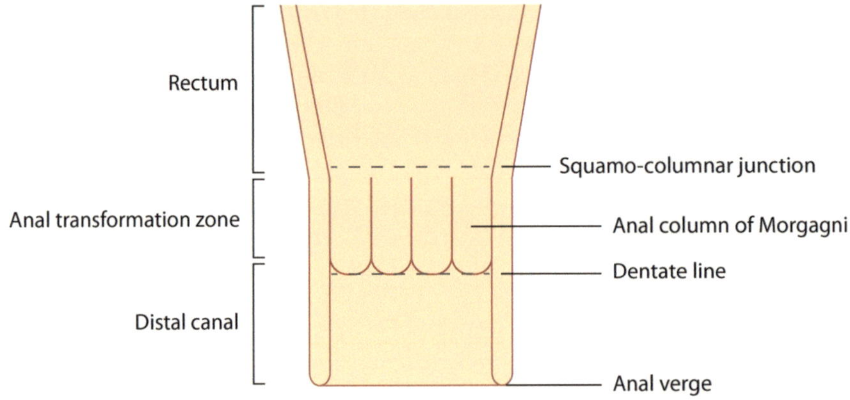

Figure 3.
Basic anatomy of the ana canal.

Subsequently, in order to aid detection of lesions that represent the source of abnormal cells on cytology screening a 4 × 4 gauze swab with acetic acid (3 or 5%) and Lugol iodine solutions should be applied. The anal verge is viewed with 10× magnification, but most of the visualization of the anal canal is done under 16× magnification. Specific areas of interest can be observed under 25× magnification for better characterization [40].

The anoscopic changes most often associated with HSIL include acetowhite change (acetic acid produces a white appearance in areas of abnormal transitional epithelium) on flat/slightly raised or thickened epithelium, with or without abnormal blood vessels (mosaic pattern/punctuation). Regarding Lugol iodine staining, lesions considered highly suspicious for HSIL do not take up Lugol stain.

After the HRA technique, a detailed report should be performed describing all highly suspicious lesions observed and those that were submitted to macrobiopsy. Lesions must be described concerning localization that must be independent of the position of the patient. The use of "o'clock" terminology should be avoided wherever possible as it depends on the patient's position (left lateral, prone, or lithotomy position). Therefore, the correct description must include the following topographies: anterior, posterior, left/right lateral, or left/right anterior/posterior. Lesion location can additionally be recorded in the anal canal concerning its proximal/distal extent as at/near the squamocolumnar junction, mid-canal, distal canal, and perianal area. Lesions should also be described considering contour, margins, acetic acid-induced whitening, Lugol's staining, epithelial pattern, and vascular pattern (mosaic pattern, punctation, warty vessels, and atypical) [40].

5.3 Molecular diagnostics

Despite the potential of molecular diagnostic tests like hr-HPV DNA detection, HPV E6/E7 mRNA analysis, and P16INK4a and Ki-67 immunostaining, their superiority over anal cytology in diagnosing anal HSIL has not been proven in the most studied risk groups (MSM and MSMLWH). Thus, their use is not recommended in these populations. However, these tests may be more effective in other at-risk groups with a lower prevalence of anal hr-HPV. In such cases, a significant number of individuals would test negative for hr-HPV and would not require further evaluation.

Considering the limitations of anal cytology, there has been significant interest in using molecular techniques to identify anal HSIL. Testing for hr-HPV subtypes has been extensively researched; however, it does not seem to improve HSIL detection and should not replace anal cytology as a standard screening test for HIV-infected MSM [41]. Moreover, a meta-analysis published in 2019 showed that hr-HPV DNA detection had poor specificity and positive predictive value, making it unsuitable for triage [38]. Recently, Chiao EY et al. demonstrated that 2 hr-HPV tests (Aptima and Hybrid Capture 2 method) showed similar sensitivity to abnormal anal cytology in predicting anal HSIL in females with HIV [42].

Besides not being included in AC screening techniques, it is important to highlight the value of patient education. Healthcare providers should educate high-risk individuals about the signs and symptoms of AC, emphasizing the importance of reporting any abnormalities promptly. Common symptoms may include anal bleeding, persistent anal itching, pain or pressure in the anal area, and changes in bowel habits.

6. Interpretation of screening results: how to manage a patient

Anal dysplasia screening has relied on cytology as the initial screening test. Cytology is reported, in order of increasing severity, as negative for squamous intraepithelial lesions, atypical squamous cells of undetermined significance (ASCUS), low-grade squamous intraepithelial lesions (LSIL), and high-grade squamous intraepithelial lesions (HSIL).

Anal cytology has a sensitivity of 70% for the detection of squamous intraepithelial lesions or the presence of any abnormality [43]. However, it has a low specificity (34%) for HSIL prediction in a subsequent biopsy, meaning it cannot determine that the lesion

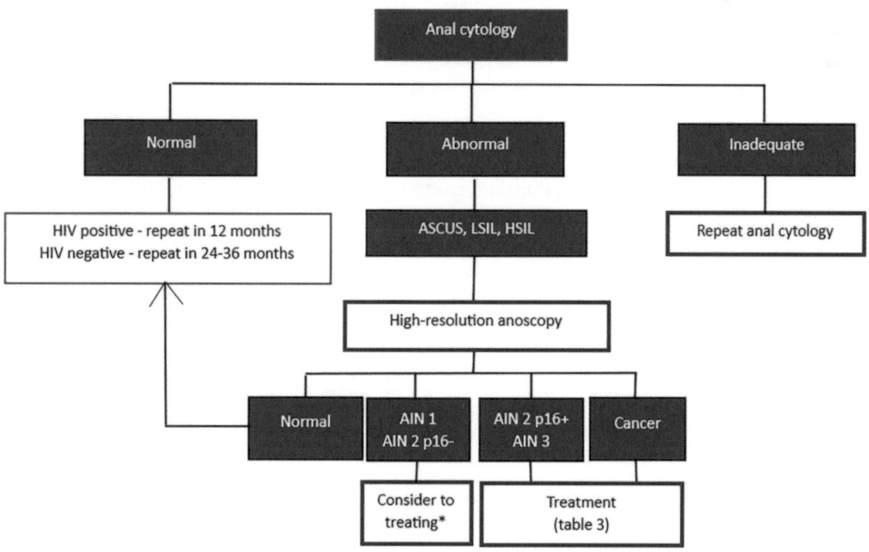

Figure 4.
*Algorithm for anal dysplasia screening. HIV—Human immunodeficiency virus, ASCUS—Atypical squamous cells of undetermined significance, LSIL—Low-grade squamous intraepithelial lesions, HSIL—High-grade squamous intraepithelial lesions, AIN—Anal intraepithelial neoplasia. *if the patient has symptoms (burning, itching, bleeding) or anxiety about the conservative strategy.*

will not be high-grade on histology. Indeed, a cytologic diagnosis of ASCUS and LSIL may have a significant risk (60 to 91%) of anal high-grade dysplasia at biopsy [44].

Therefore, an abnormal anal cytology screening test should be followed by an HRA for a diagnostic biopsy [16]. The grading of anal intraepithelial neoplasia (AIN) can only be performed by histopathological examination. AIN I and AIN II refer to nuclear abnormalities confined to the lower one-third and lower two-thirds of the epithelium, respectively, and these lesions are considered to be low-grade dysplasia. AIN III is full-thickness involvement of the epithelium and represents high-grade dysplasia or carcinoma *in situ*. Treatment should be started according to the results obtained (*vide infra*). On the other hand, abnormal anal cytology test results without abnormal histology should prompt repeat cytologic testing (**Figure 4**).

It is also important to note that screened individuals with normal anal cytology should repeat anal cytology at regular intervals: annually in HIV-positive patients and less frequently in HIV-negative individuals [45].

7. Anal dysplasia treatment

The optimal management of AIN is difficult to determine as data on the relative efficacy of different treatment agents are limited. The decision to treat and the form of treatment also depend on the size of the lesion, the location of the lesion and the goals of treatment.

Usually, low-grade dysplasia (AIN I and AIN II p16-negative) is managed expectantly with regular follow-up [46, 47]. This conservative approach is based on the overall low rate of disease progression to invasive cancer and the increased morbidity associated with local excision. Recommendations on surveillance strategies are discordant, ranging from a 6-monthly physical examination to an annual anoscopy with biopsy [48]. Nevertheless, if the patient has symptoms (burning, itching, bleeding) or anxiety about the conservative strategy, treatment may be performed. On the other hand, when high-grade lesions are identified (AIN 2 p16-positive and AIN 3), treatment is indicated due to a higher risk of progression for cancer.

Treatment aims to minimize symptoms and prevent the development of AC [49]. It may include immunomodulation therapies, ablative therapies, or surgical excision, which should be performed by a clinician with expertise in managing anal dysplasia (**Table 3**).

	Advantages	Disadvantages
Topical therapies		
Imiquimod (5%) cream	Topical treatment self-applied by patient	Off-label use Limited data
5-fluorouracil (5%) cream	Topical treatment self-applied by patient	Off-label use
Topical trichloroacetic acid	Safe during pregnancy	Off-label use Repeated office visits Useful only for small lesions or nonbulky disease
Ablative therapies		
Electrocautery/hyfrecation	Less serious side effects compared with topical treatments	High recurrence rate

	Advantages	Disadvantages
Infrared coagulation	Effective procedure	More serious adverse side effects High rates of persistent HSIL and metachronous lesions
Argon plasma coagulation	Effective and safe procedure	High recurrence rate Equipment cost
Radiofrequency ablation	Lower rates of recurrence	Limited data
Cryotherapy	Mild side effects	High recurrence rate
Surgery	Treatment choice for carcinoma *in situ*	Risk of anal stenosis More morbidity associated

Table 3.
Treatment of anal squamous intraepithelial lesions.

7.1 Immunomodulation therapies

Topical therapies are commonly used off-label to treat HSIL. Although there are many potential side effects of local therapies, most are very well tolerated, with only minimal symptoms experienced by the patient.

Imiquimod, 5% cream, is an immune modulator that has pro-inflammatory, anti-tumor, and antiviral activity through several subcellular mechanisms [50]. There are limited reports describing the efficacy of imiquimod for the treatment of anal HSIL. Nevertheless, patient-applied imiquimod appears to have efficacy against anal HSIL and is available by prescription [51]. In fact, it has been advocated by the majority of guidelines [46, 52, 53].

Topical *5-fluorouracil cream* is a pyrimidine analog, which inhibits DNA synthesis through the inhibition of the enzyme thymidylate synthase in neoplastic tissue. The most commonly used concentration for the treatment of anal HSIL is 5%. It causes erythema and edema followed by erosion, ulceration, and necrosis. It has been shown to preferentially treat neoplasms with only an inflammatory response on adjacent healthy skin. In addition, 5-fluorouracil has shown a good initial clinical response in the treatment of HSIL (59%), but recurrence may occur in up to 50% [54].

Topical trichloroacetic acid is caustic and corrodes the skin and mucous membranes. It treats HSIL by denaturing and precipitating proteins, resulting in tissue destruction [55]. Trichloroacetic acid is provider-applied in the office setting and has the advantage over other topical treatments of not requiring patient adherence other than repeated office visits for treatments. Four or five applications are typically needed to completely treat the lesion, usually spaced 3-4 weeks apart. Topical application of trichloroacetic acid is generally well tolerated but can occasionally be painful. It is the only topical treatment that is safe to use in pregnancy. However, trichloroacetic acid is unlikely to be effective in treating extensive or bulky diseases.

7.2 Ablative therapies

Ablative therapies include electrocautery/hyfrecation, argon plasma coagulation, infrared coagulation, cryotherapy, and radiofrequency ablation. Many of these therapies suffer from high recurrence rates, perhaps due to the persistence of HPV infection and because of the deep involvement of the perianal skin, which cannot be cleared by ablation.

Electrocautery is currently the treatment of choice for intra-anal HSIL in many centers. In an open-label randomized trial, Richel and colleagues showed that 58% of patients with AIN treated with electrocautery achieved a complete or partial response [56]. Indeed, electrocautery ablation of high-grade anal intraepithelial neoplasia is a safe office-based procedure. In addition, electrocautery was found to have less serious side effects, which were shorter in length in comparison with 5-fluorouracil cream and imiquimod. However, recurrence rates are substantial. For example, in a study of electrocautery in HIV-positive men, the recurrence rate was found to be 79% in 12 months, with an estimated recurrence risk approaching 100% by 50 months [57]. A separate study noted the following risk factors for persistent HSIL following hyfrecation: multiple index lesions, HIV viremia, cigarette smoking, and the presence of HPV-16/18 DNA [58].

Argon plasma coagulation can also be used to treat anal HSIL. A pilot study showed that argon plasma coagulation is comparable to other treatment modalities in terms of efficacy and safety in anal HSIL [59]. However, it requires repeated treatment because of a high recurrence rate. Pain is the main side effect, which requires appropriate attention and analgesia to be given to the patient during the procedure and in the following week.

Treatment of anal HSIL with *infrared coagulation* consists of the direct application of a pulse of irradiation in the infrared range to the anal epithelium, which results in tissue destruction. Depth of destruction is controlled by the length of pulse and healing occurs with minimal scarring. Possible procedure-related complications include immediate and delayed bleeding and infection. Multiple studies have demonstrated the safety and efficacy of infrared coagulation in patients with HSIL. For example, an open-label, randomized, multisite clinical trial of human HIV-infected adults proved that infrared coagulation ablation of anal canal HSIL was more likely to result in complete or partial resolution than active monitoring alone (62 vs. 30% at 1 year, risk difference 32, 95% CI 13-48%) [60]. It is worth noting, however, the relatively high rates of persistent HSIL within the treatment group at 1 year and the high number of metachronous HSIL.

Cryotherapy is an old technique that consists of office-based-guided liquid nitrogen application using a spray gun. It is capable of clearing HSIL. In fact, treatment success rates are comparable with those reported for current treatment modalities [61]. Side effects are common but mostly mild, of which anal pain or tenderness and mild blood loss are reported most frequently. Similar to other ablative therapies, HSIL recurrences are frequent (68%).

Radiofrequency energy delivered *via* electrodes creates a very superficial injury to the mucosa. It was effective in a small study performed at a single center [62]. However, studies of larger numbers of patients in different centers need to be performed before this technique is widely adopted in the field.

7.3 Surgery

A local surgical approach may be appropriate for selected small lesions and for carcinoma *in situ* [46]. Localized or focal AIN is defined as <30% anal circumference involved, whereas extensive AIN involves more than 30% circumference. Localized or focal AIN can be simply excised with the resulting wound left to granulate or sutured as appropriate. AIN III lesions involving more than 30% of the anal margin or canal cannot be excised as the risk of severe anal stenosis is significant, but excision of the most symptomatic area is possible. The remaining areas can then be observed at regular follow-up intervals.

Most studies describe preoperative mapping before excision, but this does not preclude recurrence. Indeed, recurrence of AIN III after local excision may appear to be more likely when resection margins are incomplete, but recurrence may occur even after microscopically complete excision. It is also important to note that aggressive treatment such as wide local excision can result in significant morbidity and therefore conservative management has been favored.

7.4 Chemoradiotherapy

Radiotherapy with concurrent chemotherapy is the current standard of care for patients with localized squamous cell cancer of the anal canal. The British guidelines state that extensive AIN III and AIN II at the margin of invasive cancers treated by chemoradiation disappear, suggesting that this treatment may have a place in patients with extensive AIN but risks causing anal stenosis [46]. Nevertheless, there is currently no literature on its use in AIN.

7.5 Anal cancer

The management of AC is beyond the scope of this chapter. Treatment modalities for AC may include radiation therapy, chemotherapy, excision, or combined modalities. The recommendations on the management of AC include the ESMO Clinical Practice Guidelines [63] and the American Society of Colon and Rectal Surgeons Clinical Practice Guidelines [17].

7.6 Surveillance

Due to the high rates of recurrence and evolving anal squamous intraepithelial lesions, surveillance is required following initial treatment. The appropriate follow-up of these patients remains an active area of investigation. Some authors suggest a follow-up in 4-6 months, including a repeat biopsy of the treatment site if there is lesion persistence. Anal cytology may also be useful as an adjunctive test to confirm lesion clearance [16].

8. Emerging trends and future directions in AC screening

A significant barrier to establishing recommendations for AC screening is the lack of evidence showing that it can reduce AC-associated morbidity and mortality. There are also few trials evaluating the efficacy of current treatment modalities as well as potential side effects and complications. Cost-effectiveness studies are also needed to justify implementing screening programs.

Identifying individuals at the highest risk of developing AC is crucial for effective screening. Researchers are exploring various risk stratification models based on factors such as HPV status, HIV infection, sexual behaviors, and immune status. These models aim to optimize screening protocols by tailoring them to individuals with the greatest likelihood of developing AC. Targeted screening strategies have the potential to improve the efficiency and cost-effectiveness of screening programs.

Screening for HPV infection has gained considerable attention as a potential method for early detection and prevention of AC [64]. Current research focuses on optimizing HPV testing methods and developing new approaches such as self-sampling kits for individuals who may feel uncomfortable with traditional sampling techniques. These advancements aim to increase screening uptake and improve the accuracy of HPV detection, ultimately reducing the burden of AC.

Advancements in imaging technologies, such as optical coherence tomography and molecular imaging, are being explored for their potential role in AC screening [65, 66]. These techniques offer noninvasive and real-time visualization of the anal canal, enabling the detection of early-stage lesions. Additionally, the identification of specific biomarkers associated with AC may aid in risk assessment and screening [67]. Ongoing research focuses on identifying reliable biomarkers that can be detected through minimally invasive methods.

As AC is strongly linked to HPV infection, the widespread administration of HPV vaccines presents an opportunity for primary prevention [68]. While HPV vaccination has primarily been promoted for the prevention of cervical cancer, its potential impact on AC prevention is significant. By reducing the prevalence of high-risk HPV infections, widespread HPV vaccination has the potential to substantially decrease the incidence of AC, particularly among populations at higher risk. Integrating HPV vaccination efforts with AC screening programs can further enhance the effectiveness of prevention strategies. Vaccination can complement screening by reducing the number of high-risk HPV infections, thereby lowering the incidence of precancerous and cancerous lesions in the anal canal. This combination approach of vaccination and screening holds promise for a comprehensive approach to AC prevention.

Continued research and collaboration between healthcare professionals, researchers, and policymakers are crucial to ensure the successful implementation of these emerging trends and the reduction of the global burden of AC.

9. Conclusion

Anal dysplasia screening plays a crucial role in the early detection and prevention of AC, particularly in high-risk populations. Identification of precancerous lesions will probably allow for a reduction in the incidence and mortality associated with AC. Anal cytology and high-resolution anoscopy have emerged as valuable tools for early detection and screening of this type of cancer. These methods have shown promise in identifying precancerous lesions and can guide further management, including the use of ablative or surgical treatments.

The implementation of anal dysplasia screening programs requires not only increased awareness among healthcare providers and patients but also the development of standardized guidelines for screening and management. Additionally, addressing barriers such as stigma, discomfort, and lack of knowledge is essential in promoting wider acceptance and uptake of screening practices. Through collaborative efforts and a commitment to research, we can make significant progress in preventing and managing anal dysplasia, thereby improving the health outcomes of at-risk populations.

Author details

Isabel Garrido[1,2*†], João Afonso[1,2†], Rosa Coelho[1,2] and Guilherme Macedo[1,2]

1 Gastroenterology and Hepatology Department, Centro Hospitalar Universitário de São João, Porto, Portugal

2 World Gastroenterology Organization (WGO) Porto Training Center, Porto, Portugal

*Address all correspondence to: isabelmng@hotmail.com

† Both authors contributed equally to the manuscript

IntechOpen

© 2023 The Author(s). Licensee IntechOpen. This chapter is distributed under the terms of the Creative Commons Attribution License (http://creativecommons.org/licenses/by/3.0), which permits unrestricted use, distribution, and reproduction in any medium, provided the original work is properly cited.

References

[1] Siegel RL, Miller KD, Wagle NS, Jemal A. Cancer statistics, 2023. CA: A Cancer Journal for Clinicians. 2023;**73**(1):17-48

[2] Damgacioglu H, Lin YY, Ortiz AP, Wu CF, Shahmoradi Z, Shyu SS, et al. State variation in squamous cell carcinoma of the anus incidence and mortality, and association with HIV/AIDS and smoking in the United States. Journal of Clinical Oncology: Official Journal of the American Society of Clinical Oncology. 2023;**41**(6):1228-1238

[3] Machalek DA, Poynten M, Jin F, Fairley CK, Farnsworth A, Garland SM, et al. Anal human papillomavirus infection and associated neoplastic lesions in men who have sex with men: A systematic review and meta-analysis. The Lancet Oncology. 2012;**13**(5):487-500

[4] Silverberg MJ, Lau B, Achenbach CJ, Jing Y, Althoff KN, D'Souza G, et al. Cumulative incidence of cancer among persons with HIV in North America: A cohort study. Annals of Internal Medicine. 2015;**163**(7):507-518

[5] Barroso LF, Stier EA, Hillman R, Palefsky J. Anal cancer screening and prevention: Summary of evidence reviewed for the 2021 centers for disease control and prevention sexually transmitted infection guidelines. Clinical Infectious Diseases: An Official Publication of the Infectious Diseases Society of America. 2022;**74**(Suppl_2):S179-SS92

[6] Bean SM, Chhieng DC. Anal-rectal cytology: The other PAP test. Laboratory Medicine. 2010;**41**(3):168-171

[7] Darragh TM, Colgan TJ, Thomas Cox J, Heller DS, Henry MR, Luff RD, et al. The lower Anogenital squamous terminology standardization project for HPV-associated lesions: Background and consensus recommendations from the College of American Pathologists and the American Society for Colposcopy and Cervical Pathology. International Journal of Gynecological Pathology: Official Journal of the International Society of Gynecological Pathologists. 2013;**32**(1):76-115

[8] Sung H, Ferlay J, Siegel RL, Laversanne M, Soerjomataram I, Jemal A, et al. Global cancer statistics 2020: GLOBOCAN estimates of incidence and mortality worldwide for 36 cancers in 185 countries. CA: A Cancer Journal for Clinicians. 2021;**71**(3):209-249

[9] Islami F, Ferlay J, Lortet-Tieulent J, Bray F, Jemal A. International trends in anal cancer incidence rates. International Journal of Epidemiology. 2017;**46**(3):924-938

[10] Daling JR, Weiss NS, Klopfenstein LL, Cochran LE, Chow WH, Daifuku R. Correlates of homosexual behavior and the incidence of anal cancer. Journal of the American Medical Association. 1982;**247**(14):1988-1990

[11] Melbye M, Coté TR, Kessler L, Gail M, Biggar RJ. High incidence of anal cancer among AIDS patients. The AIDS/cancer working group. Lancet (London, England). 1994;**343**(8898):636-639

[12] Cress RD, Holly EA. Incidence of anal cancer in California: Increased incidence among men in San Francisco, 1973-1999. Preventive Medicine. 2003;**36**(5):555-560

[13] Slesser AA, Bhangu A, Bower M, Goldin R, Tekkis PP. A systematic review of anal squamous cell carcinoma in inflammatory bowel disease. Surgical Oncology. 2013;**22**(4):230-237

[14] Wisniewski A, Fléjou JF, Siproudhis L, Abramowitz L, Svrcek M, Beaugerie L. Anal neoplasia in inflammatory bowel disease: Classification proposal, epidemiology, carcinogenesis, and risk management perspectives. Journal of Crohn's & Colitis. 2017;**11**(8):1011-1018

[15] Frisch M, Johansen C. Anal carcinoma in inflammatory bowel disease. British Journal of Cancer. 2000;**83**(1):89-90

[16] Hirsch BE, McGowan JP, Fine SM, Vail R, Merrick ST, Radix A, et al. New York State Department of Health AIDS institute clinical guidelines. In: Screening for Anal Dysplasia and Cancer in Adults with HIV [Internet]. Baltimore (MD): Johns Hopkins University; 2022 Aug 9

[17] Stewart DB, Gaertner WB, Glasgow SC, Herzig DO, Feingold D, Steele SR. The American Society of Colon and Rectal Surgeons clinical practice guidelines for anal squamous cell cancers (revised 2018). Diseases of the Colon and Rectum. 2018;**61**(7):755-774

[18] Chin-Hong PV, Reid GE. Human papillomavirus infection in solid organ transplant recipients: Guidelines from the American Society of Transplantation infectious diseases community of practice. Clinical Transplantation. 2019;**33**(9):e13590

[19] AIDS Study Group (GeSIDA) of the Spanish Society of Infectious Diseases and Clinical Microbiology. Executive summary of the GeSIDA consensus document on control and monitoring of HIV-infected patients. Enfermedades Infecciosas Microbiologia Clinica (English ed). 2019;**37**(7):467-475

[20] Thompson MA, Horberg MA, Agwu AL, Colasanti JA, Jain MK, Short WR, et al. Primary care guidance for persons with human immunodeficiency virus: 2020 update by the HIV medicine association of the infectious diseases society of America. Clinical infectious Diseases: An Official Publication of the Infectious Diseases Society of America. 2021;**73**(11):e3572-ee605

[21] Clifford GM, Georges D, Shiels MS, Engels EA, Albuquerque A, Poynten IM, et al. A meta-analysis of anal cancer incidence by risk group: Toward a unified anal cancer risk scale. International Journal of Cancer. 2021;**148**(1):38-47

[22] Arnold JD, Byrne ME, Monroe AK, Abbott SE. The risk of anal carcinoma after anogenital warts in adults living with HIV. JAMA Dermatology. 2021;**157**(3):283-289

[23] Holly EA, Whittemore AS, Aston DA, Ahn DK, Nickoloff BJ, Kristiansen JJ. Anal cancer incidence: Genital warts, anal fissure or fistula, hemorrhoids, and smoking. Journal of the National Cancer Institute. 1989;**81**(22):1726-1731

[24] Deshmukh AA, Suk R, Shiels MS, Sonawane K, Nyitray AG, Liu Y, et al. Recent trends in squamous cell carcinoma of the anus incidence and mortality in the United States, 2001-2015. Journal of the National Cancer Institute. 2020;**112**(8):829-838

[25] Brogden DRL, Kontovounisios C, Mandalia S, Tekkis P, Mills SC. The role of demographics, social deprivation and ethnicity on anal squamous cell carcinoma incidence in England. Journal of Clinical Medicine. 2021;**10**(16):3621

[26] Critchlow CW, Surawicz CM, Holmes KK, Kuypers J, Daling JR, Hawes SE, et al. Prospective study of high grade anal squamous intraepithelial neoplasia in a cohort of homosexual men: Influence of HIV infection, immunosuppression and human papillomavirus infection. AIDS (London, England). 1995;**9**(11):1255-1262

[27] Brzeziński M, Stukan M. Anal cancer and anal intraepithelial neoplasia risk among patients treated for HPV-related Gynecological diseases—A systematic. Review. 2023;**12**(13):4216

[28] Lin C, Franceschi S, Clifford GM. Human papillomavirus types from infection to cancer in the anus, according to sex and HIV status: A systematic review and meta-analysis. The Lancet Infectious Diseases. 2018;**18**(2):198-206

[29] Wilkin TJ, Chen H, Cespedes MS, Leon-Cruz JT, Godfrey C, Chiao EY, et al. A randomized, placebo-controlled trial of the quadrivalent human papillomavirus vaccine in human immunodeficiency virus-infected adults aged 27 years or older: AIDS clinical trials group protocol A5298. Clinical Infectious Diseases: An Official Publication of the Infectious Diseases Society of America. 2018;**67**(9):1339-1346

[30] Cerejeira A, Cunha S, Coelho R, Macedo G, Barkoudah E, Azevedo F, et al. Perianal warts as a risk marker for anal high-risk-human papillomavirus (HPV) detection and HPV-associated diseases. Journal of the European Academy of Dermatology and Venereology: JEADV. 2020;**34**(11):2613-2619

[31] Albuquerque A, Stirrup O, Nathan M, Clifford GM. Burden of anal squamous cell carcinoma, squamous intraepithelial lesions and HPV16 infection in solid organ transplant recipients: A systematic review and meta-analysis. American Journal of Transplantation: Official Journal of the American Society of Transplantation and the American Society of Transplant Surgeons. 2020;**20**(12):3520-3528

[32] Larsen HK, Hædersdal M, Thomsen LT, Hertzum-Larsen R, Lok TT, Bonde J, et al. Risk of anal high-grade squamous intraepithelial lesions among renal transplant recipients compared with immunocompetent controls. Clinical infectious Diseases: An Official publication of the Infectious Diseases Society of America. 2021;**73**(1):21-29

[33] Tseng HF, Morgenstern H, Mack TM, Peters RK. Risk factors for anal cancer: Results of a population-based case-control study. Cancer Causes & Control: CCC. 2003;**14**(9):837-846

[34] Daling JR, Sherman KJ, Hislop TG, Maden C, Mandelson MT, Beckmann AM, et al. Cigarette smoking and the risk of anogenital cancer. American Journal of Epidemiology. 1992;**135**(2):180-189

[35] Celie KB, Jackson C, Agrawal S, Dodhia C, Guzman C, Kaufman T, et al. Socioeconomic and gender disparities in anal cancer diagnosis and treatment. Surgical Oncology. 2017;**26**(2):212-217

[36] Wilbur DC, Nayar R. Bethesda 2014: Improving on a paradigm shift. Cytopathology: Official Journal of the British Society for Clinical Cytology. 2015;**26**(6):339-342

[37] Chin-Hong PV, Berry JM, Cheng SC, Catania JA, Da Costa M, Darragh TM, et al. Comparison of patient- and clinician-collected anal cytology samples to screen for human papillomavirus-associated anal intraepithelial neoplasia in men who have sex with men. Annals of Internal Medicine. 2008;**149**(5):300-306

[38] Dias Gonçalves Lima F, Viset JD, Leeflang MMG, Limpens J, Prins JM, de Vries HJC. The accuracy of anal swab-based tests to detect high-grade anal intraepithelial neoplasia in HIV-infected patients: A systematic review and meta-analysis. Open forum. Infectious Diseases. 2019;**6**(5):ofz191

[39] Palefsky JM. Practising high-resolution anoscopy. Sexual Health. 2012;**9**(6):580-586

[40] Hillman RJ, Cuming T, Darragh T, Nathan M, Berry-Lawthorn M, Goldstone S, et al. 2016 IANS international guidelines for practice standards in the detection of anal cancer precursors. Journal of Lower Genital Tract Disease. 2016;**20**(4):283-291

[41] Burgos J, Hernández-Losa J, Landolfi S, Guelar A, Dinares M, Villar J, et al. The role of oncogenic human papillomavirus determination for diagnosis of high-grade anal intraepithelial neoplasia in HIV-infected MSM. AIDS (London, England). 2017;**31**(16):2227-2233

[42] Chiao EY, Lensing SY, Wiley DJ, Deshmukh AA, Lee J, Darragh TM, et al. Screening strategies for the detection of anal high-grade squamous intraepithelial lesions in women living with HIV. AIDS (London, England). 2020;**34**(15):2249-2258

[43] Nathan M, Singh N, Garrett N, Hickey N, Prevost T, Sheaff M. Performance of anal cytology in a clinical setting when measured against histology and high-resolution anoscopy findings. AIDS (London, England). 2010;**24**(3):373-379

[44] Darragh TM, Winkler B. Anal cancer and cervical cancer screening: Key differences. Cancer Cytopathology. 2011;**119**(1):5-19

[45] Smyczek P, Singh AE, Romanowski B. Anal intraepithelial neoplasia: Review and recommendations for screening and management. International Journal of STD & AIDS. 2013;**24**(11):843-851

[46] Scholefield JH, Harris D, Radcliffe A. Guidelines for management of anal intraepithelial neoplasia. Colorectal Disease: The Official Journal of the Association of Coloproctology of Great Britain and Ireland. 2011;**13**(Suppl 1):3-10

[47] Svidler López L, La Rosa L. Human papilloma virus infection and anal squamous intraepithelial lesions. Clinics in Colon and Rectal Surgery. 2019;**32**(5):347-357

[48] Alam NN, White DA, Narang SK, Daniels IR, Smart NJ. Systematic review of guidelines for the assessment and management of high-grade anal intraepithelial neoplasia (AIN II/III). Colorectal Disease: The Official Journal of the Association of Coloproctology of Great Britain and Ireland. 2016;**18**(2):135-146

[49] Palefsky JM, Lee JY, Jay N, Goldstone SE, Darragh TM, Dunlevy HA, et al. Treatment of anal high-grade squamous intraepithelial lesions to prevent anal cancer. The New England Journal of Medicine. 2022;**386**(24):2273-2282

[50] Gkegkes ID, Iavazzo C, Stamatiadis AP. Intra-anal use of imiquimod: What is the clinical evidence? International Journal of STD & AIDS. 2019;**30**(10):1018-1024

[51] Kreuter A, Hochdorfer B, Stücker M, Altmeyer P, Weiland U, Conant MA,

et al. Treatment of anal intraepithelial neoplasia in patients with acquired HIV with imiquimod 5% cream. Journal of the American Academy of Dermatology. 2004;**50**(6):980-981

[52] Steele SR, Varma MG, Melton GB, Ross HM, Rafferty JF, Buie WD. Practice parameters for anal squamous neoplasms. Diseases of the Colon and Rectum. 2012;**55**(7):735-749

[53] Giani I, Mistrangelo M, Fucini C. The treatment of squamous anal carcinoma: Guidelines of the Italian Society of Colo-Rectal Surgery. Techniques in Coloproctology. 2013;**17**(2):171-179

[54] Richel O, Wieland U, de Vries HJ, Brockmeyer NH, van Noesel C, Potthoff A, et al. Topical 5-fluorouracil treatment of anal intraepithelial neoplasia in human immunodeficiency virus-positive men. The British Journal of Dermatology. 2010;**163**(6):1301-1307

[55] Megill C, Wilkin T. Topical therapies for the treatment of anal high-grade squamous intraepithelial lesions. Seminars in Colon & Rectal Surgery. 2017;**28**(2):86-90

[56] Richel O, de Vries HJ, van Noesel CJ, Dijkgraaf MG, Prins JM. Comparison of imiquimod, topical fluorouracil, and electrocautery for the treatment of anal intraepithelial neoplasia in HIV-positive men who have sex with men: An open-label, randomised controlled trial. The Lancet Oncology. 2013;**14**(4):346-353

[57] Chang GJ, Berry JM, Jay N, Palefsky JM, Welton ML. Surgical treatment of high-grade anal squamous intraepithelial lesions: A prospective study. Diseases of the Colon and Rectum. 2002;**45**(4):453-458

[58] Gaisa MM, Liu Y, Deshmukh AA, Stone KL, Sigel KM. Electrocautery ablation of anal high-grade squamous intraepithelial lesions: Effectiveness and key factors associated with outcomes. Cancer. 2020;**126**(7):1470-1479

[59] de Pokomandy A, Rouleau D, Lalonde R, Beauvais C, de Castro C, Coutlée F. Argon plasma coagulation treatment of anal high-grade squamous intraepithelial lesions in men who have sex with men living with HIV: Results of a 2-year prospective pilot study. HIV Medicine. 2018;**19**(2):81-89

[60] Goldstone SE, Lensing SY, Stier EA, Darragh T, Lee JY, van Zante A, et al. A randomized clinical trial of infrared coagulation ablation versus active monitoring of intra-anal high-grade dysplasia in adults with human immunodeficiency virus infection: An AIDS malignancy consortium trial. Clinical Infectious Diseases: An Official Publication of the Infectious Diseases Society of America. 2019;**68**(7):1204-1212

[61] Siegenbeek van Heukelom ML, Gosens KCM, Prins JM, de Vries HJC. Cryotherapy for intra- and perianal high-grade squamous intraepithelial lesions in HIV-positive men who have sex with men. American Journal of Clinical Dermatology. 2018;**19**(1):127-132

[62] Goldstone RN, Hasan SR, Drury S, Darragh TM, van Zante A, Goldstone SE. A trial of radiofrequency ablation for anal intraepithelial neoplasia. International Journal of Colorectal Disease. 2017;**32**(3):357-365

[63] Rao S, Guren MG, Khan K, Brown G, Renehan AG, Steigen SE, et al. Anal cancer: ESMO clinical practice guidelines for diagnosis, treatment and follow-up(☆). Annals of Oncology: Official Journal of the European Society for Medical Oncology. 2021;**32**(9):1087-1100

[64] Clarke MA, Wentzensen N. Strategies for screening and early detection of anal cancers: A narrative and systematic review and meta-analysis of cytology, HPV testing, and other biomarkers. Cancer Cytopathology. 2018;**126**(7):447-460

[65] Zeng Y, Xu S, Chapman WC Jr, Li S, Alipour Z, Abdelal H, et al. Real-time colorectal cancer diagnosis using PR-OCT with deep learning. Theranostics. 2020;**10**(6):2587-2596

[66] Sekhar H, Kochhar R, Carrington B, Kaye T, Tolan D, Saunders MP, et al. Three-dimensional (3D) magnetic resonance volume assessment and loco-regional failure in anal cancer: Early evaluation case-control study. BMC Cancer. 2020;**20**(1):1165

[67] Mathias-Machado MC, Peixoto RD, Moniz CMV, Jácome AA. Biomarkers in anal cancer: Current status in diagnosis, disease progression and therapeutic strategies. Biomedicine. 2022;**10**(8):2029

[68] Berry J, Glasgow SC. Vaccinations for anal squamous cancer: Current and emerging therapies. Clinics in Colon and Rectal Surgery. 2018;**31**(6):321-327

Chapter 2

Anal Cancer: A Comprehensive Review of Epidemiology, Clinical Manifestations, and Therapeutic Approaches

Mihai-Teodor Georgescu

Abstract

In this chapter, we present a comprehensive review of anal cancer, focusing on its epidemiology, clinical manifestations (semiology), and therapeutic approaches. We delve into the global incidence and prevalence rates of anal cancer, exploring significant trends and risk factors associated with the disease. We discuss the etiology and pathogenesis of anal cancer, with a particular emphasis on the role of high-risk HPV types and other contributing factors. The chapter provides a detailed analysis of the clinical presentation, diagnosis, and staging of anal cancer, shedding light on the importance of early detection and appropriate screening methods. Furthermore, we thoroughly examine the various treatment modalities available, including surgery, radiation therapy, chemotherapy, and the emerging role of immunotherapy. A multidisciplinary management approach, involving different specialists and tumor boards, is emphasized. The chapter also addresses the follow-up and survivorship care for patients, including potential treatment-related complications and psychosocial support. Finally, we discuss ongoing research efforts and future directions in the field, highlighting the need for continued investigation and optimization of treatment strategies.

Keywords: anal cancer, epidemiology, treatment, follow-up, perspectives

1. Introduction

Anal cancer stands as a significant global health concern, demanding a thorough understanding of its intricacies for effective management. This chapter offers an in-depth exploration of anal cancer, encompassing its epidemiology, clinical manifestations, treatment modalities, and future perspectives. With a focus on comprehensive understanding, the chapter addresses critical aspects ranging from disease incidence and risk factors to advanced treatment strategies and ongoing research endeavors. Through an intricate interplay of data, clinical insights, and future outlooks, this chapter endeavors to equip readers with a comprehensive understanding of anal cancer. By delving into its multifaceted dimensions, we strive to contribute to the collective knowledge that informs clinical practice and shapes the landscape of anal cancer research and care.

2. Anatomy and embryology

The anal canal is the last part of the digestive tract and extends from the rectum to the anus. It is approximately 3–4 cm long and is divided into three parts: the upper third, middle third, and lower third. The upper third is lined by columnar epithelium, while the middle and lower thirds are lined by squamous epithelium [1].

Early in embryonic development, during the third week of gestation, the developing embryo undergoes a process known as gastrulation. This process gives rise to three primary germ layers: the ectoderm, mesoderm, and endoderm. The endoderm is the innermost layer and plays a pivotal role in the formation of the digestive and urogenital systems. By the fourth week of gestation, a crucial structure called the cloaca begins to take shape. The cloaca is a transient structure that serves as a common chamber for both urinary and digestive functions. It is divided into three parts: the anterior part, which will become the future urogenital sinus; the middle part, which will give rise to the anal canal; and the posterior part, which will form the vestibule of the vagina in females or the bulb of the penis in males. Around the seventh week of gestation cloacal septation occurs. This process involves the formation of a vertical partition within the cloaca, dividing it into two distinct canals: the anterior urogenital sinus and the posterior anal canal. The partitioning is a complex process driven by the interaction of various signaling molecules and transcription factors. The anal membrane, a thin layer of tissue that separates the primitive anal canal from the exterior, also plays a critical role. It undergoes programmed cell death, allowing communication between the anal canal and the outside world [2, 3].

As development progresses, the anal canal continues to elongate and differentiate. The upper part of the anal canal develops from the hindgut endoderm and eventually becomes lined with columnar epithelium. The lower part of the canal, closer to the exterior, forms from the ectoderm and is lined with stratified squamous epithelium. This transition in epithelial types is essential for the functional distinction between the upper and lower portions of the anal canal [2, 3].

3. Histology and epidemiology

According to the World Health Organization (WHO), anal cancer is classified into two main types: squamous cell carcinoma (SCC) and adenocarcinoma. Other rare variants include basaloid carcinoma, neuroendocrine tumors, and small cell carcinoma. SCC is the most common type of anal cancer, accounting for approximately 80% of all cases. Adenocarcinoma accounts for approximately 15% of all cases and is more commonly associated with a history of inflammatory bowel disease [1].

Within the landscape of anal cancer, the epidemiological panorama offers a profound understanding of its reach and impact on a global scale. By providing insight into the incidence and prevalence rates of anal cancer across diverse regions and populations, we gain a comprehensive view of the disease's intricate nature. This section delves into these epidemiological figures, unveiling notable trends and variations that can be discerned among different communities.

Anal cancer, although relatively rare compared to other malignancies, presents distinct patterns in its distribution. Incidence rates exhibit geographical disparities, with higher occurrences documented in certain regions. For instance, according to the American Cancer Society, in the United States alone, there were an estimated 8590 new cases of anal cancer and 1280 deaths from the disease in 2021 [4]. Similarly, in the United Kingdom, the Office for National Statistics reported that there were 1174 new cases of anal cancer registered in 2019 [5].

Notably, developed countries often report elevated rates, possibly attributed to improved surveillance, diagnosis, and reporting mechanisms. However, anal cancer is a global concern. The International Agency for Research on Cancer (IARC), a part of the World Health Organization (WHO), reports that in Europe, there were approximately 13,000 new cases of anal cancer and 3400 deaths attributed to the disease in 2020 [6]. This data underscore the significance of understanding the epidemiology of anal cancer not only within high-income nations but also across a spectrum of socioeconomic settings.

Moreover, the epidemiology of anal cancer intersects with demographic factors. Gender-based variations are noteworthy, as the disease tends to affect women more frequently than men. This gender discrepancy can be linked to the higher prevalence of HPV-associated anal cancer in women. Furthermore, the influence of age is evident, with the disease typically manifesting in individuals during their later years [7].

Understanding these epidemiological nuances is crucial for several reasons. First and foremost, these statistics serve as a foundation for public health initiatives. Accurate and up-to-date data inform the allocation of resources, facilitating targeted interventions in regions with higher prevalence. Additionally, epidemiological insights guide screening and early detection efforts. By identifying groups with increased vulnerability, healthcare professionals can tailor screening protocols and diagnostic strategies to enhance the timely identification of the disease.

Beyond the medical realm, epidemiological data play a pivotal role in raising awareness. Public health campaigns and educational initiatives are fortified with this knowledge, enabling effective communication with the general populace. Heightened awareness about the risk factors and symptoms of anal cancer empowers individuals to seek medical attention promptly, potentially leading to improved outcomes through early diagnosis and intervention.

In essence, the epidemiology of anal cancer is a cornerstone of our understanding of the disease. It uncovers the complex interplay between geographical, demographic, and behavioral factors that shape its prevalence. This knowledge equips healthcare providers, researchers, and policymakers with the tools needed to formulate strategic plans, allocate resources, and foster public awareness. By delving into the epidemiological intricacies, we pave the way for a more informed and proactive approach to combating anal cancer on a global scale.

4. Etiology and pathogenesis

The etiology of anal cancer unveils a complex interplay of factors, with high-risk human papillomavirus (HPV) infection at its core. This section delves into the mechanisms underlying the development of anal cancer, spotlighting the pivotal role of HPV and its intricate interactions within the human body.

Role of High-Risk HPV Types: The association between HPV infection and anal SCC, and a study showed that 88% of patients with anal cancer were diagnosed with HPV infection [5]. High-risk HPV types, notably HPV-16 and HPV-18, stand as primary instigators in the genesis of anal cancer. HPV infection of the anal canal and perianal leads to the formation of anal squamous intraepithelial lesions (SIL). Persistent HPV infection can lead to the cancer precursor anal high-grade SIL (HSIL). A small proportion of anal HSIL, in turn, will progress to invasive anal squamous cell carcinoma [8]. The progression from intraepithelial neoplasia to cancer is caused by HPV penetrating the transformation area in the columnar mucosa of the rectum, distal to the dentate line, and increasing from the squamous junction to the proximal side [1]. Similar to cervical cancer, anal cancer is preceded by high-grade squamous intraepithelial lesions (HSILs). Treatment for cervical HSIL reduces progression to cervical cancer; however, data from prospective studies of treatment for anal HSIL to prevent anal cancer are lacking. A phase 3 trial conducted at 25 U.S. sites showed that treatment for anal HSIL reduces progression to anal cancer [9].

These viruses enter the body through mucosal surfaces, including the anal canal, and integrate their genetic material into host cells. This integration disrupts cellular control mechanisms, leading to uncontrolled growth and progression toward malignancy. The oncoproteins produced by high-risk HPV types, E6 and E7, are central players in this process. They interfere with the host cell's regulatory pathways, promoting cell division and inhibiting natural tumor suppression mechanisms. This aberrant cell behavior culminates in the development of precancerous lesions that, if left unchecked, can evolve into full-fledged anal cancer [10, 11].

Influence of Chronic Inflammation: Chronic inflammation emerges as another critical contributor to the pathogenesis of anal cancer. In the presence of persistent irritants or infections, the body's immune response becomes sustained, creating an environment conducive to cellular damage and DNA alterations. Inflammatory mediators and cytokines, designed to combat infection, can inadvertently stimulate cell proliferation and impair the DNA repair machinery. This persistent inflammation can amplify the impact of HPV infection, enhancing the risk of cellular transformation and cancer development. Moreover, chronic inflammation can lead to tissue damage, necessitating ongoing cell turnover and repair—a process that further increases the chances of genetic errors and tumor formation [12, 13].

In sum, the etiology of anal cancer is a multifaceted interplay between high-risk HPV infection and chronic inflammation. These factors converge to disrupt the delicate balance of cellular regulation, driving the progression from normal tissue to precancerous lesions and ultimately to anal cancer. A deeper comprehension of these mechanisms enhances not only our understanding of the disease but also illuminates potential avenues for targeted interventions and preventive strategies.

5. Risk factors

The etiology of anal cancer is intricate and multifaceted, influenced by a spectrum of risk factors that contribute to its development. This section unravels the web of the main risk factors, shedding light on their influence on the incidence and progression of anal cancer.

High-Risk HPV Infection: Human papillomavirus (HPV) stands as a critical player in the genesis of anal cancer. Particularly, high-risk HPV types, such as HPV-16 and HPV-18, have been implicated in the majority of anal cancer cases. These viruses can lead to cellular changes, promoting the transformation of normal anal tissue into cancerous growths. Individuals with high-risk HPV infections have a substantially elevated risk of developing anal cancer compared to those who are HPV-negative [14].

Immunosuppression: Conditions that compromise the immune system, such as HIV/AIDS, significantly amplify the susceptibility to anal cancer. Immunosuppression weakens the body's ability to control viral infections like HPV, allowing them to persist and foster malignant changes. Individuals with HIV/AIDS are estimated to face an anal cancer risk that is approximately 80 times higher than the general population [15].

Smoking: Smoking, a well-established risk factor for various cancers, including lung cancer, is also linked to anal cancer. The harmful components in tobacco smoke can trigger DNA damage and impair the body's defense mechanisms, creating an environment conducive to cancer development. Studies have demonstrated a twofold increase in the risk of anal cancer among smokers [16].

Anal Intercourse: Engaging in receptive anal intercourse is associated with an elevated risk of anal cancer. This behavior can introduce HPV and other pathogens directly to the anal mucosa, increasing the likelihood of viral persistence and cellular transformation. Those who engage in anal intercourse are estimated to have a higher risk of anal cancer compared to individuals who do not practice this behavior [17].

History of Other Cancers: A history of certain gynecological cancers, such as cervical, vaginal, or vulvar cancer, can elevate the risk of anal cancer. This linkage is particularly relevant due to the shared etiological role of high-risk HPV strains. Prior history of these cancers indicates a heightened susceptibility to HPV-related malignancies, including anal cancer.

Age and Gender: Age and gender exert considerable influence on anal cancer risk. Incidence rates tend to increase with age, with the majority of cases occurring in individuals over the age of 50 [18]. Gender also plays a role, with women being more prone to anal cancer than men. This higher incidence among women is attributed to the presence of the cervix, which provides an additional site for HPV infection [14].

6. Clinical presentation and diagnosis

The spectrum of symptoms and clinical manifestations associated with anal cancer underscores the urgency of early recognition for effective management. This section delves into the common indicators of anal cancer, emphasizing the crucial role of timely detection. Additionally, it explores a range of diagnostic approaches, encompassing physical examination, anoscopy, and biopsy, all supported by relevant references.

Common Symptoms and Clinical Manifestations: The intricate clinical landscape of anal cancer often comprises subtle yet significant symptoms. Persistent bleeding, a symptom frequently attributed to hemorrhoids, can serve as an early warning sign of anal cancer—especially if accompanied by pain or discomfort. The anal region's discomfort might arise from tumor infiltration or nerve involvement. Itching, often dismissed as a minor concern, can emerge as an initial indication of anal cancer, underscoring the need to investigate even seemingly innocuous symptoms. Altered bowel habits, encompassing changes in stool caliber, or prolonged diarrhea, might signal the presence of anal cancer. The palpation of a mass or lump near the anus during a physical examination can further raise clinical suspicion [19, 20].

Importance of Early Detection: The paramount significance of early anal cancer detection cannot be overstated. The anatomical intricacies of the anal region and the potential subtlety of its symptoms can lead to delayed diagnosis. Early identification not only enhances the prospects of successful treatment but also mitigates the need for aggressive interventions that might become imperative in advanced stages.

Thus, healthcare providers play a pivotal role in recognizing potential symptoms and advocating for appropriate diagnostic strategies [21].

Diagnostic Methods: The diagnostic trajectory for anal cancer embraces a multipronged approach, guided by well-established techniques. Physical examination by healthcare professionals can unveil palpable masses, ulcers, or other anomalies. Anoscopy, facilitated by an anoscope equipped with light and magnification, enables direct visualization of the anal canal's interior, facilitating lesion identification. Biopsy, a definitive diagnostic modality, involves procuring tissue samples from suspicious areas for in-depth pathological examination. Biopsies can be seamlessly integrated into anoscopy procedures, supported by imaging or endoscopic guidance. Histopathological analysis of biopsy samples confirms cancer cell presence and delivers pivotal staging and treatment information [22–24].

7. Staging

The staging process for anal cancer is a pivotal aspect of its clinical management, offering insights into disease extent, guiding treatment decisions, and predicting outcomes. One of the most widely used staging systems is the TNM classification, which systematically evaluates the Tumor (T), regional Lymph Nodes (N), and presence of distant Metastasis (M). This classification system aids in categorizing anal cancer into distinct stages, each with specific implications for prognosis and therapeutic planning.

Stage 0 (Carcinoma in *Situ*): This stage represents a localized abnormality where cancer cells are confined to the surface layer of anal tissue. Often termed high-grade squamous intraepithelial lesion (HSIL), this stage is typically considered a precancerous state with a favorable prognosis [22].

Stage I: At this stage, the tumor is confined to the anal canal lining without extending into deeper layers or involving nearby lymph nodes or distant sites [25].

Stage II: The tumor progresses further, potentially infiltrating deeper layers of the anal wall. Nonetheless, lymph node involvement and distant metastasis are absent [25].

Stage IIIA: The cancer advances beyond the anal wall into adjacent tissues, such as the perianal skin or neighboring organs. Lymph node involvement may or may not be present, but distant spread is not observed [25].

Stage IIIB: In this stage, the tumor has reached nearby lymph nodes but has not metastasized to distant organs [25].

Stage IIIC: Here, the cancer extends to nearby lymph nodes and may involve surrounding tissues as well [25].

Stage IV: The most advanced stage, Stage IV, signifies the cancer's spread to distant organs or distant lymph nodes. This stage is further classified into subcategories IVA (local invasion into nearby organs or lymph nodes) and IVB (distant organ involvement) [25].

Staging involves a comprehensive evaluation, including physical examination, imaging studies such as anoscopy, computer tomography, magnetic resonance imaging, positron emission tomography, and sometimes lymph node biopsies. The stage assigned using the TNM system informs treatment strategies and patient prognosis. It's important to recognize that variations in staging may exist among medical institutions and guidelines. Consulting with healthcare professionals is essential to tailor treatment plans based on precise staging assessments and individual patient characteristics.

8. Treatment

The management of anal cancer has evolved significantly over the years, witnessing the emergence of diverse treatment modalities that offer improved outcomes and enhanced patient quality of life. This comprehensive exploration delves into the intricacies of treatment options for anal cancer, underpinned by a robust foundation of clinical evidence and multidisciplinary collaboration.

Surgery: Surgical intervention remains a cornerstone in the management of anal cancer, particularly in the context of early-stage tumors and those amenable to local excision. Procedures range from wide local excisions to more extensive abdominoperineal resections, with the selection guided by factors such as tumor size, depth of infiltration, and nodal involvement [26]. Local excision, often coupled with adjuvant therapy, is suitable for small tumors confined to the anal canal lining. On the other hand, abdominoperineal resections, involving removal of the anus and rectum, are employed for larger tumors or those extending beyond the anal canal [27]. Surgical management aims to achieve complete tumor removal while preserving anal function and maintaining an optimal quality of life.

Radiation Therapy: Radiation therapy plays a pivotal role in both curative and palliative settings for anal cancer. External beam radiation therapy (EBRT) delivers targeted radiation to the tumor site and surrounding tissues, eradicating cancer cells and preventing their proliferation. EBRT can be employed as a primary treatment for early-stage cancers or in conjunction with surgery for advanced cases. Brachytherapy, a specialized form of radiation therapy, involves placing radioactive sources directly into or near the tumor site. This approach enables a high dose of radiation to be delivered precisely to the tumor, minimizing damage to surrounding healthy tissue [28]. Radiation therapy offers an organ-preserving approach, particularly beneficial for patients concerned about maintaining normal bowel and sexual function.

Chemotherapy: Chemotherapy, often combined with radiation therapy (chemoradiotherapy), has become a standard of care for locally advanced anal cancer. The synergy between chemotherapy and radiation therapy enhances tumor response and local control. A common regimen involves the administration of fluorouracil (5-FU) and mitomycin-C concurrently with radiation. This regimen has shown substantial improvements in disease control and overall survival rates [29]. Chemotherapy works by targeting rapidly dividing cancer cells, impeding their growth and promoting cell death. This combination therapy is particularly effective in eradicating microscopic cancer cells that might remain after surgery.

Targeted Therapy: The emergence of targeted therapies has introduced a novel dimension to anal cancer treatment. Targeted therapies aim to disrupt specific molecular pathways involved in cancer growth and progression. Agents such as cetuximab, an epidermal growth factor receptor (EGFR) inhibitor, have shown promise in clinical trials for advanced or recurrent anal cancer [30]. These therapies are tailored to the individual patient's tumor characteristics, allowing for a more personalized and effective approach.

Immunotherapy: Immunotherapy is an evolving frontier in cancer treatment that has begun to show promise in anal cancer. Immune checkpoint inhibitors, such as pembrolizumab and nivolumab, enhance the body's immune response against cancer cells by blocking inhibitory signals. This novel approach has demonstrated encouraging results in clinical trials, offering a potential option for patients who have exhausted conventional treatment options [31].

Multidisciplinary Approach: A multidisciplinary approach is indispensable in the management of anal cancer. Collaboration among various specialists, including radiation oncologists, medical oncologists, surgeons, pathologists, radiologists, and nurses, ensures a holistic evaluation and comprehensive treatment plan. These experts bring their unique perspectives to the table, collectively tailoring treatment strategies based on individual patient characteristics and disease stages. Multidisciplinary tumor boards facilitate in-depth discussions, enabling informed decisions that optimize patient outcomes [32].

9. Follow-up

Completing treatment for anal cancer marks a significant milestone, yet the journey toward optimal health and well-being continues post-treatment. Ongoing follow-up care, coupled with attention to potential complications and psychosocial support, forms a vital triad in the survivorship phase, ensuring patients' holistic needs are addressed.

The Imperative of Follow-up Care: Post-treatment surveillance is essential to monitor for disease recurrence, identify potential treatment-related complications, and promote overall health. Regular follow-up appointments provide opportunities for healthcare professionals to assess treatment outcomes, address any lingering concerns, and offer guidance on maintaining a healthy lifestyle. A structured follow-up schedule allows for timely intervention if new issues arise, enhancing long-term prognosis [33]. The transition from active treatment to follow-up care signifies a shift from battling cancer to focusing on preserving health and embracing a new chapter of life.

Recommendations for Follow-up Care: Based on current guidelines, such as those outlined by the National Comprehensive Cancer Network (NCCN), a recommended follow-up program for anal cancer survivors includes regular visits to an oncologist or healthcare provider. The frequency of follow-up appointments may be more frequent in the first few years after treatment and then become less frequent over time, but ongoing monitoring is essential. Surveillance imaging, such as CT scans or MRIs, may be conducted periodically to detect any signs of recurrence or new lesions. Blood tests and physical examinations are also crucial components of follow-up care. In addition, survivorship care plans may include recommendations for healthy lifestyle habits, emotional well-being support, and management of treatment-related complications [33].

Managing Treatment-Related Complications: Treatment modalities for anal cancer, including surgery, radiation therapy, and chemotherapy, may result in various side effects that can impact patients' well-being. Radiation therapy, for instance, can lead to skin irritation, fatigue, and changes in bowel habits. Chemotherapy-related complications might include fatigue, nausea, and neuropathy. Surgical procedures may give rise to wound healing challenges or changes in bowel function [34]. Recognizing these potential complications, healthcare providers tailor follow-up plans to monitor and manage these side effects, offering guidance on strategies to alleviate discomfort and maintain quality of life.

Psychosocial Support in Survivorship: Beyond physical well-being, addressing the psychosocial needs of anal cancer survivors is of paramount importance. The journey through diagnosis and treatment can evoke a range of emotions, and the transition to survivorship may come with its own set of challenges. Patients might grapple with anxiety about recurrence, body image issues, or changes in relationships. Psychosocial support, through counseling, support groups, or individual therapy, offers a safe space for patients to voice their concerns and receive coping strategies [35]. Recognizing the emotional toll and offering tailored support enhances patients' overall well-being and resilience.

Holistic Survivorship Care: A comprehensive survivorship care plan encompasses medical surveillance, addressing treatment-related complications, and nurturing psychosocial health. Oncology teams collaborate with various specialists, such as oncologists, surgeons, nurses, psychologists, and dietitians, to provide a holistic approach to care. Regular check-ups, imaging studies, and blood tests facilitate early detection of recurrence or new health issues. Health education empowers survivors to adopt healthy habits, including proper nutrition, physical activity, and smoking cessation [36].

10. Future perspectives

The landscape of anal cancer research is undergoing a dynamic transformation, driven by the relentless pursuit of improved outcomes and quality of life for patients. As our understanding of the disease deepens and novel technologies emerge, a promising array of future perspectives is unfolding, guided by available literature data and ongoing clinical trials.

Refining Personalized Therapies: Advances in molecular profiling and genomic analyses are poised to revolutionize the field of anal cancer treatment. Tailoring therapies based on individual tumor characteristics hold great promise in optimizing treatment efficacy while minimizing adverse effects. The identification of predictive biomarkers, such as molecular alterations or gene expression patterns, may guide treatment selection, ensuring that patients receive interventions most likely to benefit them. As ongoing research unravels the intricate molecular landscape of anal cancer, targeted therapies could become even more precise, ushering in an era of personalized medicine [37].

Immunotherapy's Expanding Horizons: Immunotherapy, marked by immune checkpoint inhibitors and immune stimulants, is reshaping the landscape of cancer treatment. While its role in anal cancer is still evolving, ongoing clinical trials are exploring its potential. Emerging data suggest that harnessing the immune system's power to target and eliminate cancer cells holds promise in a subset of patients. As researchers unravel the complex interplay between tumors and the immune microenvironment, the integration of immunotherapeutic agents into treatment algorithms could become a reality, potentially enhancing outcomes for advanced or refractory anal cancer [38].

Enhanced Imaging and Early Detection: In the realm of imaging, cutting-edge technologies are on the horizon, poised to refine the early detection of anal cancer and guide treatment strategies. Novel imaging modalities, such as functional magnetic resonance imaging (MRI) and positron emission tomography (PET) scans, offer unprecedented insights into tumor metabolism, microenvironment, and response to treatment. These techniques may enable oncologists to assess treatment efficacy more accurately and detect recurrences at earlier stages. Moreover, the integration of artificial intelligence and machine learning algorithms into image analysis could streamline diagnosis, staging, and treatment planning, ultimately enhancing patient outcomes [39].

Exploring Innovative Combination Therapies: The synergy between various treatment modalities remains a fertile ground for exploration. Emerging clinical trials are investigating the potential benefits of combining traditional treatments with targeted therapies, immunotherapies, or even novel agents. The aim is to exploit complementary mechanisms of action to achieve greater treatment efficacy while minimizing toxicities. By leveraging these innovative combinations, researchers envision a future where patients receive tailored, multidimensional treatment regimens that address the complex nature of anal cancer [40].

Precision Medicine and Clinical Trials: The era of precision medicine is ushering in a paradigm shift in clinical trial design and patient recruitment. Trials are becoming more refined, targeting specific patient subsets based on molecular or genetic signatures. This approach enhances not only the likelihood of identifying therapeutic benefits but also ensures that patients are exposed to interventions that align with their disease characteristics. Adaptive clinical trial designs, allowing for real-time adjustments based on emerging data, hold the potential to accelerate the translation of novel therapies from bench to bedside [41].

11. Conclusions

As we bring this comprehensive exploration of anal cancer to a close, several key insights emerge, underscoring the significance of a multidimensional understanding of this complex disease. From epidemiology to treatment modalities, the journey through the realm of anal cancer reveals the dynamic interplay of factors that shape its course. This chapter's structured approach has provided a roadmap, shedding light on critical aspects and pointing toward future horizons.

Epidemiology and Risk Factors:

The global incidence of anal cancer serves as a reminder that this disease transcends borders, necessitating a concerted public health effort. High-risk HPV infection, immunosuppression, smoking, anal intercourse, and a history of certain cancers emerge as modifiable risk factors that merit attention. Awareness campaigns and targeted interventions could potentially curb the burden of anal cancer, reinforcing the importance of early detection.

Etiology and Pathogenesis:

The central role of high-risk HPV types in anal cancer underscores the need for preventive measures and vaccination strategies. Additionally, the intricate interplay between viral factors and chronic inflammation sheds light on potential avenues for targeted therapeutic interventions, presenting opportunities for future research and innovation.

Clinical Presentation and Diagnosis:

Timely diagnosis hinges on recognizing the nuances of clinical manifestations, emphasizing the pivotal role of healthcare providers in accurate assessment. Physical examinations, anoscopy, and biopsies play essential roles in guiding treatment strategies, reaffirming the value of a thorough diagnostic approach.

Staging and Treatment:

The TNM staging system has provided a standardized framework for stratifying disease severity and guiding treatment decisions. Surgical interventions, radiation therapy, chemotherapy, targeted therapies, and immunotherapy collectively form a comprehensive armamentarium that empowers clinicians to tailor treatments to individual patients.

Follow-up and Survivorship Care:

The post-treatment phase warrants meticulous attention, with follow-up care serving as a crucial bridge to sustained health. Vigilant monitoring for treatment-related complications, coupled with psychosocial support, cultivates an environment conducive to holistic well-being for survivors.

Future Perspectives:

As the curtain rises on the horizon of anal cancer research, promising prospects beckon. The integration of precision medicine, immunotherapy, enhanced imaging, and innovative combination therapies augurs well for patient outcomes. Ongoing clinical trials stand as testaments to the field's commitment to advancing knowledge and refining treatment paradigms.

In essence, this chapter encapsulates the multifaceted nature of anal cancer, delving into its epidemiology, etiology, clinical presentation, diagnosis, staging, treatment, and beyond. By navigating this intricate landscape, healthcare professionals, researchers, and advocates can collectively steer the trajectory of anal cancer toward improved patient outcomes, heightened awareness, and the realization of a future where this disease is better understood, managed, and ultimately prevented.

Funding

This work received no funding.

Conflict of interest

The authors declare no conflict of interest.

Author details

Mihai-Teodor Georgescu[1,2]

1 "Carol Davila" University of Medicine and Pharmacy, Bucharest, Romania

2 "Prof. Dr. Al. Trestioreanu" Oncology Institute, Bucharest, Romania

*Address all correspondence to: mihai.georgescu@umfcd.ro

IntechOpen

© 2024 The Author(s). Licensee IntechOpen. This chapter is distributed under the terms of the Creative Commons Attribution License (http://creativecommons.org/licenses/by/3.0), which permits unrestricted use, distribution, and reproduction in any medium, provided the original work is properly cited.

References

[1] Yamada K, Shiraishi K, Takashima A, et al. Characteristics of anal canal squamous cell carcinoma as an HPV-associated cancer in Japan. International Journal of Clinical Oncology. 2023;**28**(4):990-998

[2] Hollinshead WH. Embryology and anatomy of the anal canal and rectum. Diseases of the Colon and Rectum. 1962;**5**:18-22. DOI: 10.1007/BF02616406

[3] Kruepunga N, Hikspoors JPJM, Mekonen HK, Mommen GMC, Meemon K, Weerachatyanukul W, et al. The development of the cloaca in the human embryo. Journal of Anatomy. 2018;**233**(6):724-739. DOI: 10.1111/joa.12882

[4] American Cancer Society. Cancer Facts and Figures 2021. Atlanta: American Cancer Society; 2021

[5] Office for National Statistics. Cancer Registration Statistics. England: Office of National Statistics (ONS); 2019. Available from: https://www.ons.gov.uk/peoplepopulationandcommunity/healthandsocialcare/conditionsanddiseases/datasets/cancerregistrationstatisticscancerregistrationsengland

[6] International Agency for Research on Cancer (IARC). Cancer today. Available from: https://gco.iarc.fr/today/home

[7] Hoots BE, Palefsky JM, Pimenta JM, Smith JS. Human papillomavirus type distribution in anal cancer and anal intraepithelial lesions. International Journal of Cancer. 2009;**124**(10):2375-2383. DOI: 10.1002/ijc.24215

[8] Anal Pre-Cancer: Squamous Intraepithelial Lesions [Internet]. USA: University of California; 2023. Available from: https://ancre.ucsf.edu/anal-pre-cancer-squamous-intraepithelial-lesions [Accessed: Sep 13, 2023]

[9] HPV and anal cancer: What you should know [Internet]. Dana-Farber Cancer Institute. 2023 [Accessed: Sep 14, 2023]. Available from: https://blog.dana-farber.org/insight/2023/08/hpv-and-anal-cancer-what-you-should-know/ [Accessed: Sep 13, 2023]

[10] Muñoz N, Bosch FX, de Sanjosé S, et al. Epidemiologic classification of human papillomavirus types associated with cervical cancer. The New England Journal of Medicine. 2003;**348**(6):518-527

[11] Stanley M. Pathology and epidemiology of HPV infection in females. Gynecologic Oncology. 2010;**117**(Suppl. 2):S5-S10

[12] Coussens LM, Werb Z. Inflammation and cancer. Nature. 2002;**420**(6917):860-867

[13] Balkwill F, Mantovani A. Inflammation and cancer: Back to Virchow? Lancet. 2001;**357**(9255):539-545

[14] de Martel C, Plummer M, Vignat J, Franceschi S. Worldwide burden of cancer attributable to HPV by site, country and HPV type. International Journal of Cancer. 2017;**141**(4):664-670

[15] Silverberg MJ, Lau B, Justice AC, et al. Risk of anal Cancer in HIV-infected and HIV-uninfected individuals in North America. Clinical Infectious Diseases. 2012;**54**(7):1026-1034

[16] Daling JR, Madeleine MM, Schwartz SM, et al. A population-based study of squamous cell vaginal cancer:

HPV and cofactors. Gynecologic Oncology. 2002;**84**(2):263-270

[17] Daling JR, Weiss NS, Hislop TG, Maden C, Coates RJ, Sherman KJ, et al. Sexual practices, sexually transmitted diseases, and the incidence of anal cancer. The New England Journal of Medicine. 1987;**317**(16):973-977

[18] Glynne-Jones R, Nilsson PJ, Aschele C, et al. Anal cancer: ESMO-ESSO-ESTRO clinical practice guidelines for diagnosis, treatment and follow-up. Radiotherapy and Oncology. 2014;**111**(3):330-339

[19] ACG Clinical Guideline. Anal Cancer screening and surveillance in human immunodeficiency virus–positive patients. The American Journal of Gastroenterology. 2018;**113**(6):899-909

[20] Goldstone RN, Goldstone AB. Modern Management of Anal Cancer. Surgical Oncology Clinics of North America. 2020;**29**(2):291-310

[21] National Comprehensive Cancer Network. Anal Carcinoma (Version 2.2021). Available from: https://www.nccn.org/professionals/physician_gls/pdf/anal.pdf

[22] Palefsky JM. Anal cancer prevention in HIV-positive men and women. Current Opinion in Oncology. 2009;**21**(5):433-438

[23] Schiffman M, Castle PE, Jeronimo J, Rodriguez AC, Wacholder S. Human papillomavirus and cervical cancer. Lancet. 2007;**370**(9590):890-907

[24] Palefsky JM, Holly EA, Ralston ML, Da Costa M, Bonner H, Jay N, et al. High incidence of anal high-grade squamous intra-epithelial lesions among HIV-positive and HIV-negative homosexual and bisexual men. AIDS. 1998;**12**(5):495-503

[25] American Joint Committee on Cancer (AJCC). AJCC Cancer Staging Manual. 8th ed. New York: Springer; 2017

[26] Northover J, Glynne-Jones R, Sebag-Montefiore D, James R, Meadows H, Wan S, et al. Chemoradiation for the treatment of epidermoid anal cancer: 13-year follow-up of the first randomized UKCCCR anal cancer trial (ACT I). British Journal of Cancer. 2010;**102**(7):1123-1128

[27] Glimelius B, Påhlman L, Cervantes A. Rectal cancer: ESMO clinical practice guidelines for diagnosis, treatment and follow-up. Annals of Oncology. 2013;**24**(Suppl. 6):vi81-vi88

[28] Sphincter preservation in anal cancer: A randomized controlled trial of radiation therapy with 5-Fluorouracil and Mitomycin-C with or without salvage radical surgery (transanal endoscopic microsurgery) for conservative management of early-stage T1-T2 N0 M0 anal canal carcinoma. ClinicalTrials.gov Identifier: NCT02002694

[29] Ajani JA, Winter KA, Gunderson LL, Pedersen J, Benson AB 3rd, Thomas CR Jr, et al. Fluorouracil, mitomycin, and radiotherapy vs fluorouracil, cisplatin, and radiotherapy for carcinoma of the anal canal: A randomized controlled trial. Journal of the American Medical Association. 2008;**299**(16):1914-1921

[30] Karydis I, Chan DS, Constantinidou A, Maraka S, Nikolaou S, Petkar I, et al. Anti-epidermal growth factor receptor (EGFR) monoclonal antibodies for the treatment of metastatic anal canal squamous cell carcinoma: Toxicity and survival from a large retrospective cohort. Journal of Cancer Research and Clinical Oncology. 2017;**143**(7):1271-1276

[31] Eng C, Chang GJ, You YN, Das P, Rodriguez-Bigas M, Xing Y, et al. The role of systemic chemotherapy and multidisciplinary management in improving the overall survival of patients with metastatic squamous cell carcinoma of the anal canal. Oncotarget. 2014;**75**(7):736-744

[32] Smith JJ, Strombom P, Chow OS, Roxburgh CS, Lynn P, Eaton A, et al. Assessment of a watch-and-wait strategy for rectal cancer in patients with a complete response after Neoadjuvant therapy. JAMA Oncology. 2019;**5**(4):e185896

[33] American Cancer Society. Follow-up care after treatment for anal cancer. Available from: https://www.cancer.org/cancer/anal-cancer/after-treatment/follow-up.html

[34] Caravatta L, Padula GD, Macchia G, Morganti AG, Deodato F, Massaccesi M, et al. Acute skin toxicity management in head and neck cancer patients treated with radiotherapy and chemotherapy or EGFR inhibitors: Literature review and consensus. Critical Reviews in Oncology/Hematology. 2015;**96**(1):167-182

[35] Mehnert A, Koch U. Psychological comorbidity and health-related quality of life and its association with awareness, utilization, and need for psychosocial support in a cancer register-based sample of long-term breast cancer survivors. Journal of Psychosomatic Research. 2008;**64**(4):383-391

[36] Alfano CM, Mayer DK, Bhatia S, Maher J, Scott JM, Nekhlyudov L, et al. Implementing personalized pathways for cancer follow-up care in the United States: Proceedings from an American Cancer Society-American Society of Clinical Oncology summit. CA: A Cancer Journal for Clinicians. 2019;**69**(6):438-450

[37] Chakravarthy AB, Shabason JE, Czito BG. Multidisciplinary management of anal cancer: The way of the future? Oncology (Williston Park, N.Y.). 2020;**34**(12):531-532

[38] Garcia-Martinez E, Loupakis F, Fakih M. Ready for primetime? The use of immunotherapy for the treatment of anal cancer. Journal of Gastrointestinal Oncology. 2021;**12**(Suppl. 1):S33-S45

[39] Nougaret S, Reinhold C, Mikhael HW, Rouanet P, Bibeau F, Brown G. The use of MR imaging in treatment planning for patients with rectal carcinoma: Have you checked the "DISTANCE"? Radiology. 2013;**268**(2):330-344

[40] Rao AD, Patel KP, Skapek SX, et al. Pediatric patients with solid tumors enrolled onto phase I trials have outcomes similar to their adult counterparts. Cancer. 2017;**123**(18):3657-3665

[41] Schilsky RL. Implementing personalized cancer care. Nature Reviews. Clinical Oncology. 2014;**11**(7):432-438

Section 2

Anal Disorders

Chapter 3

Care of Post-Operative Altered Bowel Function in Colorectal Cancer Patients

Ling-Chun Lu

Abstract

Rectal cancer patients with postoperative altered bowel function have poorer quality of life than colon rectal cancer patients with it. The altered bowel function symptoms were named low anterior resection syndrome. Mechanisms of these symptoms associated with removing rectum and receptors on its internal wall, creating neorectum, and destroying pelvic neuro-plexus by analsaving surgery. Due to the low anterior resection syndrome, patients suffered from physical, psychological and social impacts on quality of life. Three options are used to treat low anterior resection syndrome, including self-care strategies, clinician-initiated interventions, and creating a permanent stoma. The self-care strategies contain diet modification, lifestyle changes, and spiritual sublimation. The clinician-initiated interventions include prescribed medication, trans-anal irrigation, pelvic floor rehabilitation, neuromodulation, and so on. Creating a permanent stoma is the eventual choice due to anastomotic restriction. Altered bowel function may follow postoperative rectal cancer patients for whole life; however, flexibly using these care strategies may help them adjust.

Keywords: colorectal cancer, altered bowel function, low anterior resection syndrome, consequence of anal-saving surgery, care strategies of low anterior resection syndrome

1. Introduction

Altered bowel function is a common consequence in postoperative colorectal cancer patients and may impact patients' quality of life for years [1–3]. In the population, rectal cancer patients had worse long-term quality of life than colon cancer patients, which may relate to severer bowel dysfunction after they received anal-saving surgery [2, 4]. Improving the dysfunction in rectal cancer patients may effectively promote the quality of life in colorectal cancer patients [5]. The postoperative altered bowel function in rectal cancer patients with anal-saving surgery was named low anterior resection syndrome [6, 7]. This chapter will focus on definition of low anterior resection syndrome, the mechanisms of the dysfunction, its impactions on quality of life, and management strategies of low anterior resection.

IntechOpen

2. Definition of low anterior resection syndrome

Under a consensus combined in the 17th European Colorectal Congress, low anterior resection syndrome was defined as a series of bowel dysfunction symptoms after patients received anal-saving surgery, such as anterior resection, low anterior resection, ultralow anterior resection, total mesorectal excision, and so forth [4, 6]. These symptoms and their incidence included small frequent stool (70–94.4%), altered anal sense (12–98%), fecal incontinence (12–97%), fecal urgency (67%), evacuator dysfunction (47%), varied stool forms (37.6%), and gas-stool discrimination (34%) [4, 6–9]. These symptoms gradually spontaneously improved in the postoperative period but seldom totally recovered over years [4, 8–11].

3. Mechanisms of low anterior resection syndrome

A mechanism of defecation includes a series of processes (see **Figure 1**): (1) When feces move into and distend the rectum, they stimulate stretch receptors in the wall of rectum, and the receptors transmit signals along afferent fibers to spinal cord neurons; (2) A spinal reflex is initiated in which parasympathetic motor fibers (efferent fibers) stimulate the contraction of the rectum and sigmoid colon and relaxation of the internal anal sphincter; (3) When it is convenient to defecate, voluntary motor neurons are inhibited, which allow the external anal sphincter to relax, and then feces may pass [12].

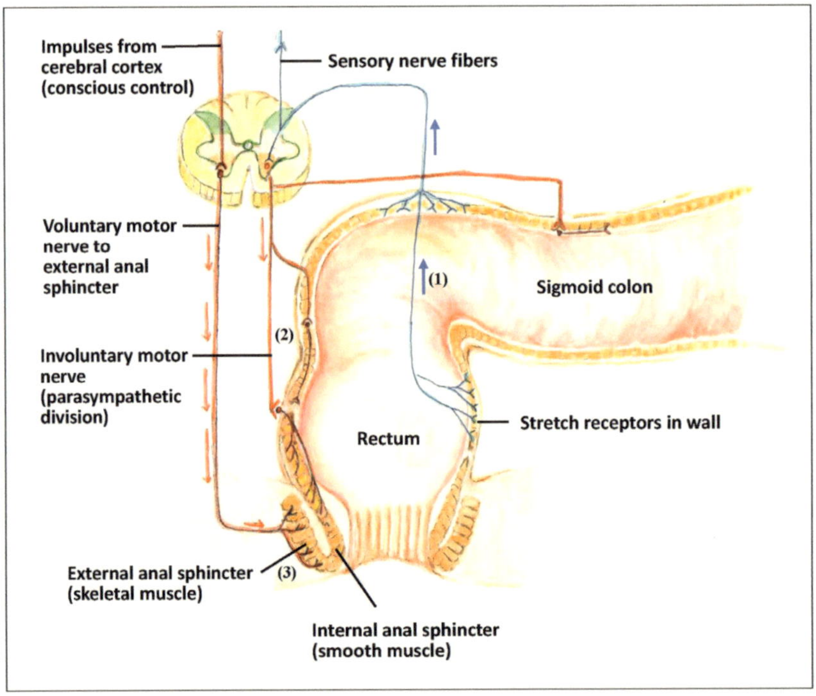

Figure 1.
The mechanism of defecation. (1) When feces move into and distend the rectum, they stimulate stretch receptors in the wall of rectum, and the receptors transmit signals along afferent fibers to spinal cord neurons, (2) A spinal reflex is initiated in which parasympathetic motor fibers (efferent fibers) stimulate the contraction of the rectum and sigmoid colon, and relaxation of the internal anal sphincter, (3) When it is convenient to defecate, voluntary motor neurons are inhibited, which allow the external anal sphincter to relax, and then feces may pass.

The purpose of anal-saving surgery is to save the anal sphincters and to avoid receiving abdominoperineal resection with permanent stoma [13]. When patients received anal-saving surgery, it may resect distal sigmoid, whole rectum, total mesorectum and partial or/and total internal sphincter or/and external sphincter,

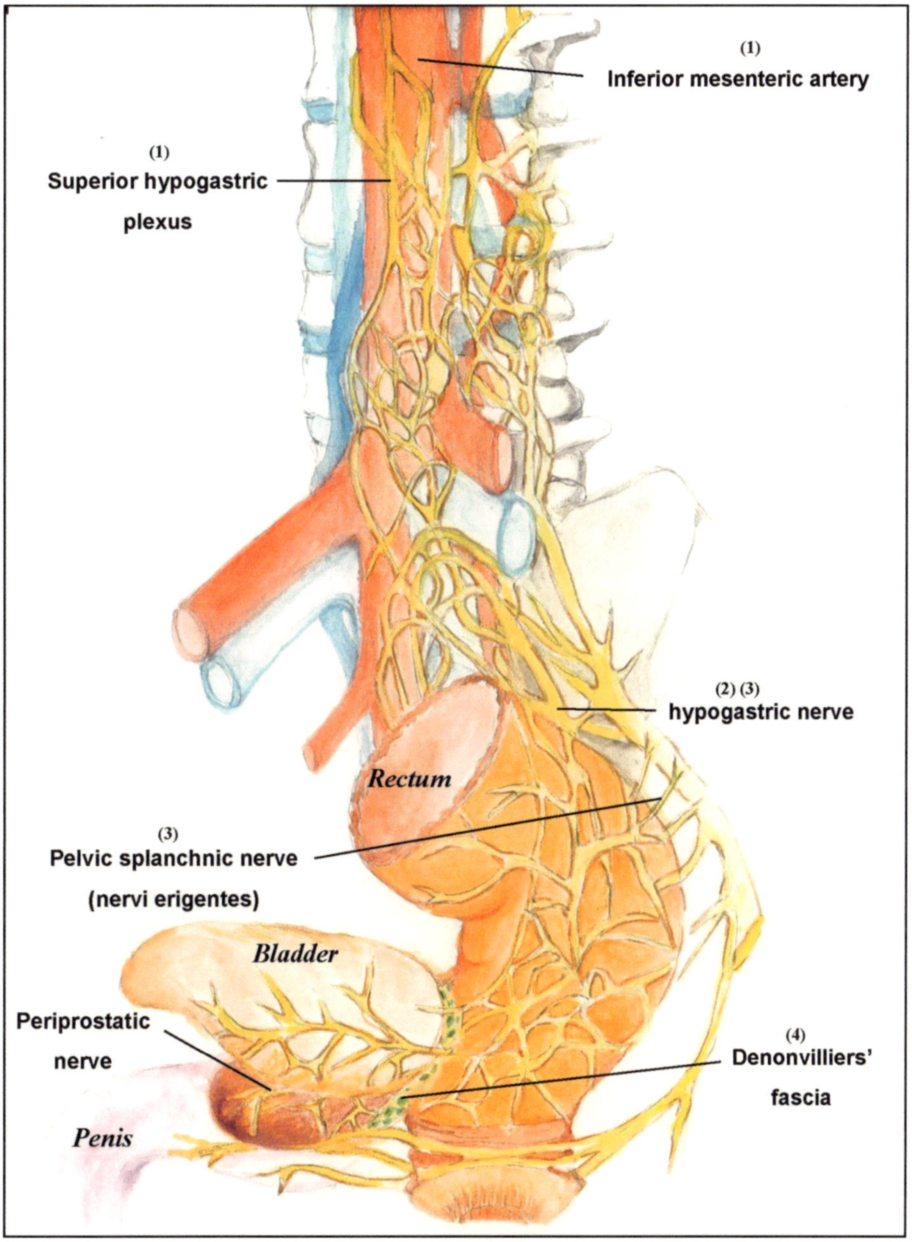

Figure 2.
Potential points of pelvic nerve injury during rectal dissection include. (1) Damage to the superior hypogastric plexus from tension or high division of the inferior mesenteric artery. (2) Injury to the main trunks of the hypogastric nerve during retrorectal dissection. (3) Injury to the inferior hypogastric plexus and nervi erigentes during the mobilization of lateral stalks. (4) Injury to the periprostatic plexus during the dissection of Denonvilliers' fascia.

as well as straight down the stump of colon to create a colon-to-colon or coloanal anastomosis for bowel continuum [13–15]. Potential points of pelvic nerve injury during rectal dissection include (see **Figure 2**): (1) Damage to the superior hypogastric plexus from tension or high division of the inferior mesenteric artery, (2) Injury to the main trunks of the hypogastric nerve during retrorectal dissection; (3) Injury to the inferior hypogastric plexus and nervi erigentes during the mobilization of lateral stalks, and (4) injury to the periprostatic plexus during the dissection of Denonvilliers' fascia [16–18].

When rectum was resected, the stump of colon was straightdown to form a neorectum [19]. Because of the neorectum with smaller volume and with decreasing available eastability following chemoradiotherapy, the mechanic change may induce small frequent stool and varied stool forms; smaller volume of neorectum and resection of the stretch receptors in the wall of rectum may lead to fecal urgency, evacuator dysfunction, altered anal sense, and gas-stool discrimination; resection of rectal receptors, destroying of pelvic neuro-plexus and resection of anal sphincter may cause fecal incontinence [13, 15, 19].

4. The symptom distress and impactions on quality of life related to low anterior resection syndrome

After rectal cancer patients received anal-saving surgery or reversal of temporary stoma, they experienced varied symptoms of altered bowl function [20–22]. They were often preoccupied with these uncontrolled excrement symptoms, which easily disturb their physical function, compel them to experience emotional distress, and interfere with their social activities [7, 20–24]. Additionally, a multicenter correctional study revealed patients with the major low anterior resection syndrome had significantly worse quality of life than the those with minor and moderate syndrome [25].

In the domain of physical function, interruption of daily activities (e.g., eating, householding, and sleep), consequent distraction in daytime, and decreased sexual behavior often related to small frequent defection, urgency, and fecal incontinence [20, 22]. Under the disturbance of sleep, there may be difficulty in falling asleep, interruption of sleep due to intent to defecate, difficulty in falling asleep post broken sleep at midnight, and poor quality of sleep [7, 20]. On the intimacy behaviors, patients and their couples may choose other methods (e.g. hug, kiss, and spiritual empathy, etc.) to replace sexual behaviors [7].

In the domain of psychological function, patients often develop varied negative moods due to uncontrolled excrement, such as distress, depress, upset, botheration, irritation, helplessness, loneness, hopelessness, and so on [7, 20, 23]. They feel tie to toilet due to frequent go to restroom, experience struggle in living because of relieving from stoma but falling in destructive bowel habits, though it is a price to survive from cancer, and mark stigma related to uncontrolled incontinence [20, 26, 27]. They often fear the spread of poor odor and feel embarrassment due to fecal incontinence [27], which lead to concern over the availability of restroom [7].

In the domain of social function, patients do not dare to go outside or dinning, compete to go to restroom with family members, are forced to change mode of work, decrease travel, and give up enjoyment [7, 20]. Their lifestyle changes may bother their family, and they may suffer from loneness because their family cannot totally understand their feeling [7, 23]. Their life style changed, thus, they feel they become a different person, in the other ward, their body image was changed [7, 26, 28]. At the same time, they also suffered from social isolation [20, 21, 26].

5. The management strategies of low anterior resection syndrome

Although management of low anterior resection syndrome remains equivocal, some strategies are mentioned [5, 29–34]. The strategies involve in three options: self-care strategies, clinician-initiated interventions, and creating a permanent stoma [29–31, 35].

5.1 Self-care strategies

The self-care strategies for treating low anterior resection syndrome contain diet modification, lifestyle changes, and spiritual sublimation [29].

Diet modification is the commonest strategy to treat the altered bowel function in postoperative rectal cancer patients [32]. Some types of foods leading to aggravation of bowel dysfunction were advised, including greasy foods, liquid foods, gas-inducing foods, sweet foods, and stimulating foods [32, 33, 36]. These foods easily increase the frequency of defecation and possibly induce diarrhea, urgency, fecal incontinence, or/and gas-stool discrimination [32]. Notably, the mechanism may be supported by a correlative study, which revealed some nutrients aggravate bowel dysfunction; for example, the consumption of protein, cholesterol, and fruit increases the frequency and urgency of defecation; the consumption of fruit decreases the abnormal sense of defecation, but the interaction of wheats and milk leads to an abnormal sense of defecation [37]. The consumption of high-fiber foods remained equivocal; some studies mentioned that it may increase the risk of diarrhea and frequency of bowel movement, but it also may decrease the incidence of fecal incontinence when taken an amount of 25 g in a day [31–33]. Although patients' motivation of diet modification is usually driven by burden of low anterior resection syndrome, they often have a trial-and-error process, need to overcome general habits, and face social interfering factors before forming new eating habits, such the availability of diet preparation, the time and amount of eating regularly, and so on [38].

Lifestyle change is a consequence of suffering from low anterior resection syndrome and also is a strategy of treating it [32, 39]. To have a supply of anal skin-care products and use sitz bath can decease perianal soreness related to frequent defecation [29]. When patients go outside, using wipes or pads, carrying spare clothes, and confirming the availability of restroom can help them to manage the embarrassment related to fecal incontinence [7, 29]. Participating some activities to divert patients' attention from defecation is a useful method to control bowel symptoms, such as walking, jogging, going work, joining religion ceremony, and so on [33, 40]. Minor patients note that special body position can improve evacuator function; additionally, some patients change their schedule or mode of jobs for return-to-work [33].

In spiritual sublimation, building up a confidence of managing low anterior resection and feeling normality, constructing positive or thankful life attitude, accepting the dysfunction as part of them, and seeking reason to be strong usually help patients to adjust their altered bowel function and cancer disease [7, 23, 33]. In clinical practice, healthcare professionals can find that symptoms did not disappear, but positive attitude and thinking can promote patients' perception and quality of life [7, 24]. Acceptability and sharing experiences with other rectal cancer patients with low anterior resection syndrome can decrease patients' loneness and helplessness [23, 24].

5.2 Clinician-initiated interventions

The clinician-initiated interventions for managing low anterior resection syndrome include prescribed medication, trans-anal irrigation, pelvic floor rehabilitation (such as pelvis floor exercise, biofeedback, functional electrostimulation, and rectal balloon training), and neuromodulation (percutaneous/transcutaneous tibial nerve stimulation and sacral nerve stimulation), and so forth [29, 41].

Some prescribed medications are usually used to improve these altered bowel function [29, 32]. Phenylephrine gel twice a day or once every 8 hours may increase the anal sphincter resting pressure and decrease fecal incontinence, and Botox-A may relieve anal neuropathic pain [26, 38]. Loperamide is the most commonly prescribed oral anti-diarrhea agent to treat low anterior resection syndrome, which can activate the resting tone of internal anal sphincter and reduce episodes of defecation [31]. In clinical practice, the dose of anti-diarrhea medicine is often used by patients' self-judgment [32].

Indication of trans-anal irrigation is suggested for use in postoperative rectal cancer patients with severe or chronic low anterior resection syndrome [31]. The procedure of irrigation is usually undertaken with a rectal catheter or an anal cone and using 500 to 1500 mL daily or three to four time a week; patients usually train by clinicians or using a training video, and then they are also supervised the outcomes at least 4 weeks to 6 months [29]. The volume of irrigation, intervals between irrigation procedure, and choice of irrigation device remained equivocal and depend on patients' or educators' judgment [31, 39]. Under patients' perception, trans-anal irrigation can improve symptoms of low anterior resection, control the time of defecation, and promote their quality of life; however, patients may feel stressful and have intent of refusal due to conduct the procedure with catheterization [39].

The mechanism of pelvic floor muscle rehabilitation focuses on training coordination, sensory function, and strength of pelvis floor muscle to improve fecal incontinence [31]. The methods may consist of: (1) Pelvis floor muscle training depends on steady contraction of pelvis floor muscles to increase maximum strength, extend the duration of contractions, and improve coordination of pelvic floor muscles (a recommended frequency of the contraction is 25-40 times for three sections a day); (2) Biofeedback allows patients to directly visualize the effects of contraction and relaxation of the pelvis floor muscle and helps them to maintain habitually high-quality pelvic floor movement; (3) Functional electrostimulation induces construction of pelvis floor, and then, patients relearn and optimize the contractions by sensory feedback of this artificial contraction; and (4) Rectal balloon training depends on putting a balloon into rectum to stimulate intent of defecation, and then, patients are trained to resist the urge to defecate [29, 30, 42–44]. Varied studies validate the effectiveness of the contents of intervention, which include pelvis floor muscle training alone, biofeedback with pelvis floor muscle training, electromyography biofeedback, rectal balloon biofeedback, or all of them [45]. Although the better benefits seem to be proved on multimodalities than the single one, but the conclusion remained equivocal because of several risks of bias, including low quality across all studies due to small sample sizes, insufficient long-term follow-up, lack of randomized and blinding assessment, and heterogeneity of outcome [31, 45]. Additionally, patients' satisfaction remained unclear [46].

Neuromodulation included percutaneous tibial nerve stimulation, transcutaneous tibial nerve stimulation, and sacral nerve stimulation, which can restore neural pathway by continuous neural stimulation to treating various forms of urinary and fecal incontinence by activating nerve potentials to contract anal sphincter [31]. Percutaneous tibial nerve stimulation is applying a needle electrical stimulation into the tibial nerve at ankle, and is undertaking for 12, 17, or 20 sessions each lasting for 30 minutes; the undertaken intervals are more frequently initially, either once or twice a week, decreasing to weekly, fortnightly, monthly or sixmonthly [29]. The transcutaneous tibial nerve stimulation is to undertake a similar method of transcutaneous one, but it is using a cutaneous pad to substitute the needle electrical stimulation [31]. The procedure of sacral nerve stimulation is to put a lead of temporary external stimulator at the level of S2, S3, or S4 under general anesthesia, connecting it to a sacral nerve stimulation device and fixing its positions in a subcutaneous gluteal pocket; the setting divides the test and permanent stage, and the permanent implementation is conducted after confirming effective response during test stage [47]. The benefits of neuromodulation were revealed in previous studies, however, they still remained biases due to the results from researches with small sample sizes and lack of long-term follow-up [29, 31].

5.3 Creating a permanent stoma

Anastomosis stricture may develop in postoperative rectal cancer survivor, which may relate to previous radiation and surgery and aggravate symptoms of altered bowel function [30, 35]. When reconstruction of anastomosis is a contraindication to patients, creating a permanent stoma should be the eventual choice [30].

6. Conclusion

Altered bowel function is a consequence of anal-saving surgery. The symptoms impact patients' physical, psychological, and social domains of quality of life and may follow postoperative rectal cancer patients for whole life. Flexibly using these care strategies may help them rebalance on a new road.

Acknowledgements

I am sincerely thankful for the all kind help from our editing team and the opportunity to share knowledge. The figures in this chapter were created by Li-Hua Fang, a pharmacist from the Department of Pharmacy at the Koo-Foundation Sun Yet-Sen Cancer Centre in Taipei, Taiwan. All correspondence to Li-Hua Fang can be addressed to fang500301@gmail.com.

Conflict of interest

The author has no conflicts of interest relevant to this article.

Author details

Ling-Chun Lu
Second Degree of Science in Nursing, College of Medicine, National Taiwan University, Taipei, Taiwan

*Address all correspondence to: lulingchun@ntu.edu.tw

IntechOpen

© 2024 The Author(s). Licensee IntechOpen. This chapter is distributed under the terms of the Creative Commons Attribution License (http://creativecommons.org/licenses/by/3.0), which permits unrestricted use, distribution, and reproduction in any medium, provided the original work is properly cited.

References

[1] Korai T, Akizuki E, Okita K, Nishidate T, Okuya K, Sato Y, et al. Defecation disorder and anal function after surgery for lower rectal cancer in elderly patients. Annals of Gastroenterological Surgery. 2021;**6**(1):101-108

[2] Jansen L, Herrmann A, Stegmaier C, Singer S, Brenner H, Arndt V. Health-related quality of life during the 10 years after diagnosis of colorectal cancer: A population-based study. Journal of Clinical Oncology. 2011;**29**(24):3263-3269

[3] Su J, Liu Q, Zhou D, Yang X, Jia G, Huang L, et al. The status of low anterior resection syndrome: Data from a single-center in China. BMC Surgery. 2023;**23**(1):1-9

[4] Knowles G, Haigh R, McLean C, Phillips HA, Dunlop MG, Din FV. Long term effect of surgery and radiotherapy for colorectal cancer on defecatory function and quality of life. European Journal of Oncology Nursing. 2013;**17**(5):570-577

[5] Laursen BS, Sørensen GK, Majgaard M, Jensen LB, Jacobsen KI, Kjær DK, et al. Coping strategies and considerations regarding low anterior resection syndrome and quality of life among patients with rectal cancer; a qualitative interview study. Frontiers in Oncology. 2022;**12**:1040462

[6] Keane C, Wells C, O'Grady G, Bissett IP. Defining low anterior resection syndrome: A systematic review of the literature. Colorectal Disease: the Official Journal of the Association of Coloproctology of Great Britain and Ireland. 2017;**19**(8):713-722

[7] Lu LC, Huang XY, Chen CC. The lived experiences of patients with post-operative rectal cancer who suffer from altered bowel function: A phenomenological study. European Journal of Oncology Nursing. 2017;**31**:69-76

[8] Maris A, Penninckx F, Devreese AM, Staes F, Moons P, Van Cutsem E, et al. Persisting anorectal dysfunction after rectal cancer surgery. Colorectal Disease. 2013;**15**(11):e672-e679

[9] Chatwin NAM, Ribordy M, Givel JC. Clinical outcomes and quality of life after low anterior resection for rectal cancer. The European Journal of Surgery - Acta chirurgica. 2002;**168**(5):297-301

[10] Li C, Tang H, Zhang Y, Zhang Q, Yang W, Yu H, et al. Experiences of bowel symptoms in patients with rectal cancer after sphincter-preserving surgery: A qualitative meta-synthesis. Supportive Care in Cancer: Official Journal of the Multinational Association of Supportive Care in Cancer. 2022;**31**(1):23

[11] Varghese C, Wells CI, O'Grady G, Christensen P, Bissett IP, Keane C. The longitudinal course of low anterior resection syndrome: An individual patient meta-analysis. Annals of Surgery. 2022;**276**(1):46-54

[12] Martin F, Nath J, Bartholomew E. Fundamentals of Anatomy & Physiology. 12th ed. Pearson; 2023

[13] Pucciani F. A review on functional results of sphincter-saving surgery for rectal cancer: The anterior resection syndrome. Updates in Surgery. 2013;**65**(4):257-263

[14] Barisic G, Markovic V, Popovic M, Dimitrijevic I, Gavrilovic P, Krivokapic Z. Function after intersphincteric resection

for low rectal cancer and its influence on quality of life. Colorectal Disease. 2011;**13**(6):638-643

[15] Wallace MH. Glynne-Jones R: Saving the sphincter in rectal cancer: Are we prepared to change practice? Colorectal Disease. 2007;**9**(4):302-308; discussion 308-309

[16] Chew MH, Yeh YT, Lim E, Seow-Choen F. Pelvic autonomic nerve preservation in radical rectal cancer surgery: Changes in the past 3 decades. Gastroenterology Report (Oxford). 2016;**4**(3):173-185

[17] Sanghyun A, Ik Yong K. Pelvic anatomy for distal rectal cancer surgery. In: John C-B, editor. Current Topics in Colorectal Surgery. Rijeka: IntechOpen; 2021. Ch. 7

[18] Varghese C, Wells CI, Bissett IP, O'Grady G, Keane C. The role of colonic motility in low anterior resection syndrome. Frontiers in Oncology. 2022;**12**:975386

[19] Chen SC, Futaba K, Leung WW, Wong C, Mak T, Ng S, et al. Functional anorectal studies in patients with low anterior resection syndrome. Neurogastroenterology & Motility. 2022;**34**(3):1-10

[20] Taylor C, Bradshaw E. Tied to the toilet: Lived experiences of altered bowel function (anterior resection syndrome) after temporary stoma reversal. Journal of Wound, Ostomy & Continence Nursing. 2013;**40**(4):415-421

[21] Reinwalds M, Blixter A, Carlsson E. A descriptive, qualitative study to assess patient experiences following stoma reversal after rectal cancer surgery. Ostomy/Wound Management. 2017;**63**(12):29-37

[22] Tsui H, Huang XY. Experiences of losing bowel control after lower anterior resection with sphincter saving surgery for rectal cancer: A qualitative study. Cancer Nursing. 2022;**45**(6):E890-E896

[23] Pape E, Decoene E, Debrauwere M, Van Nieuwenhove Y, Pattyn P, Feryn T, et al. The trajectory of hope and loneliness in rectal cancer survivors with major low anterior resection syndrome: A qualitative study. European Journal of Oncology Nursing. 2022;**56**:102088

[24] Buergi C. It has become a part of me: Living with low anterior resection syndrome after ostomy reversal: A phenomenological study. Journal of Wound, Ostomy, and Continence Nursing. 2022;**49**(6):545-550

[25] Juul T, Ahlberg M, Biondo S, Espin E, Jimenez LM, Matzel KE, et al. Low anterior resection syndrome and quality of life: An international multicenter study. Diseases of the Colon and Rectum. 2014;**57**(5):585-591

[26] Reinwalds M, Blixter A, Carlsson E. Living with a resected rectum after rectal cancer surgery-struggling not to let bowel function control life. Journal of Clinical Nursing. 2018;**27**(3-4):e623-e634

[27] Desnoo L, Faithfull S. A qualitative study of anterior resection syndrome: the experiences of cancer survivors who have undergone resection surgery. European Journal of Cancer Care (England). 2006;**15**(3):244-251

[28] Hirpara DH, Azin A, Mulcahy V, Le Souder E, O'Brien C, Chadi SA, et al. The impact of surgical modality on self-reported body image, quality of life and survivorship after anterior resection for colorectal cancer – A mixed methods study. Canadian Journal of Surgery. 2019;**62**(4):235-242

[29] Burch J, Swatton A, Taylor C, Wilson A, Norton C. Managing bowel symptoms after sphincter-saving rectal cancer surgery: A scoping review. Journal of Pain and Symptom Management. 2021;**62**(6):1295-1307

[30] Sarcher T, Dupont B, Alves A, Menahem B. Anterior resection syndrome: What should we tell practitioners and patients in 2018? Journal of Visceral Surgery. 2018;**155**(5):383-391

[31] Rosen H, Sebesta CG, Sebesta C. Management of low Anterior Resection Syndrome (LARS) following resection for rectal cancer. Cancers. 2023;**15**(3):778

[32] Yin L, Fan L, Tan R, Yang G, Jiang F, Zhang C, et al. Bowel symptoms and self-care strategies of survivors in the process of restoration after low anterior resection of rectal cancer. BMC Surgery. 2018;**18**(1):35

[33] Liu W, Xia HO. Can I control my bowel symptoms myself? The experience of controlling defaecation dysfunction among patients with rectal cancer after sphincter-saving surgery: A qualitative study. International Journal of Qualitative Studies on Health & Well-Being. 2022;**17**(1):1-13

[34] Pape E, Van Haver D, Lievrouw A, Van Nieuwenhove Y, Van De Putte D, Van Ongeval J, et al. Interprofessional perspectives on care for patients with low anterior resection syndrome: A qualitative study. Colorectal Disease. 2022;**24**(9):1032-1039

[35] Zeman M, Czarnecki M, Chmielarz A, Idasiak A, Grajek M, Czarniecka A. Assessment of the risk of permanent stoma after low anterior resection in rectal cancer patients. World Journal of Surgical Oncology. 2020;**18**(1):207

[36] Harji D, Fernandez B, Boissieras L, Berger A, Capdepont M, Zerbib F, et al. A novel bowel rehabilitation programme after total mesorectal excision for rectal cancer: The BOREAL pilot study. Colorectal Disease. 2021;**23**(10):2619-2626

[37] Liu W, Xu JM, Zhang YX, Lu HJ, Xia HO. The relationship between food consumption and bowel symptoms among patients with rectal cancer after sphincter-saving surgery. Frontiers in Medicine. 2021;**8**:642574

[38] Liu W, Xu JM, Zhang YX, Lu HJ, Xia HO. The experience of dealing with defecation dysfunction by changing the eating behaviours of people with rectal cancer following sphincter-saving surgery: A qualitative study. Nursing Open. 2021;**8**(3):1501-1509

[39] McCutchan GM, Hughes D, Davies Z, Torkington J, Morris C, Cornish JA. Acceptability and benefit of rectal irrigation in patients with low anterior resection syndrome: A qualitative study. Colorectal Disease. 2017;**20**:O76-O84

[40] Nakagawa H, Sasai H, Tanaka K. Defecation dysfunction and exercise habits among survivors of rectal cancer: A pilot qualitative study. Healthcare (Basel). 2022;**10**(10):2029

[41] Rodrigues BDS, Rodrigues FP, Buzatti KCLR, Campanati RG, Profeta da Luz MM, Gomes da Silva R, et al. Feasibility study of transanal irrigation using a colostomy irrigation system in patients with low anterior resection syndrome. Diseases of the Colon and Rectum. 2022;**65**(3):413-420

[42] van der Heijden JAG, Kalkdijk-Dijkstra AJ, Pierie JPEN, van Westreenen HL, Broens PMA, Klarenbeek BR. Pelvic floor rehabilitation after rectal cancer surgery. A Multicenter randomized clinical trial (FORCE trial). Annals of Surgery. 2022;**276**(1):38-45

[43] Sacomori C, Lorca LA, Martinez-Mardones M, Salas-Ocaranza RI, Reyes-Reyes GP, Pizarro-Hinojosa MN, et al. A randomized clinical trial to assess the effectiveness of pre- and post-surgical pelvic floor physiotherapy for bowel symptoms, pelvic floor function, and quality of life of patients with rectal cancer: CARRET protocol. Trials. 2021;**22**(1):1-11

[44] Asnong A, D'Hoore A, Van Kampen M, Wolthuis A, Van Molhem Y, Van Geluwe B, et al. The role of pelvic floor muscle training on low anterior resection syndrome: A Multicenter randomized controlled trial. Annals of Surgery. 2022;**276**(5):761-768

[45] Chan KYC, Suen M, Coulson S, Vardy JL. Efficacy of pelvic floor rehabilitation for bowel dysfunction after anterior resection for colorectal cancer: A systematic review. Supportive Care in Cancer: Official Journal of the Multinational Association of Supportive Care in Cancer. 2021;**29**(4):1795-1809

[46] Li H, Guo C, Gao J, Yao H. Effectiveness of biofeedback therapy in patients with bowel dysfunction following rectal cancer surgery: A systemic review with meta-analysis. Therapeutics & Clinical Risk Management. 2022;**18**:71-93

[47] De Meyere C, Nuytens F, Parmentier I, D'Hondt M. Five-year single center experience of sacral neuromodulation for isolated fecal incontinence or fecal incontinence combined with low anterior resection syndrome. Techniques in Coloproctology. 2020;**24**(9):947-958

Chapter 4

Perspective Chapter: Obstructed Defecation – From Diagnosis to Treatment

Chris Gillespie

Abstract

Obstructed defecation is a common, disabling condition, with significant crossover to other functional gastrointestinal disorders as well as pelvic floor problems. It requires a comprehensive assessment as it involves functional, behavioural, psychological and anatomical aspects. This chapter will address the broad aspects of obstructed defecation including an in-depth discussion of concepts of normal and abnormal defecation, pathophysiology, and appropriate use of investigations. A summary of nonoperative therapies including biofeedback and irrigation will feature, along with an update on the evidence for surgical options in obstructed defecation.

Keywords: obstructed defecation, constipation, rectopexy, rectocele, rectal prolapse

1. Introduction

Obstructed defecation is a widely accepted term used to define the symptoms of anorectal outlet obstruction; it is a symptom complex and not a diagnosis.

Despite the Rome IV criteria classifying functional defaecation disorders, there is currently no specific accepted strict definition for obstructed defecation; the most widely used criteria, however, are those defining the subset of functional constipation in Rome IV [1]. These include two or more of the following occurring in more than 25% of defecations:

1. Straining

2. Lumpy or hard stool

3. A sensation of incomplete evacuation

4. A sensation of anorectal obstruction or blockage

5. Manual manoeuvres to facilitate defecation (e.g. rectal/vaginal/perineal support).

The other components for a diagnosis of functional constipation include less than three spontaneous bowel movements per week and the absence of or infrequent loose stool without the use of laxatives.

To make a diagnosis of a functional defaecation disorder, patients must also have objective evidence of impaired evacuation in two of the below tests:

1. Abnormal balloon expulsion test.

2. Abnormal anorectal evacuation pattern with manometry or anorectal EMG.

3. Impaired rectal evacuation by imaging.

2. The symptom complex and associated problems

Obstructed defaecation can be an extremely debilitating condition with frequent coexisting and associated symptoms. Presentation is often delayed due to embarrassment or a perceived lack of treatment options. It is a chronic problem, well established in having a significant impact on quality of life, with some experiencing severe symptoms interfering with their daily activities or social functioning. The impairment is at least as significant as medical chronic conditions such as diabetes, depression and neurological diseases [2].

Many patients report abdominal pain and/or significant bloating, and potentially even nausea or food avoidance, and often this is their main complaint [3]. This can divert attention away from outlet obstruction symptoms and lead to a diagnosis of irritable bowel syndrome (IBS), which currently has a different treatment algorithm. It is now becoming increasingly recognised, however, that functional constipation and irritable bowel syndrome are a spectrum of disease, rather than entirely distinct entities, as per the update to Rome IV [4]. Essentially, the diagnostic criteria between irritable bowel syndrome with constipation (IBS-C) and functional constipation are very similar, differing only in the presence of abdominal pain in IBS-C. A 2021 cohort study using machine learning to compare patients with functional constipation and IBS-C supported the concept of the two disorders being a one-dimensional spectrum rather than two disparate diseases [5]. Mechanistically, this is plausible, with an outlet/emptying disorder likely to lead to a high-pressure colon and visceral pain, although IBS may feature additional visceral hypersensitivity requiring other modes of analgesia [3].

There is a significant crossover between symptoms amongst functional gastrointestinal disorders, with more than one third of patients having symptoms overlapping with another disorder [6] as alluded to above. The clinician should obtain a complete pelvic floor history as well as screening for symptoms of irritable bowel syndrome, which often coexist. In general, symptomatic relief is the primary goal of treatment along with improvement in quality of life, and treatments that are known to be effective for functional constipation have been shown to improve quality of life and symptoms in IBS-C [7]. Therefore, the distinction or segregation between these functional gastrointestinal (GI) disorders is less clinically relevant.

Over half of all patients presenting to a pelvic floor unit with functional constipation will also have symptoms of faecal incontinence. This may include passive faecal leakage or urge incontinence, and the coexistence of symptoms is missed by over 85% of referring clinicians [8]. In fact, the progression of longstanding obstructed defaecation to faecal incontinence is widely acknowledged, and an area of ongoing longitudinal research—these patients often have signs of mechanical dysfunction including perineal descent [9], presumably from excessive straining over years.

With the multicompartment nature of pelvic floor disorders, it is also important for the clinician to uncover symptoms of vaginal prolapse and urinary symptoms such as incomplete voiding or urinary incontinence, often related to the same underlying pathophysiology.

A history of sexual abuse can be important to appraise as only 17% of victims disclose this history to their doctor, and a psychologist or psychiatrist is an important member of the multidisciplinary team supporting these people [10]. There is a strong association with functional gastrointestinal disorders and chronic pain and those with constipation may have worse symptoms and quality of life [11], although anorectal physiology findings are similar to those without this history [12].

Haemorrhoids are also a common complaint in patients with obstructed defaecation along with rectal bleeding. Amongst patients undergoing haemorrhoidectomy, a Saudi Arabian study found 24.2% had obstructed defaecation syndrome and this was shown to have a negative correlation with postoperative patient satisfaction [13]. A Chinese study also showed that a higher obstructed defaecation score was significantly associated with recurrence of haemorrhoids postoperatively and less satisfaction with surgery [14]—both studies supporting the importance of treating the underlying defaecatory disorder, along with its consequent haemorrhoids.

3. Prevalence and epidemiology

The precise epidemiology of obstructed defaecation is poorly understood because there is no unified definition of the syndrome. The literature varies widely depending on the definition and the population studied, but its prevalence estimates range from 2 to 30%. It is particularly prevalent in multiparous postmenopausal women and more frequently observed after hysterectomy [15].

An Australian population-based study using market research analysed the prevalence of functional constipation [16]. In 2376 respondent's representative of the Australian population, 24% had chronic functional constipation based on Rome III criteria and 59% self-reported constipation in the last 12 months. The most common symptoms participants described were straining, hard stool and the feeling of incomplete evacuation, with each reported by about 80% of those with constipation.

4. Normal and abnormal defaecation

An understanding of obstructed defaecation first requires an appreciation of the mechanism of normal defaecation.

Normal defaecation requires the following:

1. The delivery of soft-formed stool to the rectum.

2. Normal cognitive/behavioural elements in toileting and normal childhood defaecatory acquisition.

3. Psychosocial aspects including access to toilets and appropriate response to the call to stool.

4. Dietary aspects/gastrocolic reflex.

5. Colonic motor activity and propulsive force.

6. Rectal and anal compliance/elasticity.

7. Intact neural pathways.

8. Intact pelvic supports.

9. Normal coordination of the abdominopelvic cylinder during the defecation manoeuvre.

Normal defaecation is a complex mechanism with functional, physiological and psychosocial elements.

The delivery of soft-formed stool to the rectum is achieved with an intact colon with normal transit. In general, fibre supplementation is a useful adjunct to optimising stool consistency and a routine part of assessment, using the Bristol stool chart. The assistance of a dietitian can be invaluable.

The development of a normal defaecatory reflex occurs during early childhood but is poorly understood. Certainly, the effect of childhood physical, emotional and sexual abuse cannot be underestimated during this critical time of neuroplasticity [10]. Problems often initially manifest as paediatric GI disorders, with people going on to continue to suffer with symptoms into adulthood.

Issues with toileting behaviour such as a timely response to the call to stool, and access to toilets, form the basis for a lot of the intervention that pelvic floor physiotherapists make. Psychological stress or distress may lead to disordered defaecation and avoidance of public/school toilets [17] and other lifestyle or vocational issues may disrupt a normal toileting pattern. These are often underestimated and understudied elements of defaecatory dysfunction that can be easily addressed.

A normal defaecatory manoeuvre requires coordinated movement of the entire abdominopelvic cylinder and anal opening, with complex dynamic muscular changes in the pelvis to facilitate a smooth, effective evacuation. A proctographic study of 20 females demonstrated a bidirectional pull on the anal canal during defecation, with the posterior wall of the anorectum moving posteriorly and the anterior wall moving ventrally, thereby increasing the anal canal to twice its diameter during defaecation, mechanistically facilitating evacuation [18]. The musculoelastic theory of defaecation suggests that the passive contraction of the puborectalis muscle against the opposing pull of the levator plate maintains the anorectal angle, and thereby continence. During defaecation, puborectalis relaxes, but the pubococcygeus muscle contracts, pulling the anterior rectal wall open against the opposing contraction of the levator plate, which can now pull the anorectal wall posteriorly, unopposed. This theory would be concordant with the observed changes during normal proctography and result in less resistance to faecal flow [19]. Normal defaecation may therefore involve both relaxation and activation components in pelvic floor muscular activity.

Effective pelvic floor muscular function also requires integrity to its ligamentous supports. A large European multicentre prospective series of over 650 females with coexisting vaginal apical prolapse and other pelvic floor symptoms underwent a gynaecological transvaginal surgery, with reconstruction of the uterosacral and cardinal ligaments [20]. Amongst those with faecal and urinary incontinence, there was a statistically significant improvement in symptoms with this gynaecological surgery, illustrating the importance of these ligaments in anorectal and bladder function. A retrospective study also demonstrated an improvement in anorectal function with transvaginal surgery for vaginal prolapse (sacrospinous fixation), including a statistically significant improvement in the obstructed defaecation and constipation scoring system scores [21]. These studies support the concept of pelvic ligamentous integrity being an important element of normal anorectal function (**Figure 1**).

The gradual progression in grades of rectal prolapse that has been previously demonstrated [22] leads to high-grade internal rectal prolapse with potential plugging of the anal canal, causing obstruction of defaecation. With a loss of fascial supports also comes a loss of effective force vector for push, with this dissipating into a rectocoele or causing loss of pelvic floor mechanical advantage. About 74% improvement in obstructed defaecation observed with rectopexy surgery [23] again supports the concept of a restoration of rectal supports improving obstructed defaecation in some patients due to an improvement in the mechanics of defaecation (**Figure 2**).

Another very important element in normal defaecation is normal coordination of the defaecatory manoeuvre. Dyssynergia refers to a lack of coordination of the abdominal and pelvic floor muscles during defaecation, leading to an inability to evacuate stool. This affects approximately 50% of all constipated patients [24]. The elements of dyssynergia include the following [25]:

1. Inadequate rectal propulsion.

2. Paradoxical anal closure.

3. Inadequate anal opening.

4. Impaired rectal sensation.

Dyssynergic defecation remains controversial, but is considered an entity in the Rome IV criteria [1]. It is common and has a significant effect on quality of life, with the majority of patients being female [25].

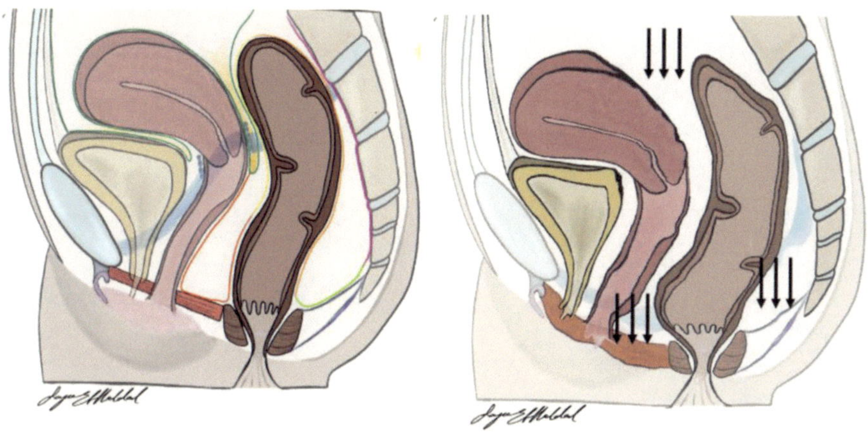

Figure 1.
Normal pelvic anatomy (left) and mechanical pelvic floor dysfunction with loss of pelvic ligamentous integrity (right) (illustrated by Joyce El-Haddad).

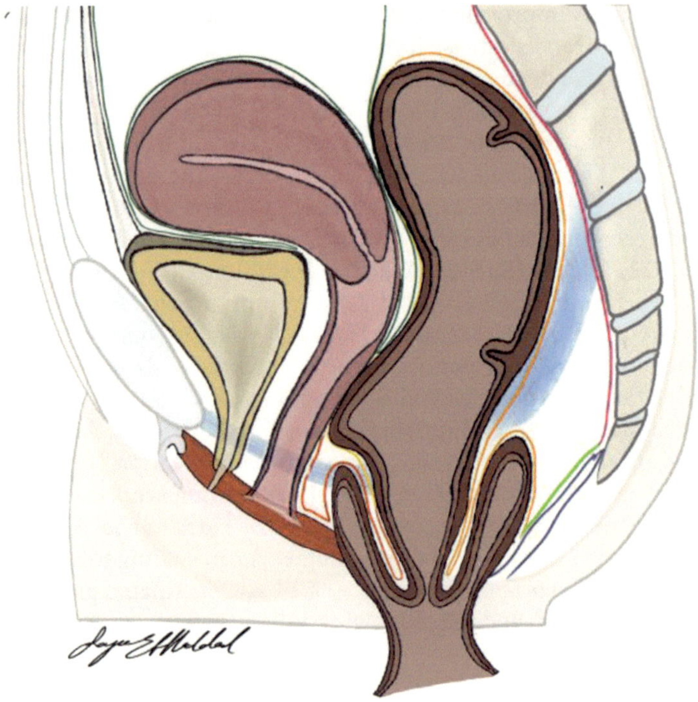

Figure 2.
Mechanical pelvic floor dysfunction with high-grade internal rectal prolapse (illustrated by Joyce El-Haddad).

Many patients with dyssynergia describe straining and incomplete evacuation, but abdominal pain and bloating are also frequent symptoms [25]. There is a high rate of physical and sexual abuse in this cohort [26]. As a cause of chronic functional outlet obstruction, it can be associated with slow colonic transit in longstanding cases, particularly when constipation goes back to childhood or where there is laxative

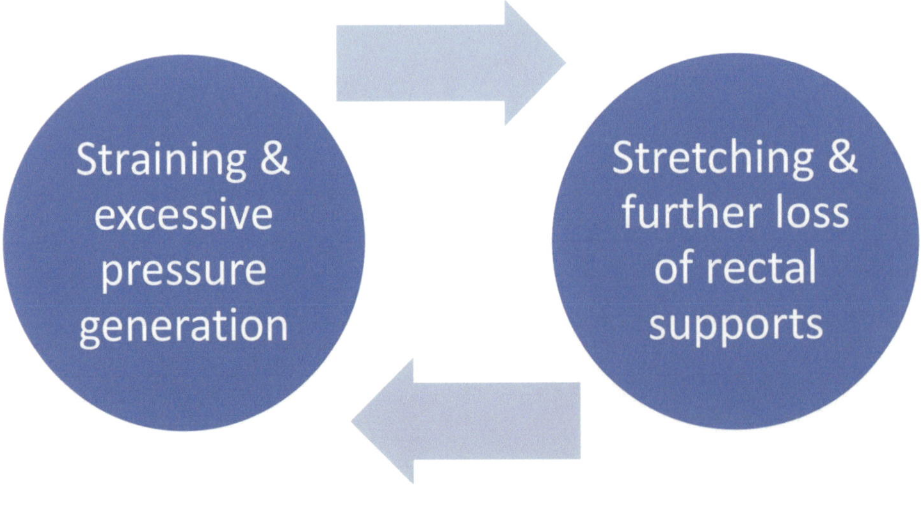

Figure 3.
Concepts in the pathophysiology of obstructed defecation.

dependence [27]. As with the other causes of obstructed defaecation, there is a significant overlap with IBS features and in fact, IBS patients benefit similarly from biofeedback therapy to patients with isolated dyssynergia [7]. Biofeedback therapy has also been shown to improve transit time in patients with defaecatory disorders [28], making evaluation and treatment for dyssynergia in constipated patients important.

The majority of patients with obstructed defecation have a combination of both anatomical and functional derangements—requiring a cautious approach and judicious use of investigations. Excessive pressures from straining and ineffective defecation may lead to stretching of supportive tissue and prolapse; equally impaired mechanics and loss of pelvic supports from obstetric trauma or surgery may lead to straining to better effect defecation. A vicious cycle of excessive straining may then lead to further deterioration—perhaps explaining the gradual progression from pure obstructed defecation to that combined with faecal incontinence (**Figure 3**).

5. Investigations for obstructed defecation

The assessment of obstructed defecation serves the purposes of both facilitating diagnosis and treatment, as well as exclusion of other pathology, albeit rare. There are no studies to guide the clinician but in general, blood tests including screening for biochemical or metabolic disorders are acceptable, including full blood count, renal and thyroid function and serum calcium [29]. The astute clinician will keep an open mind in considering other diseases such as cauda equina syndrome or neurological/endocrine disease, which may masquerade as obstructed defecation.

A digital rectal examination is mandatory and can be used to both exclude local disease and evaluate during dynamic movements for the presence of rectocoele, haemorrhoids and prolapse.

The yield of colonoscopy in this cohort is low, although an endoscopic assessment can provide reassurance and will often diagnose adenomatous polyps, although at a rate similar to the general population [30].

Colonic transit studies aim to distinguish slow transit from obstructed defecation and require the patient to come off laxatives for the study. The diagnosis of slow colonic transit may lead to treatment options such as stimulant treatment or surgery, but slow transit also improves with biofeedback therapy [28], a mainstay of treatment for obstructed defecation. Transit studies should therefore be deferred until patients have had biofeedback, and slow transit has not been shown to affect the results of surgery for obstructed defecation [31].

Anorectal manometry has not been validated for its role in the workup for obstructed defecation, but remains an extremely useful tool in the investigation of obstructed defecation. Widespread variance in practice has led to the International Anorectal Physiology Working Group providing a consensus statement regarding the role of physiological tests in anorectal structure and function, and a protocol for performing anorectal manometry [32]. Certainly, anorectal physiology tests are well tolerated by patients, and can direct treatment including diagnosis of altered rectal sensation, hypotonia, dyssynergia and an absent recto-anal inhibitory reflex, which could lead to consideration of Hirschsprung's disease [33]. It is recommended as a comprehensive evaluation of anorectal function by the European Society of Neurogastroenterology and Motility guidelines on functional constipation [34].

Proctography, either fluoroscopic or magnetic resonance, allows a dynamic assessment of anorectal function and is considered the current "gold-standard" in the diagnosis of high-grade internal rectal prolapse. It also assesses for other pelvic floor anatomical abnormalities such as enterocoele, cystocoele and vaginal vault prolapse. The presence of an enterocoele predicts a good response to ventral mesh rectopexy and therefore adds clinical utility to this test [35]. A Cochrane review reported an 89% sensitivity and specificity of 92% for the diagnosis of rectal prolapse, although this did not separate internal and external rectal prolapse and include low-grade internal rectal prolapse, generally not considered clinically relevant [36]. Similar to anorectal manometry, wide variations in reporting have led to a consensus statement regarding the performance of proctography, with this report acknowledging the results are often dependent on patient and radiographer factors [37].

The role of an examination under anaesthetic in the diagnosis of rectal prolapse, which may detect occult high-grade internal rectal prolapse in a false-negative proctogram, requires further evaluation [38].

6. Non-operative therapies

A holistic approach to obstructed defecation, with identification of both anatomical derangement and functional and behavioural contributers, is important and more likely to lead to symptom improvement. Overall, treatment should be targeted at symptoms and aimed to improve quality of life, rather than correcting anatomy or proctographic abnormalities.

The benefit of a multidisciplinary approach to functional constipation has been shown over single specialist care [39], with initial treatment including dietary modification, laxatives/medication, psychological therapy and pelvic floor biofeedback.

Fibre has the benefit of potentially modulating gut dysbiosis as well as achieving a softer, more manageable, stool consistency. Most evidence for fibre supplementation is behind soluble fibre, such as psyllium husks; however, its use can be limited by the development of bloating or abdominal pain in those with IBS-C symptomatology [40]. In some patients, particularly those with coexisting slow transit, reducing fibre improves symptoms [41, 42].

The input of a dietitian can provide expert advice and is common practice, although there is not much evidence supporting dietetic intervention in obstructed defecation. An Australian study pooled 126 patients referred to a colorectal pelvic floor clinic, 44% of whom presented with obstructed defecation, to dietitian-led input including a healthy eating programme and fibre supplementation. Overall, 25% of the 126 patients had complete resolution of symptoms, with a high degree of satisfaction [42]. Dietitians are also more likely to recognise patients who have an eating disorder, with 24% of these patients suffering from functional constipation [43].

Exercise and fluid intake are also considered part of basic management, although again there is paucity in the literature to support this. A NICE review from 2021 found only low to very low-level evidence supporting exercise, fluid intake and dietary intake measures in preventing pelvic floor symptoms, and there were no studies on obstructed defecation specifically [44].

In terms of laxative therapy, there have been more placebo-controlled trials over the last 15 years and a recent systematic review showed the strongest evidence base in treatment of constipation with polyethyene glycol and senna [45]. Docusate, a commonly prescribed laxative, had no recommendation as there is surprisingly little evidence for its use, with no clinical studies published since 2004.

Psychological therapy may have a role in those patients with IBS-C symptoms, with systematic reviews demonstrating improvements in IBS symptoms, particularly with cognitive-behavioural therapy and gut-directed hypnotherapy [46]. As the crossover between IBS and functional constipation is more recognised, these therapies may play a role in improving quality of life in obstructed defecation patients.

7. Biofeedback therapy

Specialist pelvic floor physiotherapists with further training in defaecatory physiotherapy are able to provide a holistic approach to optimising lifestyle around toileting and defaecatory technique. This includes the timing of defaecation, improving lifestyle measures pertaining to toileting, dietary advice and laxative advice. Specifically, positioning and toileting technique are improved. There is evidence that the "squatting" technique for defaecation leads to a better evacuation, hence the benefit of using a stool when on a Western toilet [47].

Biofeedback therapy refers to reinstitution of a more "normal" defaecatory technique with the use of visual feedback to the patient. Expert physiotherapists are also able to perform volumetric rehabilitation to treat altered sensitivity in the rectum.

A randomised study comparing biofeedback therapy and polyethylene glycol for obstructed defaecation showed an improvement in clinical symptoms in the biofeedback group [48]. There is randomised evidence for a benefit over standard care in pelvic floor dyssynergia [28] and an improvement in constipation symptoms and patients with internal rectal prolapse [49]. Long-term follow-up from the well-known Poppy trial has shown that patients who underwent pelvic floor physiotherapy treatment were less likely to require hospital treatment for pelvic floor disorders such as faecal incontinence for a period of over 10 years [50].

The benefits of specialist pelvic floor physiotherapy cannot be overstated as a safe and non-invasive measure with clear evidence of an improvement in patients with obstructed defaecation and the potential to avoid surgery.

8. Irrigation

Transanal irrigation, first developed by Christensen et al., allows patients to better manage defecatory dysfunction with regular rectal irrigation and controlled bowel emptying. Its safety is well established, and randomised data has shown its efficacy in neurogenic bowel dysfunction and low anterior resection syndrome [51–55]. In obstructed defecation, there is no randomised data [56], but improvements in symptom severity and quality of life are well documented. Importantly, 50–60% of patients are no longer using the device after 12 months, indicating a significant dropout rate or potentially less efficacy or satisfaction [57, 58].

There is limited long-term data in obstructed defecation, and the therapy does require significant education, patient investment and time, but transanal irrigation clearly has a place in the treatment algorithm for obstructed defecation.

Antegrade colonic irrigation, something well recognised in children, has a role in the treatment of adult defecatory dysfunction although the data on results is limited. There are no comparative studies, but a systematic review in 2016 was able to analyse results in over 400 patients, 209 of whom had constipation, and found a 67.7% pooled success rate for constipated patients, at a median follow-up of 39 months. This included the Malone procedure, ileal neoappendicostomy, open caecostomy and percutaneous endoscopic caecostomy. There was a notably significant surgical morbidity [59]. For patients with intractable severe defecatory difficulties despite maximal treatment, antegrade colonic irrigation is something to be considered if transanal irrigation is not feasible or the patient chooses this over a colostomy.

9. Rectocoele repair

A rectocoele repair aims to address the impairment in biomechanics created by a rectocoele. A rectocoele is thought to form from traumatic detachment of the pericervical ring from the rectovaginal septum during labour [60]. Further pressure or straining can lead to herniation of the rectum and septum anteriorly, ultimately creating a pocket for stool and a loss of effective defecatory vector. Patients often are aware of a bulge and defecatory difficulties, and may even be aware of stool becoming trapped in the rectocoele.

The difficulty in the management of rectocoeles is in determining in which patients is the rectocoele the main player in the impaired defecatory mechanics. Successful surgery is only likely if the rectocoele is the main driver of symptoms.

Small (<2 cm) rectocoeles are a common finding, and 80% of parous females are diagnosed with a rectocoele on proctogram [61]. Over 30% of women with pelvic organ prolapse will have a rectocoele [62]; the difficulty is not in identifying a rectocoele, but in determining its significance. There is no universally accepted grading system for rectocoeles, with most measuring the maximal anterior extent of the rectocoele beyond the "normal" rectovaginal septum position. Gynaecological assessment assesses the extent of the rectocoele in relation to the vaginal introitus, the reference point for the POP-Q system. In general, only rectocoeles greater than 3 cm are considered potentially significant.

About 60% of rectocoeles occur in the setting of dyssynergia, and in these patients, initial treatment should be directed at the functional element with the usual strategy of supportive therapy and biofeedback. The excessive straining and impaired defecation from dyssynergia may well have accelerated the development of the rectocoele, and two case series have demonstrated worse surgical outcomes for rectocoele repair in patients with dyssynergia [63, 64].

The formation of a rectocoele represents a loss of suspensory ligamentous support and rarely occurs in isolation. A degree of internal rectal prolapse will be present in 80%, and some may also have symptomatic vaginal prolapse. The decision between rectocoele repair and rectopexy to address the internal rectal prolapse component is contentious and often based on the grade and anatomy of the internal rectal prolapse. In one series, rectal intussusception was predictive of a poorer result to the anterior Delormes operation [64].

In general, transanal rectocoele repair is more likely to be successful in patients who vaginally digitate, with a New Zealand study showing an 80% success for this group, who were the most likely to benefit from the surgery in their cohort [64]. The other factor is the rectocoele, which does not empty on proctography [65], although other papers have not shown any correlation between success and rectocoele size or contrast trapping [66].

Transanal repair includes a plication of the defective rectal muscularis layer, as well as excision of redundant mucosa. It is termed a Delormes operation in some parts of the world, and can be performed circumferentially, isolated to the anterior rectal wall where the rectocoele is, or tailored to the prolapse. It is very well tolerated, with minimal morbidity, and good outcomes at short-term follow-up. Over time, recurrence of the rectocoele may occur with some studies reporting recurrence rates approaching 50% by 5 years [64, 67]. In terms of functional results, long-term follow-up studies have demonstrated persisting benefits at 5 years, with sustained significant reductions in the Constipation Scoring System, Obstructed Defecation Score and Patient Assessment of Constipation Quality of Life scores [68, 69]. A persisting symptom improvement is more likely in patients who receive postoperative pelvic floor physiotherapy, and these patients are more likely to be satisfied [69]. There are concerns about potential worsening of faecal incontinence due to the anal stretch required for the procedure, although this is controversial. Some studies report up to 1/3 of previously continent women suffering gas or liquid incontinence at 5 years [67], but other more recent papers report a long-term improvement in faecal incontinence, with a 50% reduction in the Faecal Incontinence Severity Index in 2/3 of patients [68].

Transvaginal repair is usually performed by the gynaecologist and now includes a defect-specific repair of the damaged rectovaginal septum, perhaps better addressing the pathophysiology of the rectocoele. It results in significant improvement in obstructed defecation symptoms, including a reduced odds ratio of postoperative straining and incomplete emptying of 0.17 and 0.1 specifically [70]. Predictors of failure include residual rectocoele postoperatively, a higher preoperative Wexner score [71], shorter functional anal canal length and seepage on proctography [72]. There is, however, a high rate of sexual dysfunction [73]. Long-term results demonstrate a persisting benefit at 5 years, with a national register-based cohort study using patient reported outcome measures reporting over 70% 'cure' and over 75% satisfaction with the surgery [74].

Transperineal rectocele repair involves a curvilinear incision between the anal verge and posterior fourchette, and a dissection in the rectovaginal plane to allow its direct repair. Concomitant levatorplasty to restore the vaginal hiatus, and a sphincter repair if needed, can also be performed *via* this approach, along with a perineorrhaphy. Mesh or other implants have been used. There are only a small number of studies in the literature, reporting a median 72.7% improvement in symptoms and improvement in quality of life [75], but no long-term data is available.

A pelvic floor multidisciplinary team (MDT) meeting may assist in decision making as to the best surgical approach for each patient. A British team reported their experience with a pelvic floor MDT, with all 7 of their cases of prolapse and obstructed defecation having a change in management team [76].

In 2017, Grossi et al. published a systematic review encompassing an extensive literature review including transanal, trans-vaginal and trans-perineal approaches to rectocoele. This concluded with an overall low level of evidence and an inability to sufficiently compare procedures [77].

10. Stapled transanal procedures

Stapled transanal procedures for obstructed defecation followed Longo's development of the technique in 2004 [78], with the concept of excision of the internally prolapsing rectum and redundant wall of the rectocoele leading to an improvement in anatomical derangement and thereby function. The procedure involves excision of rectal wall and creation of a stapled anastomosis. The STARR procedure involves separate excisions of the anterior and posterior prolapsing rectum, and the subsequent Trans-STARR procedure allows a more tailored excision of the prolapse using a Contour Transtar stapler. Specific exclusion criteria include an enterocoele at rest and anal incontinence with Wexner score > 7 [79]. Of 47 papers in a 2018 systematic review, all reported an improvement in constipation symptoms when recorded, with >50% improvement in ODS score, along with high rates of patient satisfaction [80]. No conclusions were able to be made regarding superiority of STARR vs. Trans-STARR.

In terms of safety, the systematic review by Mercer-Jones analysed the results of 8340 patients from multiple studies, with acceptably low morbidity. Postoperative bleeding occurred in 1.6%, sepsis in 0.2%, and anastomotic dehiscence in 0.3%, with very low rates of other serious complications. Postoperative pain was variably reported, but had an overall rate of 0.7% beyond 6 months. Urgency, often cited as a concern for the STARR procedure, was reported in 5.2% although how much of this was truly new urgency was debateable [80].

A more recent study of long-term outcomes out to 10 years, however, was somewhat concerning, with persisting pain and a significant rate of urgency reported as featured in the European STARR registry [81] and the 2010 NICE recommendation [82]. Amongst 60 patients at 10 years follow-up after STARR surgery, 38% had persisting perineal pain, 22% had urgency and 21% would not select STARR again [83].

11. Botulinum toxin injection for obstructed defecation

Dyssnergic defecation, now a recognised functional gastrointestinal disorder, can cause significant suffering, including symptoms of incomplete evacuation and straining as well as urgency and abdominal symptoms. Biofeedback, laxatives and improving toileting habits and lifestyle are standard basic treatment, usually beneficial in 70% of cases. Botulinum toxin-A targeted at specific hypertonic or non-relaxing muscles can improve symptoms when standard initial treatments fail [84]. Disordered defecation may respond to denervation of dysfunctional muscles, and biofeedback may be rendered more effective through a less paradoxical or less functionally obstructed defecation. Whilst the effect is temporary, the 2–3 month effect is an opportunity to take advantage of the alteration in defecatory manoeuvre and reinstitute a more physiologically "normal" coordination of the defecatory reflex [85, 86].

Subjective improvement has been reported in 30–100% with a reduction in the Constipation Severity Score [87–89], although the approach to injection and dosing is highly variable across institutions [85]. Dosages range from 12 to 200 units, with most studies targeting both puborectalis and the anal sphincter muscle. Techniques including palpation and ultrasound or electromyographic guidance, and the majority of procedures are performed either without anaesthesia or with sedation.

Serious complications are rare [90], with aggregated rates of faecal incontinence of 6.9% and flatal incontinence of 4.1% [85]. Not surprisingly, the finding of high-grade internal rectal prolapse may render Botulinum toxin less effective [91].

12. Rectopexy for obstructed defecation

Rectopexy for functional anorectal symptoms is centred around the premise of treating high-grade rectal intussusception and its effect on anorectal biomechanics, leading to an improvement in symptoms of obstructed defecation, quality of life and the often coexisting faecal leakage. In general, the main indication is high-grade internal rectal prolapse, with the rectopexy aiming to prevent the intussuscipiens from "plugging" the anal canal or activating the rectoanal inhibitory reflex. The rectocoele is also considered "treated" with better rectal wall support and creation of scar in the rectovaginal septum.

Traditionally used to treat external rectal prolapse, rectopexy has undergone many iterations over time, including the traditional posterior sutured rectopexy, resection rectopexy and the widely used ventral mesh rectopexy. Ventral mesh rectopexy, originally described by Andre d'Hoore, has the advantage of sparing the posterolateral dissection of the rectum—complete circumferential rectal mobilisation is thought to be responsible for the rates of *de novo* constipation reported, *via* division of lateral rectal ligaments and accompanying autonomic nerves [92].

Unfortunately, the evidence base for rectopexy for internal rectal prolapse and obstructed defecation remains low level, with only retrospective series published with varying quality and measurement of results. There are four papers on resection rectopexy, the most recent published in 2006, and multiple case series on ventral mesh rectopexy. With a lack of comparative papers, any conclusions regarding superiority between the surgical techniques have not been able to be confidently made [93]. Serious complications were rare, with Grossi's systematic review suggesting a trend to a higher rate of surgical complications with resection rectopexy, although another systematic review by Emile et al. did not find difference [23]. Concerns regarding the use of mesh for functional GI disorders were addressed by the European Society of Coloproctology (ESCP) who published a guidance paper following rigorous literature review [94]. Mesh-related complications are serious but uncommon, reported in 1.1% of ventral mesh rectopexies for internal rectal prolapse [23]. The ESCP guidance document recommended mesh rectopexy be considered in the management of internal rectal prolapse, rectocoele and enterocoele, when conservative management is maximised and the condition continues to have a strong negative impact on quality of life.

In the medium term, 68% of patients report a subjective improvement in symptoms at a median of 44 months [95], and this corresponds to a significant improvement in symptom severity scores, with a significant drop in ODS scores sustained at 2 years [96]. Ventral mesh rectopexy is shown to improve constipation in 76.6%, with resection rectopexy improving 68.6% of patients. Concomitantly, and importantly, faecal incontinence symptoms improved in 62.5 and 52.7%, respectively [23].

Solitary rectal ulcer syndrome may be treated with ventral mesh rectopexy, with successful healing in 78% of patients [93].

Anatomical recurrence occurs in 2–7% of patients [93] and although this correlates with outcome, symptomatic recurrence is more relevant to patients and the true outcome in terms of function for this surgery will be borne out with longer-term follow-up and improved patient-reported outcome measures.

13. Conclusions

Obstructed defecation is a common, disabling condition with significant symptom crossover to other functional GI disorders as well as other pelvic floor problems. It requires a broad assessment as it involves functional, behavioural, psychological and anatomical aspects. Treatment is aimed at improving symptoms and quality of life and patients benefit from a multidisciplinary approach aiming to address all aspects of the dysfunction.

Supportive treatment and biofeedback therapy are a mainstay of patient management, with biofeedback also potentially improving the satisfaction and outcomes of any surgery. Surgery, in carefully selected cases after exhaustion of nonoperative treatment, is generally safe and carries good results although we still lack adequate data in the literature on important patient-reported outcomes, particularly in the longer term.

Author details

Chris Gillespie
Colorectal Surgeon, University of Queensland, Queen Elizabeth II Hospital and Princess Alexandra Hospital, Brisbane, Australia

*Address all correspondence to: gillespiechris@yahoo.com.au

IntechOpen

© 2023 The Author(s). Licensee IntechOpen. This chapter is distributed under the terms of the Creative Commons Attribution License (http://creativecommons.org/licenses/by/3.0), which permits unrestricted use, distribution, and reproduction in any medium, provided the original work is properly cited.

References

[1] Lacy BE, Patel NK. Rome criteria and a diagnostic approach to irritable bowel syndrome. Journal of Clinical Medicine. 2017;**6**(11):99. DOI: 10.3390/jcm6110099

[2] Brochard C et al. Quality of life in 1870 patients with constipation and/or fecal incontinence: Constipation should not be underestimated. Clinics and Research in Hepatology and Gastroenterology. 2019;**43**(6):682-687. DOI: 10.1016/j.clinre.2019.02.011

[3] Wong MYW, Hebbard G, Gibson PR, Burgell RE. Chronic constipation and abdominal pain: Independent or closely interrelated symptoms? Journal of Gastroenterology and Hepatology. 2020;**35**(8):1294-1301. DOI: 10.1111/jgh.14970

[4] Simren M, Palsson OS, Whitehead WE. Update on Rome IV criteria for colorectal disorders: Implications for clinical practice. Current Gastroenterology Reports. 2017;**19**(4):15. DOI: 10.1007/s11894-017-0554-0

[5] Ruffle JK et al. Constipation predominant irritable bowel syndrome and functional constipation are not discrete disorders: A machine learning approach. American Journal of Gastroenterology. 2021;**116**(1):142-151. DOI: 10.14309/ajg.0000000000000816

[6] Fairlie T et al. Overlap of disorders of gut–brain interaction: A systematic review and meta-analysis. The Lancet Gastroenterology & Hepatology. 2023;**8**(7):646-659. DOI: 10.1016/S2468-1253(23)00102-4

[7] Patcharatrakul T, Gonlachanvit S. Outcome of biofeedback therapy in dyssynergic defecation patients with and without irritable bowel syndrome. Journal of Clinical Gastroenterology. 2011;**45**(7):593-598. DOI: 10.1097/MCG.0b013e31820c6001

[8] Vollebregt PF, Wiklendt L, Dinning PG, Knowles CH, Scott SM. Coexistent faecal incontinence and constipation: A cross-sectional study of 4027 adults undergoing specialist assessment. EClinicalMedicine. 2020;**27**:100572. DOI: 10.1016/j.eclinm.2020.100572

[9] Pucciani F. A theory of progression from obstructed defecation to fecal incontinence. Techniques in Coloproctology. 2015;**19**(12):713-715. DOI: 10.1007/s10151-015-1394-2

[10] Drossman DA. Sexual and physical abuse in women with functional or organic gastrointestinal disorders. Annals of Internal Medicine. 1990;**113**(11):828. DOI: 10.7326/0003-4819-113-11-828

[11] Imhoff LR, Liwanag L, Varma M. Exacerbation of symptom severity of pelvic floor disorders in women who report a history of sexual abuse. Archives of Surgery. 2012;**147**(12):1123. DOI: 10.1001/archsurg.2012.1144

[12] Hanna M, Bray G, Ding YC, Srinath H, Warwick A, Gillespie C. The effect of a sexual abuse history on symptoms and anorectal physiology findings in patients presenting to a colorectal pelvic floor service. ANZ Journal of Surgery. 2023;**93**(6):1604-1608. DOI: 10.1111/ans.18230

[13] Abd El Maksoud WM et al. Prevalence of obstructed defecation among patients who underwent hemorrhoidectomy and correlation between preoperative constipation score and postoperative patients'

satisfaction: A prospective study in two centers. Healthcare. 2023;**11**(5):759. DOI: 10.3390/healthcare11050759

[14] Li Q et al. Correlation between poor defecation habits and postoperative hemorrhoid recurrence. Frontiers in Surgery. 2022;**9**:903215. DOI: 10.3389/fsurg.2022.930215

[15] Higgins PD, Johanson JF. Epidemiology of constipation in North America: A systematic review. American Journal of Gastroenterology. 2004;**99**(4):750-759. DOI: 10.1111/j.1572-0241.2004.04114.x

[16] Werth BL, Williams KA, Fisher MJ, Pont LG. Defining constipation to estimate its prevalence in the community: Results from a national survey. BMC Gastroenterology. 2019;**19**(1):75. DOI: 10.1186/s12876-019-0994-0

[17] Laffolie J, Ibrahimi G, Zimmer K-P. Poor perception of school toilets and increase of functional constipation. Klinische Pädiatrie. 2021;**233**(1):5-9. DOI: 10.1055/a-1263-0747

[18] Petros P, Swash M, Bush M, Fernandez M, Gunnemann A, Zimmer M. Defecation 1: Testing a hypothesis for pelvic striated muscle action to open the anorectum. Techniques in Coloproctology. 2012;**16**(6):437-443. DOI: 10.1007/s10151-012-0861-2

[19] Bush M, Petros P, Swash M, Fernandez M, Gunnemann A. Defecation 2: Internal anorectal resistance is a critical factor in defecatory disorders. Techniques in Coloproctology. 2012;**16**(6):445-450. DOI: 10.1007/s10151-012-0860-3

[20] Liedl B et al. Is overactive bladder in the female surgically curable by ligament repair? Central European Journal of Urology. 2017;**70**(1):53-59. DOI: 10.5173/ceju.2017.938

[21] Colbran RE, Warwick AM, Krause HG, Goh JT, Gillespie CJ. The effect of transvaginal prolapse surgery on anorectal function. Journal of Coloproctology. 2023;**43**(1):18-23. DOI: 10.1055/s-0043-1764196

[22] Wijffels NA, Collinson R, Cunningham C, Lindsey I. What is the natural history of internal rectal prolapse? Colorectal Disease. 2009;**12**(8):822-830. DOI: 10.1111/j.1463-1318.2009.01891.x

[23] Emile SH, Elfeki HA, Youssef M, Farid M, Wexner SD. Abdominal rectopexy for the treatment of internal rectal prolapse: A systematic review and meta-analysis. Colorectal Disease. 2017;**19**(1):13-24. DOI: 10.1111/codi.13574

[24] Lestár B, Penninckx FM, Kerremans RP. Defecometry. Diseases of the Colon and Rectum. 1989;**32**(3):197-201. DOI: 10.1007/BF02554527

[25] Rao SSC, Tuteja AK, Vellema T, Kempf J, Stessman M. Dyssynergic defecation: Demographics, symptoms, stool patterns, and quality of life. Journal of Clinical Gastroenterology. 2004;**38**(8):680-685. DOI: 10.1097/01.mcg.0000135929.78074.8c

[26] Leroi A-M, Berkelmans I, Denis P, Hémond M, Devroede G. Anismus as a marker of sexual abuse. Digestive Diseases and Sciences. 1995;**40**(7):1411-1416. DOI: 10.1007/BF02285184

[27] Glia A, Lindberg G, Nilsson LH, Mihocsa L, Åkerlund JE. Clinical value of symptom assessment in patients with constipation. Diseases of the Colon and Rectum. 1999;**42**(11):1401-1408. DOI: 10.1007/BF02235036

[28] Rao SSC, Valestin J, Brown KC, Zimmerman B, Schulze K. Long-term efficacy of biofeedback therapy for dyssynergic defecation: Randomized controlled trial. American Journal of Gastroenterology. 2010;**105**(4):890-896. DOI: 10.1038/ajg.2010.53

[29] Forootan M, Bagheri N, Darvishi M. Chronic constipation: A review of literature. Medicine. 2018;**97**(20):e10631. DOI: 10.1097/MD.0000000000010631

[30] Kwan B, Gillespie C, Warwick A. Colonoscopic findings in patients with pelvic floor dysfunction. ANZ Journal of Surgery. 2023;**93**(6):1609-1612. DOI: 10.1111/ans.18258

[31] Gosselink MP et al. Impact of slow transit constipation on the outcome of laparoscopic ventral rectopexy for obstructed defaecation associated with high grade internal rectal prolapse. Colorectal Disease. 2013;**15**(12):e749-e756. DOI: 10.1111/codi.12443

[32] Carrington EV et al. The international anorectal physiology working group (IAPWG) recommendations: Standardized testing protocol and the London classification for disorders of anorectal function. Neurogastroenterology & Motility. 2020;**32**(1):e13679. DOI: 10.1111/nmo.13679

[33] Carrington EV et al. Expert consensus document: Advances in the evaluation of anorectal function. Nature Reviews. Gastroenterology & Hepatology. 2018;**15**(5):309-323. DOI: 10.1038/nrgastro.2018.27

[34] Serra J et al. European society of neurogastroenterology and motility guidelines on functional constipation in adults. Neurogastroenterology & Motility. 2020;**32**(2):e13762. DOI: 10.1111/nmo.13762

[35] Ris F et al. Rectal axis and enterocele on proctogram may predict laparoscopic ventral mesh rectopexy outcomes for rectal intussusception. Techniques in Coloproctology. 2017;**21**(8):627-632. DOI: 10.1007/s10151-017-1643-7

[36] van Gruting IMA, Stankiewicz A, Thakar R, Santoro GA, IntHout J, Sultan AH. Imaging modalities for the detection of posterior pelvic floor disorders in women with obstructed defaecation syndrome. Cochrane Database of Systematic Reviews. 2021;**9**:CD011482. DOI: 10.1002/14651858.CD011482.pub2

[37] Paquette I et al. Consensus definitions and interpretation templates for fluoroscopic imaging of defecatory pelvic floor disorders. Diseases of the Colon and Rectum. 2021;**64**(1):31-44. DOI: 10.1097/DCR.0000000000001829

[38] Bunni J, Courtney ED. Examination of the rectum under anaesthesia with a circular anal dilator is crucial before, during and after rectal prolapse correction surgery—'Getting it right first time': A video vignette. Colorectal Disease. 2021;**23**(3):758-759. DOI: 10.1111/codi.15475

[39] Basnayake C et al. Long-term outcome of multidisciplinary versus standard gastroenterologist care for functional gastrointestinal disorders: A randomized trial. Clinical Gastroenterology and Hepatology. 2022;**20**(9):2102-2111.e9. DOI: 10.1016/j.cgh.2021.12.005

[40] Singh P, Tuck C, Gibson PR, Chey WD. The role of food in the treatment of bowel disorders: Focus on irritable bowel syndrome and functional constipation. American Journal of Gastroenterology. 2022;**117**(6):947-957. DOI: 10.14309/ajg.0000000000001767

[41] Ho K-S. Stopping or reducing dietary fiber intake reduces constipation and its associated symptoms. World Journal of Gastroenterology. 2012;**18**(33):4593. DOI: 10.3748/wjg.v18.i33.4593

[42] Courtice S et al. Poster abstracts in alphabetical order. Nutrition & Dietetics. 2018;**75**:68-121. DOI: 10.1111/1747-0080.12427

[43] Boyd C, Abraham S, Kellow J. Psychological features are important predictors of functional gastrointestinal disorders in patients with eating disorders. Scandinavian Journal of Gastroenterology. 2005;**40**(8):929-935. DOI: 10.1080/00365520510015836

[44] National Institute for Health and Care Excellence. Pelvic floor dysfunction: Prevention and nonsurgical management. In: Lifestyle Factors for the Prevention of Pelvic Floor Dysfunction (NICE Guideline No. 210). London: National Institute for Health and Care Excellence (NICE); 2021

[45] Rao SSC, Brenner DM. Efficacy and safety of over-the-counter therapies for chronic constipation: An updated systematic review. American Journal of Gastroenterology. 2021;**116**(6):1156-1181. DOI: 10.14309/ajg.0000000000001222

[46] Black CJ, Thakur ER, Houghton LA, Quigley EMM, Moayyedi P, Ford AC. Efficacy of psychological therapies for irritable bowel syndrome: Systematic review and network meta-analysis. Gut. 2020;**69**(8):1441-1451. DOI: 10.1136/gutjnl-2020-321191

[47] Modi RM et al. Implementation of a defecation posture modification device. Journal of Clinical Gastroenterology. 2019;**53**(3):216-219. DOI: 10.1097/MCG.0000000000001143

[48] Chiarioni G, Whitehead WE, Pezza V, Morelli A, Bassotti G. Biofeedback is superior to laxatives for normal transit constipation due to pelvic floor dyssynergia. Gastroenterology. 2006;**130**(3):657-664. DOI: 10.1053/j.gastro.2005.11.014

[49] Hwang YH et al. Biofeedback therapy for rectal intussusception. Techniques in Coloproctology. 2006;**10**(1):11-16. DOI: 10.1007/s10151-006-0244-7

[50] Maxwell M, Berry K, Wane S. Pelvic Floor Muscle Training for Women with Pelvic Organ Prolapse: The PROPEL Realist Evaluation. Southampton (UK): NIHR Journals Library; 2020 (Health Services and Delivery Research, No. 8.47.) Chapter 7, The POPPY trial participant data linkage study. Available from: https://www.ncbi.nlm.nih.gov/books/NBK565824/

[51] Meurette G et al. Low anterior resection syndrome after rectal resection management: Multicentre randomized clinical trial of transanal irrigation with a dedicated device (cone catheter) versus conservative bowel management. British Journal of Surgery. 2023;**110**(9):1092-1095. DOI: 10.1093/bjs/znad078

[52] Pieniowski EHA et al. A randomized controlled clinical trial of transanal irrigation versus conservative treatment in patients with low anterior resection syndrome after rectal cancer surgery. Annals of Surgery. 2023;**277**(1):30-37. DOI: 10.1097/SLA.0000000000005482

[53] Rosen HR, Kneist W, Fürst A, Krämer G, Hebenstreit J, Schiemer JF. Randomized clinical trial of prophylactic transanal irrigation versus supportive therapy to prevent symptoms of low anterior resection syndrome after rectal resection. BJS Open. 2019;**3**(4):461-465. DOI: 10.1002/bjs5.50160

[54] Brochard C et al. Transanal irrigation is a better choice for bowel dysfunction

in adults with Spina bifida: A randomised controlled trial. Colorectal Disease. 2023;**25**(6):1267-1276. DOI: 10.1111/codi.16518

[55] Christensen P, et al. A randomized, controlled trial of transanal irrigation versus conservative bowel management in spinal cord -injured patients. Gastroenterology. 2006;**131**(3):738-747. DOI: 10.1053/j. gastro.2006.06.004

[56] Emmett CD, Close HJ, Yiannakou Y, Mason JM. Trans-anal irrigation therapy to treat adult chronic functional constipation: Systematic review and meta-analysis. BMC Gastroenterology. 2015;**15**(1):139. DOI: 10.1186/s12876-015-0354-7

[57] Juul T, Christensen P. Prospective evaluation of transanal irrigation for fecal incontinence and constipation. Techniques in Coloproctology. 2017;**21**(5):363-371. DOI: 10.1007/s10151-017-1635-7

[58] Vollebregt PF, Dekker L, Han-Geurts IJM, Felt-Bersma RJF. Prospective cohort study of high-volume transanal irrigation in patients with constipation and/or faecal incontinence. Colorectal Disease. 2023;**25**(8):1658-1670. DOI: 10.1111/codi.16628

[59] Chan DSY, Delicata RJ. Meta-analysis of antegrade continence enema in adults with faecal incontinence and constipation. British Journal of Surgery. 2016;**103**(4):322-327. DOI: 10.1002/bjs.10051

[60] Dixon T. Obstructed defaecation: A pathophysiological approach. In: Pelvic Floor Disorders for the Colorectal Surgeon. Oxford, United Kingdom: Oxford University Press; 2010. pp. 57-68. DOI: 10.1093/med/9780199579624.003.0005

[61] Hicks CW, Weinstein M, Wakamatsu M, Pulliam S, Savitt L, Bordeianou L. Are rectoceles the cause or the result of obstructed defaecation syndrome? A prospective anorectal physiology study. Colorectal Disease. 2013;**15**(8):993-999. DOI: 10.1111/codi.12213

[62] Collinson R. Rectocele. In: Pelvic Floor Disorders for the Colorectal Surgeon. Oxford, United Kingdom: Oxford University Press; 2010. pp. 115-126. DOI: 10.1093/med/9780199579624.003.0011

[63] Tjandra JJ, Ooi B-S, Tang C-L, Dwyer P, Carey M. Transanal repair of rectocele corrects obstructed defecation if it is not associated with anismus. Diseases of the Colon and Rectum. 1999;**42**(12):1544-1550. DOI: 10.1007/BF02236204

[64] Abbas SM, Bissett IP, Neill ME, Macmillan AK, Milne D, Parry BR. Long-term results of the anterior Delorme's operation in the management of symptomatic rectocele. Diseases of the Colon and Rectum. 2005;**48**(2):317-322. DOI: 10.1007/s10350-004-0819-1

[65] Murthy VK, Orkin BA, Smith LE, Glassman LM. Excellent outcome using selective criteria for rectocele repair. Diseases of the Colon and Rectum. 1996;**39**(4):374-378. DOI: 10.1007/BF02054049

[66] Ellis CN, Essani R. Treatment of obstructed defecation. Clinics in Colon and Rectal Surgery. 2012;**25**(1):24-33. DOI: 10.1055/s-0032-1301756

[67] Roman H, Michot F. Long-term outcomes of transanal rectocele repair. Diseases of the Colon and Rectum. 2005;**48**(3):510-517. DOI: 10.1007/s10350-004-0800-z

[68] Tsunoda A, Kusanagi H. Annual long-term functional outcomes after

transanal repair for symptomatic rectocele. Annals of Coloproctology. 2022. DOI: 10.3393/ac.2022.00283.0040

[69] Leo CA et al. Long-term functional outcome after internal Delorme's procedure for obstructed defecation syndrome, and the role of postoperative rehabilitation. Journal of Investigative Surgery. 2018;**31**(3):256-262. DOI: 10.1080/08941939.2017.1300714

[70] Gustilo-Ashby AM, Paraiso MFR, Jelovsek JE, Walters MD, Barber MD. Bowel symptoms 1 year after surgery for prolapse: Further analysis of a randomized trial of rectocele repair. American Journal of Obstetrics and Gynecology. 2007;**197**(1):76.e1-76.e5. DOI: 10.1016/j.ajog.2007.02.045

[71] Emile SH, Elfallal AH, Abdelnaby M, Balata M. Higher symptom score, larger residual rectocele, and lower rectal compliance predict failure of improvement after surgical treatment of rectocele. Journal of Coloproctology. 2022;**42**(3):245-250. DOI: 10.1055/s-0042-1756146

[72] Ferrari L et al. Preoperative predictors of success after transvaginal rectocoele repair. Techniques in Coloproctology. 2023;**27**(10):859-866. DOI: 10.1007/s10151-023-02822-1

[73] Haase P, Skibsted L. Influence of operations for stress incontinence and/or genital descensus on sexual life. Acta Obstetricia et Gynecologica Scandinavica. 1988;**67**(7):659-661. DOI: 10.3109/00016348809004283

[74] Nüssler E, Granåsen G, Bixo M, Löfgren M. Long-term outcome after routine surgery for pelvic organ prolapse—A national register-based cohort study. International Urogynecology Journal. 2022;**33**(7):1863-1873. DOI: 10.1007/s00192-022-05156-y

[75] Fathy M, Elfallal AH, Emile SH. Literature review of the outcome of and methods used to improve transperineal repair of rectocele. World Journal of Gastrointestinal Surgery. 2021;**13**(9):1063-1078. DOI: 10.4240/wjgs.v13.i9.1063

[76] Pandeva I, Biers S, Pradhan A, Verma V, Slack M, Thiruchelvam N. The impact of pelvic floor multidisciplinary team on patient management: The experience of a tertiary unit. Journal of Multidisciplinary Healthcare. 2019;**12**:205-210. DOI: 10.2147/JMDH.S186847

[77] Grossi U, Horrocks EJ, Mason J, Knowles CH, Williams AB. Surgery for constipation: Systematic review and practice recommendations. Colorectal Disease. 2017;**19**:73-91. DOI: 10.1111/codi.13781

[78] Longo A. Obstructed defecation because of rectal pathologies. Novel surgical treatment: Stapled transanal rectal resection (STARR). In: Acts of 14th International Colorectal Disease Symposium. Fort Lauderdale, FL; 2003

[79] Corman ML et al. Consensus conference on the stapled transanal rectal resection (STARR) for disordered defaecation. Colorectal Disease. 2006;**8**(2):98-101. DOI: 10.1111/j.1463-1318.2005.00941.x

[80] Mercer-Jones M, Grossi U, Pares D, Vollebregt PF, Mason J, Knowles CH. Surgery for constipation: Systematic review and practice recommendations. Colorectal Disease. 2017;**19**:49-72. DOI: 10.1111/codi.13772

[81] Jayne DG, Schwandner O, Stuto A. Stapled transanal rectal resection for obstructed defecation syndrome: One-year results of the European STARR registry. Diseases of the Colon

and Rectum. 2009;**52**(7):1205-1212. DOI: 10.1007/DCR.0b013e3181a9120f

[82] National Institute for Health and Care Excellence. Stapled Transanal Rectal Resection for Obstructed Defaecation Syndrome. United Kingdom: National Institute for Health and Care Excellence; 2010. Available from: www.nice.org.uk/guidance/ipg351; 2010 (NICE Guidelines No. 351)

[83] Schiano di Visconte M, Nicolì F, Pasquali A, Bellio G. Clinical outcomes of stapled transanal rectal resection for obstructed defaecation syndrome at 10-year follow-up. Colorectal Disease. 2018;**20**(7):614-622. DOI: 10.1111/codi.14028

[84] Carter D, Dickman R. The role of botox in colorectal disorders. Current Treatment Options in Gastroenterology. 2018;**16**(4):541-547. DOI: 10.1007/s11938-018-0205-z

[85] Chaichanavichkij P, Vollebregt PF, Scott SM, Knowles CH. Botulinum toxin type A for the treatment of dyssynergic defaecation in adults: A systematic review. Colorectal Disease. 2020;**22**(12):1832-1841. DOI: 10.1111/codi.15120

[86] Dressler D, Saberi FA, Barbosa ER. Botulinum toxin: Mechanisms of action. Arquivos de Neuro-Psiquiatria. 2005;**63**(1):180-185. DOI: 10.1590/S0004-282X2005000100035

[87] Zhang Y. Botulinum toxin type-A injection to treat patients with intractable anismus unresponsive to simple biofeedback training. World Journal of Gastroenterology. 2014;**20**(35):12602. DOI: 10.3748/wjg.v20.i35.12602

[88] Faried M, El Nakeeb A, Youssef M, Omar W, El Monem HA. Comparative study between surgical and non-surgical treatment of anismus in patients with symptoms of obstructed defecation: A prospective randomized study. Journal of Gastrointestinal Surgery. 2010;**14**(8):1235-1243. DOI: 10.1007/s11605-010-1229-4

[89] Farid M et al. Comparative study between botulinum toxin injection and partial division of puborectalis for treating anismus. International Journal of Colorectal Disease. 2009;**24**(3):327-334. DOI: 10.1007/s00384-008-0609-7

[90] Madaliński MH et al. Side effects of botulinum toxin injection for benign anal disorders. European Journal of Gastroenterology & Hepatology. 2002;**14**(8):853-856. DOI: 10.1097/00042737-200208000-00007

[91] Hompes R, Harmston C, Wijffels N, Jones OM, Cunningham C, Lindsey I. Excellent response rate of anismus to botulinum toxin if rectal prolapse misdiagnosed as anismus ('pseudoanismus') is excluded. Colorectal Disease. 2012;**14**(2):224-230. DOI: 10.1111/j.1463-1318.2011.02561.x

[92] Samaranayake CB, Luo C, Plank AW, Merrie AEH, Plank LD, Bissett IP. Systematic review on ventral rectopexy for rectal prolapse and intussusception. Colorectal Disease. 2009;**12**(6):504-512. DOI: 10.1111/j.1463-1318.2009.01934.x

[93] Grossi U, Knowles CH, Mason J, Lacy-Colson J, Brown SR. Surgery for constipation: Systematic review and practice recommendations. Colorectal Disease. 2017;**19**:37-48. DOI: 10.1111/codi.13773

[94] Maeda Y et al. European Society of Coloproctology guidance on the use of mesh in the pelvis in colorectal surgery. Colorectal Disease.

2021;**23**(9):2228-2285. DOI: 10.1111/codi.15718

[95] Mäkelä-Kaikkonen J et al. Does ventral rectopexy improve pelvic floor function in the long term? Diseases of the Colon and Rectum. 2018;**61**(2):230-238. DOI: 10.1097/DCR.0000000000000974

[96] Mandovra P, Kalikar V, Patankar RV. Laparoscopic ventral mesh rectopexy for obstructive defecation syndrome: Follow-up in the Indian population. Journal of Minimal Access Surgery. 2021;**17**(3):305-310. DOI: 10.4103/jmas.JMAS_292_19

Chapter 5

Low Anterior Resection Syndrome (LARS)

Sotirios-Georgios Popeskou and Dimitrios Christoforidis

Abstract

Rectal cancer surgery has undergone significant advancements, with a shift towards sphincter-sparing operations due to improved surgical techniques and neoadjuvant treatments. However, this has given rise to low anterior resection syndrome (LARS), characterised by various bowel functional abnormalities adversely impacting patients' quality of life. This chapter delves into the definition, risk factors, diagnosis and current treatment recommendations for LARS. The new consensus definition of LARS incorporates a range of symptoms, and their impact on mental, emotional and social well-being. The widely accepted LARS score, a patient-reported outcome measure, aids in standardising reporting but has limitations. LARS has a multifactorial aetiology involving colonic dysmotility, iatrogenic nerve damage, neorectal reservoir dysfunction, recto-anal inhibitory reflex loss, and anal sphincter dysfunction. Various risk factors, including tumour location, anastomotic leak, diverting stoma, pelvic radiotherapy and surgical approach, all contribute to LARS development. Treatment modalities encompass conservative measures such as dietary modifications, probiotics and medications, while advanced treatments include pelvic floor rehabilitation, transanal irrigation, neuromodulation and, ultimately, surgery for refractory cases. Although research has improved our understanding of LARS, further studies are essential to increase prevention and improve treatment strategies.

Keywords: low anterior resection syndrome, colorectal surgery, ano-rectal dysfunction, rectal cancer, defecation abnormalities

1. Introduction

Surgery for rectal cancer has evolved, especially for low-lying tumours. Thanks to better surgical techniques combined with the ever-advancing neoadjuvant treatments, abdominoperineal resections have decreased in favour of sphincter-sparing operations. Although these procedures assure bowel continuity and avoid the need for a permanent stoma, they come with frequent functional disturbances that can have a detrimental impact on patients' quality of life. Low anterior resection syndrome (LARS) is the term used to describe the bowel functional abnormalities following rectal surgery and consists of a constellation of symptoms, ranging from incontinence to obstructed defecation. In this chapter, we will discuss the definition, risk factors, diagnosis and current treatment recommendations.

2. Definition

Traditionally, LARS was defined as a "disordered bowel function after rectal resection, leading to a detriment in quality of life" [1]. Although this definition accurately describes the clinical picture, it makes it practically impossible to accurately identify and report LARS due to the heterogeneity of its symptoms [2, 3]. The LARS score, a validated patient-reported outcome measure, has helped the standardisation of reporting [4]. However, the LARS score may significantly underestimate the impact of evacuation dysfunction and may not accurately assess the impact of symptoms on an individual patient's quality of life. For these reasons, a recent international consensus definition of LARS has been established using input from patients, colorectal surgeons and healthcare specialists involved in the care of low anterior resection patients [5].

LARS is defined by at least one of the following symptoms resulting in at least one of the following consequences that occur after a sphincter-sparing rectal procedure (modified from 5) (**Table 1**).

3. The LARS score

The LARS score was developed to surpass discrepancies in reporting functional outcomes and was designed to be a quick clinical evaluation screening tool for patients suffering from LARS symptoms. It is a validated questionnaire for assessing a patient's bowel function after sphincter-sparing surgery and comprised mainly five questions [4]: incontinence for flatus, incontinence for liquid stool, faecal frequency (number of bowel movements per day), clustering (the need to defecate less than an hour from the last one) and urgency. The score has a scale from 0 to 42 points. Outcome is defined as no LARS (0–20), minor LARS (21–29) and major LARS (30–42). Significant differences have been found between no LARS and major LARS in nearly all functional scales of quality of life [6]. The LARS score, widely accepted by colorectal surgeons, suffers from certain disadvantages. It appears to be insensitive to evacuation dysfunction, and in some patients, it might overestimate the impact LARS symptoms have on their quality of life [7]. Furthermore, studies have shown it to have a high sensitivity but a low specificity,

Symptoms	Consequences
• Variable, unpredictable bowel function • Altered stool consistency • Increased stool frequency • Repeated painful stools • Emptying difficulties • Urgency • Incontinence • Soiling	• Toilet dependence • Preoccupation with bowel function • Dissatisfaction with bowels • Strategies and compromises • Impact on mental and emotional well-being • Impact on social and daily activities • Impact on relationships and intimacy • Impact on roles, commitments and responsibilities

Table 1.
Consensus definition of low anterior resection syndrome (LARS) (modified from Keane et al. [5]).

as it was found to exist in the general population free of any rectal procedures, in significant numbers [8].

Other scoring systems, like the MSKCC Bowel Function Instrument, have been developed but never gained wide acceptance [9].

4. Epidemiology

LARS is frequent. It is estimated that 50–90% of patients undergoing a low anterior resection will face at least some degree of bowel dysfunction [10]. The reported incidence of LARS varies in the literature. The pooled incidence of major LARS was reported to be 44% (ranging from 10 to 72%) in one of the biggest and most recent meta-analyses from 50 studies on the subject [11]. When the epidemiology of specific symptoms is reported, variation persists. Faecal incontinence is reported to occur in 6–87% of low anterior resection patients, 8–75% of patients having three or more defecations per day with 5–87% reporting urgency [12].

The previously accepted notion that LARS was a short-term phenomenon after low rectal surgery with a transitory character has been proven false, as patients report long-term effects up to 15 years after their operation with evacuatory disorders varying from 12 to 74% [1].

5. Aetiology

LARS pathophysiology remains a matter of debate and appears to be multifactorial. A combination of colonic dysmotility, neorectal reservoir dysfunction, anatomical and sensory alterations, anal sphincter dysfunction and pelvic floor function.

5.1 Colonic dysmotility

Patients with major LARS problems have been shown to have an increased postprandial response and higher neorectal pressures postprandially, suggesting that severe bowel dysfunction may be attributed to abnormal gastrointestinal motility [13]. These patients have been found to have increased bowel contractions as also increased neorectal tone compared with healthy patients [13]. Bryant et al. reported that patients after LAR have small, irregular waves at the site of the neorectum and the presence of these waves was associated with faecal soiling, urgency and multiple evacuations. Furthermore, meal-induced colonic motility reported significantly earlier contractions in patients with increased bowel frequency compared to those without [1].

5.2 Iatrogenic nerve damage

LARS might be attributed to iatrogenic nerve damage during the initial operation affecting not only colonic motility but also urinary and sexual function. The left colon starting from the distal third of the transverse to the end of the sigmoid, receives their sympathetic, parasympathetic and sensory supply via nerves from the inferior mesenteric plexus. Evidence that denervation of the left and sigmoid colon results in increased motility with shorter transit time has been shown in the literature [14–16]. The rectum receives a sympathetic nervous supply from the lumbar splanchnic nerves and superior and inferior hypogastric plexuses. Parasympathetic supply is provided from S2–4 via the pelvic splanchnic nerves and inferior hypogastric plexuses with associated afferent sensory fibres following this parasympathetic supply. The risk of pelvic nerve injury during surgery depends on the surgical technique and the underlying pathology, with pre-operative radiotherapy contributing to the potential injury. The sympathetic component may be damaged during ligation of the inferior mesenteric artery (IMA) on the aorta or while dissecting at the pelvic brim. The possible locations of parasympathetic nerve damage are during perineal dissection if the plane extends out of the mesorectal fascia, especially during lateral pelvic wall dissection. In men, the risk of injury is higher during anterior rectal dissection of the Denonvillier fascia and at the base of the prostate [17].

5.3 Neorectal reservoir dysfunction

Removal of the rectum and in particular the rectosigmoid junction, which normally is the physiologic distal control centre for the regulation of bowel transit, can leave bowel mobility without an inhibitory mechanism. This lack of distal negative feedback signals to oppose increased proximal colonic motility further exacerbates the symptoms of LARS. LARS can also be manifested with rectal evacuatory dysfunction. Symptoms include infrequent defecation, incomplete rectal emptying and excessive straining [1]. The suspected mechanism is loss of recto-anal coordination, presenting as paradoxical anal contraction and impaired rectal contraction [1]. These patients also present a lowered rectal sensation possibly due to impairment of the parasympathetic and sympathetic nerve supply to the rectum [1]. Another suspected mechanism is the neo-reservoir decreased compliance and capacity that can lead to frequent defecation. Additionally reduced capacity can lead to higher pressures in the neorectum that can itself lead to soiling even with a small amount of faecal matter present in the low anal canal [18].

5.4 Recto-anal inhibitory reflex loss (RAIR)

LARS patients can exhibit loss of their RAIR resulting in disordered evacuation due but not limited to poor sampling and impaired discrimination of liquid versus gas rectal content. It can be manifested as faecal soiling, incontinence urgency, or incomplete evacuation [12]. Patients with an absent RAIR present worse functional outcomes when associated with a lower reservoir capacity and a shortened high-pressure zone [19].

5.5 Anal sphincter dysfunction

The anal sphincter complex can sustain injury directly due to stapling during surgery [12], neoadjuvant radiotherapy, or damage to its innervation. A decrease in mean anal resting pressures and maximum squeeze pressures that do not recover over time has been shown in studies evaluating anal sphincter function after LAR [1, 18]. These changes can be transitory as they have been shown to improve after 6 months [18].

6. Risk factors

Several risk factors have been identified that may predispose patients to develop LARS after a low anterior resection. The most recent systematic review and metaanalysis including 50 studies that used the validated LARS score determined the following [11]:

6.1 Tumour location-level of anastomosis

Worse functional outcomes have been associated with a lower anastomotic distance to the anal verge. Tumour and subsequently anastomotic height were assessed as comparing Total versus partial mesorectal resections: the results showed that the risk of major LARS was significantly increased in patients after TME compared to PME (pooled OR 2.13, 95% CI 1.49–3.04) [11]. Similar results were confirmed by other studies [20]. It is therefore fundamental to retain a longer rectal remnant after ensuring radical resection for low third rectal cancer in order to improve anorectal function.

6.2 Anastomotic leak

Anastomotic leak negatively affects anorectal function, and this effect has been found to be valid when seen as a directly measured outcome in various studies and also after sensitivity analysis (OR 1.98, 95% CI 1.34–2.93) [11]. The mechanism involved suggests a combination of scarring and adhesion formation decreasing the neorectum compliance and capacity, combined with possible nerve injury due to pelvic sepsis [12, 20, 21]. Particular consideration is advised when deciding to take down a diverting stoma in these patients.

6.3 Diverting stoma

Despite the fact that stomas are not only effective in reducing the severity of anastomotic leak consequences but also protective against it [22], they have been found to negatively affect functional outcomes leading to various degrees of LARS (OR 1.89, 95% CI 1.58–2.27) [11]. A very recent paper studying patients after TME and comparing functional outcomes using the LARS score found that patients with a stoma (ileostomy or colostomy) had increased postoperative functional disturbances. These disturbances were shown to be proportional to the attending time for closure, especially for patients with ileostomy. When ileostomy closure was performed after 90 days, there was a statistically significant difference ($p = 0.05$ between 90 and 180 days and $p = 0.01$ after 180 days). The LARS score after ileostomy was significantly worse compared to patients without a stoma ($p = 0.04$), and while the trend was similar, no significance was found in the LARS score after colostomy compared with patients without a stoma ($p = 0.2$) [23]. Previous papers also confirmed better outcomes after early closure and hypothesised that the length of the excluded bowel seems to be relevant to the functional outcome, considering that patients with ileostomy may experience worse and more persistent functional dysfunction compared to those after colostomy [24]. The precise reason of stoma-related bowel dysfunction is not clear, but it is possible to be attributed to diversion colitis, enteric nervous system alterations, or changes in epithelial function of the terminal ileum, causing bile acid malabsorption, small bowel bacterial overgrowth, or bacterial recolonization of the colon after stoma reversal [23].

6.4 Pelvic radiotherapy

Irradiation-induced pelvic fibrosis combined with subsequent direct nerve and vascular injury from radiation seems to be the culprit for the functional disturbances leading to LARS [25–28]. Whether long course or short course, studies have shown that pelvic radiotherapy is consistently associated with LARS independent of the timing of administration (adjuvant vs. neoadjuvant) [11, 25–28].

6.5 Type of surgical approach and type of anastomosis

Given the high incidence of LARS after rectal resections, the different types of surgical approaches and different types of anastomoses have been studied in order to examine possible advantages. LARS after TaTME compared with LapTME showed no statistical significance as far as LARS incidence is concerned [11]. The same applies for pouch reconstruction versus straight anastomosis [11], although there are some studies that found decreased bowel frequency, reduced fragmentation and less urgency during the first year in patients with colonic J pouch compared with straight anastomosis [29, 30]. This advantage, however, seems to disappear after the first year. Side-to-side anastomosis does not seem to provide significant advantages either [31].

7. Treatment

LARS treatment, similar to its aetiology, is multimodal and can be treated with lifestyle changes, medications, trans-anal irrigation, pelvic floor rehabilitation, neurostimulation, or surgery [32]. LARS management is often empirical and symptom-based with limited evidence as most studies are observational and noncontrolled [33]. Patients with persistent functional disturbances after stoma closure or 4–6 weeks after the cardinal operation are evaluated using the LARS score and treated according to the character, variety, severity and duration of their symptoms. The colorectal surgeon should ensure that there is no underlying cause for the patient's symptoms (e.g., radiation-related mucosal lesions, anastomotic stricture and local recurrence). Conservative measures will help most of the patients with LARS up to some point, but patients presenting with major LARS (LARS score ≥ 30) typically require multimodal therapy with advanced treatments. The treatment options are reviewed hereafter.

7.1 Conservative measures

7.1.1 Diet modifications

High-fibre low-fat diet, avoidance of alcoholic beverages, cold beverages and spicy or stimulating food. However, insoluble fibre may worsen symptoms as diarrhoea, defecation frequency and bloating [34]. Based on expert opinion, bulking agents are well tolerated and may be beneficial in decreasing clustering and improving stool consistency [33].

7.1.2 Probiotics

Popular treatment used for IBS-D and IBD acts as gut microbiota modulator. A randomised control trial comparing a probiotic agent (lactobacillus plantarum) to placebo in patients with LARS did not find any significant difference in the LARS scores. The authors attributed the result in the short treatment period and the use of a single strain of beneficial bacteria instead of a multispecies one [35].

7.1.3 Loperamide

Although not specifically examined in LARS, its wide use is supported by its efficacy in treating two pathologies with similar symptoms, IBS-D and bowel dysfunction after restorative proctocolectomy. It has been evaluated in randomised trials were it was shown to be more effective when compared to placebo in decreasing frequency and improving stool consistency in patients with IBS-D [36].

7.1.4 Serotonin receptor antagonists

Serotonin (5-hydroxytryptamine (5-HT)) is a central and enteric nervous system neurotransmitter. It is an important mediator in the gut that influences gut motility and secretion, inhibiting colon mobility and causing constipation [37–39]. There is high-level evidence from randomised control trials studying Ramosetron (unavailable in European countries) vs. "conservative treatment" and recently Ondansetron versus placebo in LARS patients, suggesting that 5-HT inhibitors can lead to improvement of symptoms, decrease in LARS score and improvement in quality of life [40–42].

7.2 Advanced treatments

7.2.1 Pelvic floor rehabilitation (PFR)

PFR includes a variety of treatments consisting of biofeedback, pelvic floor muscle training, electrostimulation and volumetric/rectal balloon training. It seems to improve bowel function and quality of life, but its long-term efficacy remains under question. An RCT where pelvic floor muscle training was performed regularly, starting at 1 month after sphincter-sparing resection or ostomy closure, reported statistically significant improvement compared to the control group at 4 and 6 months, but this effect disappeared at 12 months [43]. The heterogeneity of the different protocols used in pelvic floor rehabilitation, the recommended duration of the various treatments and methods, still do not permit solid conclusions.

7.2.2 Transanal irrigation (TAI)

TAI represents one of the most efficacious treatments for LARS. It has been suggested that regular TAI (once/day or 3–4 times/week) has a mechanical effect of a high volume of water irrigating the colon and stimulating its motility [44]. Two randomised trials, one comparing TAI with posterior tibial nerve stimulation and another comparing medical treatment to TAI both reported significantly lower LARS scores and improvement in the quality of life [45, 46]. TAI was also associated with the best outcomes among all treatments reviewed in a recent systemic review and meta-analysis [32]. Perforation is a rare complication that can be avoided if a rectal and endoscopic evaluation prior to the start of the treatment excludes anatomical anomalies [33]. In case of stenosis, a soft Foley catheter can be used.

7.2.3 Neuromodulation

Sacral nerve modulation (SNM) and lately posterior tibial nerve stimulation (PTNS) are the two main methods used for patients who present with major LARS after a year of multimodular therapies. SNM decreases anterograde colonic motility while increases retrograde colonic motor activities and in the same time impairs postprandial changes in rectal motility, mechanisms important for the improvement of symptoms in LARS patients [47, 48]. SNM is an invasive procedure, which requires the placement of electrodes in the sacral foramen and the installation of an electric impulse-generating device in the subcutaneous tissue. A few studies showed promising results from the SNM application on LARS patients. They reported improvement in symptomatology and quality of life [49–52]. However, studies are small, often retrospective and with high heterogeneity. A systematic review of SNM in LARS patients showed an improvement of symptoms in the vast majority of patients with permanent implantation, with an additional improvement in quality of life and the ability to defer defecation. However, its small size (43 patients from 7 studies) does not permit definitive conclusions, and further studies are required [21]. PTNS also has been shown to reduce LARS score and faecal incontinence scores in two randomised control trials that compared it with sham simulation and medical treatment, respectively [53, 54]. Despite these promising results, a meta-analysis of these two trials failed to show any significant differences in follow-up scores or faecal incontinence scores [32].

7.2.4 Surgery

Patients with severe LARS refractory to any of the aforementioned treatment modalities will eventually benefit from a terminal stoma.

8. Conclusion

LARS is very frequent in patients undergoing surgery for rectal cancer and can lead to significant decrease in quality of life. Recent research has led to a better understanding of the underlying causative mechanisms of this syndrome, and several treatment modalities have been developed. Further research is still needed to provide better evidence for the prevention and treatment of LARS.

Author details

Sotirios-Georgios Popeskou and Dimitrios Christoforidis*
Facoltà di medicina, Department of Surgery, Ospedale Regionale di Lugano, Ente Ospedaliero Cantonale, Università della Svizzera Italiana, Switzerland

*Address all correspondence to: dimitri.christoforidis@eoc.ch

IntechOpen

© 2024 The Author(s). Licensee IntechOpen. This chapter is distributed under the terms of the Creative Commons Attribution License (http://creativecommons.org/licenses/by/3.0), which permits unrestricted use, distribution, and reproduction in any medium, provided the original work is properly cited.

References

[1] Bryant CL et al. Anterior resection syndrome. The Lancet Oncology. 2012;**13**:e403-e408

[2] Keane C et al. Defining low anterior resection syndrome: A systematic review of the literature. Colorectal Disease. 2017;**19**:713-722

[3] Chapman SJ et al. A cross-sectional review of reporting variation in postoperative bowel dysfunction after rectal cancer surgery. Diseases of the Colon and Rectum. 2017;**60**:240-247

[4] Emmertsen KJ et al. Low anterior resection syndrome score: Development and validation of a symptom-based scoring system for bowel dysfunction after low anterior resection for rectal cancer. Annals of Surgery. 2012;**255**:922-928

[5] Keane C et al. International consensus definition of low anterior resection syndrome. Diseases of the Colon and Rectum. 2020;**63**(3):274-284

[6] Emmertsen KJ et al. Impact of bowel dysfunction on quality of life after sphincter-preserving resection for rectal cancer. The British Journal of Surgery. 2013;**100**(10):1377-1387

[7] Ribas Y et al. Clinical application of the LARS score: Results from a pilot study. International Journal of Colorectal Disease. 2017;**32**:409-418

[8] Juul T et al. Normative data for the low anterior resection syndrome score (LARS score). Annals of Surgery. 2019;**269**:1124-1128

[9] Temple LK et al. The development of a validated instrument to evaluate bowel function after sphincter-preserving surgery for rectal cancer. Diseases of the Colon and Rectum. 2005;**48**:1353-1365

[10] Juul T et al. Low anterior resection syndrome and quality of life: An international multicenter study. Diseases of the Colon and Rectum. 2014;**57**:585-591

[11] Sun R et al. The incidence and risk factors of low anterior resection syndrome (LARS) after sphincter-preserving surgery of rectal cancer: A systematic review and meta-analysis. Supportive Care in Cancer. 2021;**29**(12):7249

[12] Ziv Y et al. Low anterior resection syndrome (LARS): Cause and effect and reconstructive considerations. Techniques in Coloproctology. 2012;**17**:151-162

[13] Emmertsen KJ et al. A hyperactive postprandial response in the neorectum—The clue to low anterior resection syndrome after total mesorectal excision surgery? Colorectal Disease. 2013;**15**:e599-e606

[14] Koda K et al. Denervation of the neorectum as a potential cause of defecatory disorder following low anterior resection for rectal cancer. Diseases of the Colon and Rectum. 2005;**48**(2):210-217

[15] Lee WY et al. Surgical autonomic denervation results in altered colonic motility: An explanation for low anterior resection syndrome? Surgery. 2008;**143**(6):778-783

[16] Ng KS et al. Colonic transit in patients after anterior resection: Prospective, comparative study using single-photon emission CT/CT

scintigraphy. The British Journal of Surgery. 2020;**107**(5):567

[17] Keating JP et al. Sexual function after rectal excision. ANZ Journal of Surgery. 2004;**74**:248-259

[18] Efthimiadis C et al. Manometric and clinical evaluation of patients after low anterior resection for rectal cancer. Techniques in Coloproctology. 2004;**8**:S205-S207

[19] Kakodkar R et al. Low anterior resection with total mesorectal excision for rectal cancer: Functional assessment and factors affecting outcome. Colorectal Disease. 2005;**8**:650-656

[20] Bregendahl S et al. Bowel dysfunction after low anterior resection with and without neoadjuvant therapy for rectal cancer: A population-based cross-sectional study. Colorectal Disease. 2013;**15**:1130-1139

[21] Ramage L et al. A systematic review of sacral nerve stimulation for low anterior resection syndrome. Colorectal Disease. 2015;**17**(9):762-771

[22] Phan K et al. Does a stoma reduce the risk of anastomotic leak and need for re-operation following low anterior resection for rectal cancer: Systematic review and meta-analysis of randomized controlled trials. Journal of Gastrointestinal Oncology. 2019;**10**:179-187

[23] Martelucci J et al. Ileostomy versus colostomy: Impact on functional outcomes after total mesorectal excision for rectal cancer. Colorectal Disease. 2023;**25**:1686-1693

[24] Keane C et al. Functional outcomes from a randomized trial of early closure of temporary ileostomy after rectal excision for cancer. The British Journal of Surgery. 2019;**106**:645-652

[25] Buzatti K et al. Pathophysiological aspects of the low anterior resection syndrome for treatment of rectal cancer. Revista do Colégio Brasileiro de Cirurgiões. 2017;**44**(4):397-402

[26] Chen TY et al. Bowel function 14 years after preoperative short-course radiotherapy and total mesorectal excision for rectal cancer: Report of a multicenter randomized trial. Clinical Colorectal Cancer. 2015;**14**(2):106-114

[27] Ihnát P et al. Anorectal dysfunction after laparoscopic low anterior rectal resection for rectal cancer with and without radiotherapy (manometry study). Journal of Surgical Oncology. 2018;**117**(4):710

[28] Downing A et al. Functional outcomes and health-related quality of life after curative treatment for rectal cancer: A population-level study in England. International Journal of Radiation Oncology, Biology, Physics. 2019;**103**(5):1132-1142

[29] Koch SM et al. Retrograde colonic irrigation for faecal incontinence after low anterior resection. International Journal of Colorectal Disease. 2009;**24**:1019-1022

[30] Heriot AG et al. Meta-analysis of colonic reservoirs versus straight coloanal anastomoses after anterior resection. The British Journal of Surgery. 2006;**93**:19-32

[31] Siddiqui MR et al. A meta-analysis comparing side to end with colonic J-pouch formation after anterior resection for rectal cancer. Techniques in Coloproctology. 2010;**14**:113-123

[32] Emile SH et al. Systematic review and meta-analysis of randomized clinical trials on the treatment of low anterior resection syndrome. Surgery. 2023;**173**(6):1352

[33] Christensen P et al. Management guidelines for low anterior resection syndrome - the MANUEL project. Colorectal Disease. 2021;**23**(2):461

[34] Yin L et al. Bowel symptoms and self-care strategies of survivors in the process of restoration after low anterior resection of rectal cancer. BMC Surgery. 2018;**18**:35

[35] Yoon BJ, Oh HK, Lee J, et al. Effects of probiotics on bowel function restoration following ileostomy closure in rectal cancer patients: A randomized controlled trial. Colorectal Disease. 2021;**23**(4):901-910

[36] Lazaraki G et al. Recent advances in pharmacological treatment of irritable bowel syndrome. World Journal of Gastroenterology. 2014;**20**(27):8867-8885

[37] Gershon MD et al. Review article: Serotonin receptors and transporters—roles in normal and abnormal gastrointestinal motility. Alimentary Pharmacology & Therapeutics. 2004;**20**(Suppl 7):3-14

[38] Jing F et al. Metabolic kinetics of 5-hydroxytryptamine and the research targets of functional gastrointestinal disorders. Digestive Diseases and Sciences. 2014;**59**(11):2642-2648

[39] Cremonini F et al. Efficacy of alosetron in irritable bowel syndrome: A meta-analysis of randomized controlled trials. Neurogastroenterology and Motility. 2003;**15**(1):79-86

[40] Itagaki R et al. Serotonin (5-HT3) receptor antagonists for the reduction of symptoms of low anterior resection syndrome. Clinical and Experimental Gastroenterology. 2014;**7**:47-52

[41] Ryoo SB et al. Anterior resection syndrome: A randomized clinical trial of a 5-HT3 receptor antagonist (ramosetron) in male patients with rectal cancer. The British Journal of Surgery. 2021;**108**(6):644-651

[42] Popeskou SG et al. Ondansetron for low anterior resection syndrome (LARS): A double blind, placebo controlled, cross-over, randomized study. Annals of Surgery. 2023;**279**(2):196-202. DOI: 10.1097/SLA.0000000000005995

[43] Asnong A et al. The role of pelvic floor muscle training on low anterior resection syndrome: A multicenter randomized controlled trial. Annals of Surgery. 2022;**276**(5):761

[44] Martellucci J et al. Role of transanal irrigation in the treatment of anterior resection syndrome. Techniques in Coloproctology. 2018;**22**:519-527

[45] Enriquez-Navascues JM et al. A randomized trial comparing transanal irrigation and percutaneous tibial nerve stimulation in the management of low anterior resection syndrome. Colorectal Disease. 2020;**22**:303-309

[46] EHA P et al. A randomized controlled clinical trial of transanal irrigation versus conservative treatment in patients with low anterior resection syndrome after rectal cancer surgery. Annals of Surgery. 2023;**277**:30e37

[47] Michelsen HB et al. Sacral nerve stimulation for faecal incontinence alters colorectal transport. The British Journal of Surgery. 2008;**95**(6):779-784

[48] Michelsen HB et al. Rectal motility after sacral nerve stimulation for faecal incontinence. Neurogastroenterology and Motility. 2010;**22**(1):36-41

[49] Holzer B et al. Sacral nerve stimulation in patients after rectal resection—preliminary report. Journal of Gastrointestinal Surgery. 2008;**12**:921

[50] De Miguel M et al. Sacral nerve stimulation for the treatment of faecal incontinence following low anterior resection for rectal cancer. Colorectal Disease. 2011;**13**:72

[51] Moya P et al. Sacral nerve stimulation in patients with severe fecal incontinence after rectal resection. Techniques in Coloproctology. 2012;**16**:263

[52] Schwandner O et al. Sacral neuromodulation for fecal incontinence and "low anterior resection syndrome" following neoadjuvant therapy for rectal cancer. International Journal of Colorectal Disease. 2013;**28**:665

[53] Marinello FG et al. Percutaneous tibial nerve stimulation in patients with severe low anterior resection syndrome: Randomized clinical trial. The British Journal of Surgery. 2021;**108**:380e387

[54] Cuicchi D et al. Randomized pilot trial of percutaneous posterior tibial nerve stimulation versus medical therapy for the treatment of low anterior resection syndrome: One-year follow-up. Diseases of the Colon and Rectum. 2020;**63**:1602-1609

Chapter 6

Fecal Incontinence: From Anatomy to Recent Advances

Anup Chalise, Satyadeep Bhattacharya and Bishnu P. Kandel

Abstract

The anatomy and physiology of the pelvic floor are complex. A thorough understanding of the anatomy is required to understand how we attain physiological continence. Fecal incontinence can be a life-altering condition that presents as an inability to maintain voluntary control of the passage of gas, liquid, or solid stool through the anus in patients who previously had control. The key to successfully managing a patient with fecal incontinence is to identify the underlying cause. There have been many prescribed procedures for patients requiring surgical correction to attain continence. However, the results are dismal for many patients. Recent advances have challenged these procedures with higher success rates.

Keywords: anal sphincter, continence, fecal incontinence, reconstructive surgery, perineum

1. Introduction

Fecal incontinence is a worldwide problem. The prevalence of fecal incontinence is difficult to estimate because often, this condition is underreported due to social stigma. The overall reported prevalence of fecal incontinence ranges from 2 to 21%, with a median of 7.7%. There is a significant variation depending on age. The reported prevalence of fecal incontinence is 7% in women younger than thirty, which rises to 22% in their seventh decade. In geriatric patients, its prevalence is reported as high as 25 to 35% of nursing home residents and 10 to 25% of hospitalized patients. Fecal incontinence is the second leading cause of nursing home placement in the geriatric population [1–3]. Studies have shown no difference in prevalence among males and females [1, 2]. However, this condition markedly impairs quality of life [1].

Let us discuss this topic in detail, starting from the factors that maintain continence to understand better how to diagnose and select treatment options for patients presenting with this disorder. We aim to cover the different types of surgical procedures, but describing every detail is out of the scope of this chapter.

2. Anatomy

2.1 Anatomy of the perineum

The pelvic floor is a complex structure made chiefly of muscles and tendons spanning the pelvic outlet. The majority of this musculotendinous structure comprises the levator ani (**Figure 1**, comprised of three muscles: iliococcygeus, pubococcygeus, and ischiococcygeus) lying in a symmetrically paired fashion to cover the outlet that maintains a constant tone even with changes in pressure (e.g., voiding, defecation, Valsalva maneuver), and contracts at times of acute rise in pressure (e.g., coughing, sneezing) [3, 4].

Understanding this anatomy is essential to know how physiological continence is maintained. The pubococcygeus comprises of further two parts in both males and females. In males, this muscle is split into the pubourethralis and the puborectalis, while in females, this muscle splits into the pubovaginalis and the puborectalis. When talking about fecal continence, it is important to note that the puborectalis serves in part the sphincter complex of the rectum and as a pelvic floor muscle. At rest (i.e., when not defecating or actively contracting the perineum), the 'puborectalis sling' (**Figure 2**) pulls the anorectal junction anteriorly toward the pubis. This sling forms an angulation between the rectum and anal canal, called the anorectal angle [3, 4].

2.2 Anatomy of the external anal sphincter and the internal anal sphincter

The External Anal Sphincter (EAS) is a complex of three sphincter muscles criss-crossing each other. These three muscular loops form an efficient closing mechanism. When only one loop is present, there is continence of solid stools, but not liquid stools or gas. In males, this sphincter complex is preserved in a trilaminar pattern, while in females, the transverse perineii muscle fuses with the EAS in the lower part of the perineum forming a single complex structure [3].

The trilaminar EAS comprises the following structures from in to outwards [5, 6]:

- Deep EAS, which lacks a posterior attachment and is related to the puborectalis.

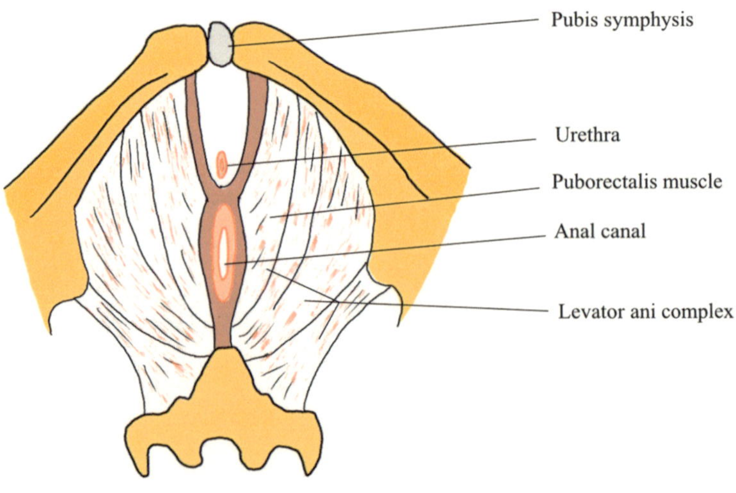

Figure 1.
The pelvic floor showing the arrangement of muscle fibers in a male patient.

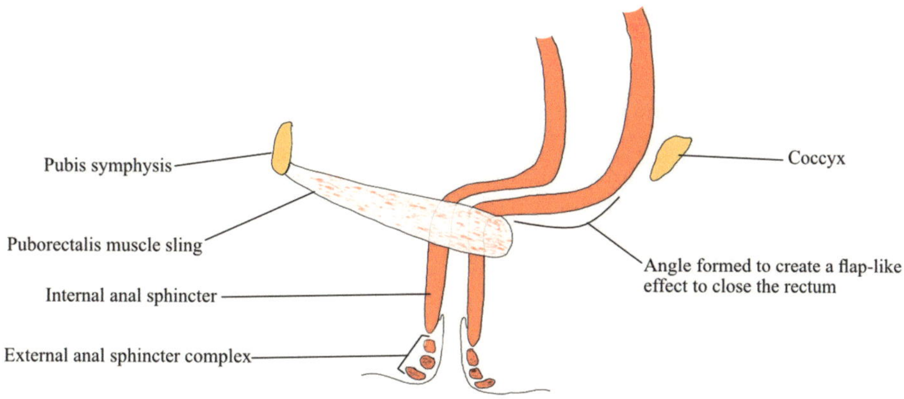

Figure 2.
The puborectalis sling that forms the anorectal angle.

- Superficial EAS, which is attached to the anococcygeal ligament posteriorly.
- Subcutaneous EAS, which is a circular structure encircling the anal canal, attached to the anococcygeal ligament posteriorly and the perineal body anteriorly.

When performing a digital rectal examination, one can feel the puborectalis sling in the posterior wall of the rectum. The sling forms the junction between the levator ani muscle and the EAS [3].

The Internal Anal Sphincter (IAS) is a fairly simple structure compared to the EAS. The IAS is a continuation of the circular smooth muscle of the rectum, ending 6–8 mm above the junction of the superficial and subcutaneous parts of the EAS with a well-defined and rounded edge [3–5].

2.3 Blood and nerve supply to the perineum

Understanding how various factors lead to incontinence also requires understanding the vascular and neural supply to the sphincter complex. The pelvic splanchnic nerves accomplish evacuation of the bowel, while the pudendal and the pelvic splanchnic nerves serve to maintain continence [3–6].

The IAS receives its motor innervation from the parasympathetic fibers of the pelvic splanchnic nerves, which inhibit contraction. In contrast, the sympathetic fibers supplying the IAS induce contraction to maintain continence [3–6].

The EAS has supply from both the inferior rectal branch of the internal pudendal nerve and the perineal branch of the fourth sacral nerve, with the levator ani supplied by branches of the S4 (S3-S5) nerve root [3–6].

3. Physiology

3.1 Definition and physiology of continence

Continence derives from the Latin word *continere* or *tenere*, which means the ability to retain a bodily discharge voluntarily. The loss of this voluntary ability leads to incontinence. Continence depends on various factors, including anatomical barriers like the pelvis, curvatures of the rectum, and transverse rectal folds, or physiological barriers like the rectal compliance and the rectoanal sensation.

The structural and functional integrity of the pelvic floor, rectum, sigmoid colon, and anus, along with the IAS and EAS, maintain continence in humans. A study has shown that the contributing factors to continence include, in descending order, nerve-induced activity in the IAS (45%), EAS (35%), anal hemorrhoid plexus (15%), and myogenic tone in IAS (10%). The IAS provides the resting tone of the sphincter, i.e., the 'resting pressure,' while the EAS provides voluntary control of the sphincter, i.e., the 'squeeze pressure' [7]. The hemorrhoidal cushion acts as a mechanical blockade to the exiting stool, contributing to continence [8].

So, when stool reaches the rectum, it gets distended. A reflexive relaxation of the IAS occurs by the process termed Recto Anal Inhibitory Reflex (RAIR) [8]. Sometimes when the person is unable to defecate (i.e., unable to find a 'safe' spot to defecate), the rectum relaxes to allow more stool to fit in, i.e., the accommodation reflex. So, RAIR leads to defecation, while accommodation leads to continence. However, this process is also influenced by the content within the rectum (i.e., solid, liquid, or gas), which is identified by the anal mucosa by the sampling reflex. Loose stool often decreases resting and squeeze pressures, leading to loss of physiological continence mechanisms [3, 8].

3.2 Definition and causes of fecal incontinence

A life-altering condition that presents with an inability to maintain voluntary control of the passage of gas, liquid, or solid stool through the anus in patients who previously had control is defined as fecal incontinence [6, 9]. Thus, most patients experience social isolation and decreased quality of life [1, 2].

Mechanisms of incontinence have been broadly classified as follows [2]:

1. Suprasphincteric dysfunction: issues with stool consistency/volume, rectal compliance and motility, defect in rectoanal inhibitory reflex, and altered rectal sensation.

2. Sphincteric dysfunction: disintegration of IAS, age-related changes, trauma (including obstetric events like forceps or vacuum delivery, anal surgery like sphincterotomy, dilatation, hemorrhoidectomy, or fistula surgery), altered EAS integrity.

3. Neurological: pudendal nerve injury, hypogastric nerve (sympathetic) injury, pelvic nerve (parasympathetic) injury, intrinsic nerve (enteric) injury.

4. Congenital: anorectal malformations, spina bifida, isolated sacral agenesis, following surgical treatment for Hirschsprung disease.

5. Central nervous system disorders: cerebrovascular accidents, Parkinson's disease, multiple sclerosis, spinal cord injury.

6. Secondary causes: dysfunctional autonomic nervous system (e.g., diabetic patients), intestinal disorders, inflammatory bowel disease, pelvic non-intestinal surgery, rectal resection, pelvic radiotherapy, and rectal prolapse.

Case summary: A 17-year-old male had initially undergone surgery for Fournier gangrene with IAS and EAS involvement. A temporary diversion loop colostomy was also made to protect the wound. However, the patient developed anal stenosis late in the course of the disease. It was difficult to admit even a finger in his anus. However, following two settings of V-Y anoplasty, and a series of post-operative anal dilatation, a finger could readily be admitted into his anus. Nevertheless, his anal tone was very weak. What would you do next?

4. Investigations

4.1 History

The following questions need to be addressed when taking a history from a patient with fecal incontinence [3]:

- History of diarrhea/loose stool and fecal urgency.
- Nature of incontinence: Is the patient aware of incontinence episodes, or is it related to stressful situations when they cannot stop even when they try?
- Degree of incontinence:
    - Is the patient incontinent only to solid, liquid, or gas?
    - How frequently does the patient experience these symptoms?

4.2 Physical examination

When examining the patient, check for soiling, erythema of perineal skin, signs indicating previous trauma, and perform a squeeze test on DRE while assessing the symmetry of closure. Also, look for the rectum/anal canal descent by asking the patient to bear down (Valsalva maneuver) and look for the anal wink or anal cutaneous reflex to assess for pudendal injury [2, 3, 6, 9].

4.3 Severity of incontinence

One can use a simple bedside scoring method called the Browning and Parks scale to assess the severity of incontinence [10]. Alternatively, the Cleveland Clinic Florida fecal incontinence (Wexner) scale can also be used [11]. Do note that leakage of solid stool is considered more severe than leakage of liquid stool or gas. Also, none of these scales will consider defecation frequency, i.e., they may underestimate incontinence in patients with lower defecation frequency.

The Browning and Parks scale assigns four categories to incontinence. Normal patients are assigned to Category 1. Those with difficulty in controlling flatus and diarrhea are assigned to Category 2. Patients with no control of diarrhea and those without control of solid stool are assigned to Categories 3 and 4, respectively [10].

4.4 Tests for incontinence

Let us discuss some commonly used tests for fecal incontinence. Basic investigations include stool and blood tests to identify commonly treatable causes. This can be followed up with a sigmoidoscopy or colonoscopy to check for any mass lesions that may lead to incontinence. Endoscopic ultrasound (EUS) can also help demonstrate lesions in the IAS and EAS, including disruptions and atrophy. An alternative to patients who do not tolerate sigmoidoscopy or colonoscopy may be evaluated using MRI defecography scans or endoanal MRI [3, 6, 12].

Among more specific tests, *anorectal manometry* is the most widely available and the best tool that tests defects in sphincter function, anal reflexes, rectal sensory function, and compliance. It is also used to assess defecatory function by the expulsion of a rectal balloon, saline continence test, and measurement of rectoanal pressures during straining [3, 6].

Rectal sensitivity is tested by a rectal balloon inflated with incremental volumes. The first detectable sensation is the rectal sensory threshold, which occurs with 30–60 mL of air or fluid. A defecation sensation or urgency occurs with 60–160 mL of air or fluid (defecatory desire volume). Pain occurs with more than 270 mL of air or fluid, with the maximum tolerable volume ranging from 160 to 70 mL of air or fluid. This adaptability of the rectum is calculated by changing rectal pressure during the distention of the balloon with air or fluid [3, 6].

Another test to assess for dyssynergia is the *balloon expulsion test*. A normal subject can expel a 50 mL balloon filled with water within a minute, but this is impaired when there is a lack of neural coordination. Other tests to identify neural injury include pudendal nerve terminal motor latency testing and electromyography (EMG) [3, 6].

5. Treatment

Once incontinence and its severity have been defined, treatment is started. There are multiple goals of treatment. Firstly, identify underlying disorders and treat them, for example, diarrhea, inflammatory bowel disease, and modification of existing medications used by the patient. Some patients benefit from adding fiber to the diet, while others benefit from including loperamide in their treatment regimen. The use of *biofeedback training* can also improve symptoms in some patients. EMG feedback devices are available to assist patients with this process. Surgery and other treatment modalities are only advised once a significant sphincter defect is identified or medical therapy fails. Let us discuss some of these treatment modalities in detail [3, 6, 8, 13].

5.1 Surgical options

Since the success rate of surgeries is low, multiple options exist for treating incontinence. These include but are not limited to [1–3, 6, 8–11, 13, 14]:

- *Restoration and improvement of residual sphincter function*

This can involve correcting a defective external anal sphincter, sphincteroplasty, correcting a defective pelvic floor, correction of anorectal deformities, Sacral Nerve Stimulation (SNS), or Posterior Tibial Nerve Stimulation (PTNS).

- *Increasing the outlet resistance of the anal sphincter*

This can involve augmentation of the anal sphincter and anal cushions (anal bulking agents), anal encirclement (Thiersch procedure), non-dynamic graciloplasty.

- *Dynamic sphincter replacement*

This involves the use of artificial anal sphincters or a dynamic graciloplasty.

- *Fecal diversion*

This is done when surgery is contraindicated for sphincter repair, i.e., fecal diversion via colostomy and ileostomy.

5.2 Creating a stoma for incontinence

The indications for forming a stoma for incontinence include [3]:

- An injury to the cloaca;
- An associated rectovaginal fistula;
- In the presence of Crohn's disease;
- A history of radiotherapy.

The absolute contraindication for surgery is gross pudendal neuropathy in women. Pudendal neuropathy is evaluated by checking for perianal numbness and examination findings of a lack of sphincter contraction in the bend of the 'U' of the divided anal sphincter [3].

6. Recent advances in treatment

6.1 Anal bulking

This procedure was started by Shafik in 1993 by injecting polytetrafluoroethylene into the submucosa. This was then developed by Kumar et al. in 1998 to glutaraldehyde cross-linked collagen (GAX). Currently, there are multiple options, like the bioplastic, silicone-based beads, carbon-coated zirconium beads (Durasphere), autologous fat, calcium hydroxylapatite (Coaptite), Zuidex, Permacol, and even stem cells. The principle behind all these bulking agents is to provide the cushion effect (as provided by the anal cushion). So, patients with failed conservative management and a structurally intact but weak anal sphincter complex benefit from these agents [14–16].

Recent advances in these agents include using Polyacrylonitrile (Hyexpan) cylinders that inflate by absorbing water. The volume of these implants increases by up to 750%, which has shown much promise in providing continence to these patients [9, 14–16]. Another recent advance uses a magnetic anal sphincter augmentation device (FENIX MAS). This device has been shown to significantly reduce weekly incontinent episodes and weekly incontinent days in a 5-year study [17].

6.2 Sacral nerve modulation

Approved by the FDA in 2011, multiple studies have shown a 50% reduction in incontinent episodes per week over 12 weeks in at least 50% of patients [18, 19]. The efficacy of this device was demonstrated first by Wexner et al., and a long-term follow-up of 3 years has shown an 86% success rate (n = 83) [20].

6.3 Clamping devices

An experimental treatment has been proposed by Han et al. with the use of prototype clamping devices that reform the anorectal angle. This helps improve continence even in the absence of a sphincter complex [21].

7. Conclusion

Fecal incontinence is a lifestyle-altering disease process. Many treatment modalities can be used to achieve continence in incontinent patients. Some of the newer modalities have shown better outcomes compared to surgical treatment. A good selection of the patient with adequate pre-operative workup is essential for a favorable outcome.

Acknowledgements

The authors do not have any acknowledgments to make.

Conflict of interest

The authors declare no conflict of interest.

DOI: http://dx.doi.org/10.5772/intechopen.1002616

Author details

Anup Chalise[1*], Satyadeep Bhattacharya[2] and Bishnu P. Kandel[3]

1 B.P. Smriti Community Co-operative Hospital Ltd., Kathmandu, Nepal

2 Nepal Mediciti Hospital Pvt. Ltd., Lalitpur, Nepal

3 Institute of Medicine, Tribhuwan University Teaching Hospital, Kathmandu, Nepal

*Address all correspondence to: anup.chalise1346@gmail.com

IntechOpen

© 2023 The Author(s). Licensee IntechOpen. This chapter is distributed under the terms of the Creative Commons Attribution License (http://creativecommons.org/licenses/by/3.0), which permits unrestricted use, distribution, and reproduction in any medium, provided the original work is properly cited.

References

[1] Ng K-S, Sivakumaran Y, Nassar N, Gladman MA. Fecal incontinence. Diseases of the Colon & Rectum. 2015;**58**(12):1194-1209. DOI: 10.1097/dcr.0000000000000514

[2] Bharucha AE, Knowles CH, Mack I, Malcolm A, Oblizajek N, Rao S, et al. Faecal incontinence in adults. Nature Reviews Disease Primers. 2022;**8**(1):53. DOI: 10.1038/s41572-022-00381-7

[3] Bharucha AE, Blandon RE. In: Ratto C, Doglietto G, editors. Fecal Incontinence: Diagnosis and Treatment. 1st ed. Italy: Wiley; 2007. pp. 3-10

[4] Ranee T, Fenner DE. In: Sultan A, Thakar R, Fenner D, editors. Perineal and Anal Sphincter Trauma: Diagnosis and Clinical Management. 1st ed. UK: Springer; 2007. pp. 1-12

[5] Yeo CJ. Shackelford's Surgery of the Alimentary Tract. Philadelphia, PA: Elsevier; 2019. pp. 1662-1675

[6] Yeo CJ. Shackelford's Surgery of the Alimentary Tract. Philadelphia, PA: Elsevier; 2019. pp. 1721-1732

[7] Penninckx F, Lestar B, Kerremans R. The internal anal sphincter: Mechanisms of control and its role in maintaining anal continence. Baillière's Clinical Gastroenterology. 1992;**6**(1):193-214. DOI: 10.1016/0950-3528(92)90027-c

[8] Brunicardi FC, Andersen DK, Billiar TR, Dunn DL, Hunter JG, Kao LS, et al. Schwartz's Principles of Surgery. 11th ed. Vol. 2. New York: McGraw-Hill; 2019. pp. 1259-1329

[9] Da Silva G, Sirany A. Recent advances in managing fecal incontinence. F1000Research. 2019;**8**(F1000 Faculty Rev):1291. DOI: 10.12688/f1000research.15270.2

[10] Browning GG, Parks AG. Postanal repair for neuropathic faecal incontinence: Correlation of clinical result and anal canal pressures. British Journal of Surgery. 1983;**70**(2):101-104. DOI: 10.1002/bjs.1800700216

[11] Jorge MJ, Wexner SD. Etiology and management of Fecal incontinence. Diseases of the Colon & Rectum. 1993;**36**(1):77-97. DOI: 10.1007/bf02050307

[12] Raizada V, Bhargava V, Karsten A, Mittal RK. Functional morphology of anal sphincter complex unveiled by high definition anal manometery and three-dimensional ultrasound imaging. Neurogastroenterology & Motility. 2011;**23**(11):1013-e460. DOI: 10.1111/j.1365-2982.2011.01782.x

[13] Person B. Advances in the surgical treatment of fecal incontinence. Surgical Innovation. 2005;**12**(1):7-21. DOI: 10.1177/155335060501200103

[14] Camilleri-Brennan J. Anal Injectable and Implantable Bulking Agents for Faecal Incontinence [Internet]. Current Topics in Faecal Incontinence. IntechOpen; 2020. DOI: 10.5772/intechopen.91952

[15] Vaizey CJ, Kamm MA. Injectable bulking agents for treating faecal incontinence. British Journal of Surgery. 2005;**92**(5):521-527. DOI: 10.1002/bjs.4997

[16] de la Portilla F. Internal anal sphincter augmentation and substitution. Gastroenterology Report. 2014;**2**(2):106-111. DOI: 10.1093/gastro/gou004

[17] Sugrue J, Lehur P-A, Madoff RD, McNevin S, Buntzen S, Laurberg S, et al. Long-term experience of magnetic anal sphincter augmentation in patients with fecal incontinence. Diseases of the Colon & Rectum. 2017;**60**(1):87-95. DOI: 10.1097/dcr.0000000000000709

[18] Lim JT, Hastie IA, Hiscock RJ, Shedda SM. Sacral nerve stimulation for fecal incontinence: Long-term outcomes. Diseases of the Colon & Rectum. 2011;**54**(8):969-974. DOI: 10.1097/dcr.0b013e31821e57c2

[19] Hull T, Giese C, Wexner SD, Mellgren A, Devroede G, Madoff RD, et al. Long-term durability of sacral nerve stimulation therapy for chronic fecal incontinence. Diseases of the Colon & Rectum. 2013;**56**(2):234-245. DOI: 10.1097/dcr.0b013e318276b24c

[20] Wexner SD, Coller JA, Devroede G, Hull T, McCallum R, Chan M, et al. Sacral nerve stimulation for fecal incontinence. Annals of Surgery. 2010;**251**(3):441-449. DOI: 10.1097/sla.0b013e3181cf8ed0

[21] Han D, Yan G, Wang Z, Jiang P, Liu D, Zhao K, et al. An artificial anal sphincter based on a novel clamping mechanism: Design, analysis, and testing. Artificial Organs. 2021;**45**(8):E293-E303. DOI: 10.1111/aor.13924

Section 3

Rectal Prolapse

Chapter 7

Internal Rectal Prolapse in Children: A Hidden Cause of Constipation Requiring Comprehensive Evaluation and Treatment

Salahedin Delshad

Abstract

Internal rectal prolapse in children is a significant cause of persistent constipation that is resistant to medication. This condition, characterized by mucosal folds in the distal rectum, leads to obstructive constipation, rectal dilation, and potential fecal incontinence if not promptly diagnosed and treated. Symptoms include drug-resistant constipation, pain, facial flushing, sweating, crying, avoidance of the toilet, and straining during defecation. In advanced stages, loss of appetite and rectal bleeding may occur. Despite unsuccessful treatment with various laxatives, specialized pediatric gastroenterologists are unable to improve the condition. This study compared 153 pediatric patients with internal rectal prolapse to a control group of hospitalized children without the condition. Diagnosis and treatment approaches are discussed, emphasizing the importance of distinguishing this condition from other causes of constipation, such as Hirschsprung's disease. Radiological findings and a classification system based on the thickness of prolapsed mucosa are also presented. Treatment options include sclerotherapy for lower-grade prolapse. However, the abstract should provide a more concise and accurate summary of the article.

Keywords: internal rectal prolapse, constipation, pediatric, surgical procedures, rectum

1. Introduction

Constipation functional constipation is a prevalent condition in childhood, about 29.6% worldwide. In the United States, represents 3–5% of pediatric visits and a considerable annual healthcare cost.

Constipation in children has various causes. Some of them are treated by pediatricians with medication and dietary changes. Others are treated by pediatric surgeons with various surgical procedures. According to available statistics, more than one-third of children referred to pediatric gastroenterologists are due to constipation. One of the unknown causes of constipation in children is internal rectal prolapse, which has been less discussed in books on pediatric diseases and surgery. Therefore, we also encounter it less frequently in articles in pediatric and gastrointestinal journals. ASMAN first described this issue in adults in 1957 [1].

Internal rectal prolapse (IRP) is a condition where the rectum, the lowest part of the large intestine, slides inside itself during defecation. It can cause symptoms such as fecal incontinence, difficulty in emptying the bowel, anal pain and bleeding [2]. The prevalence and incidence of IRP are not well known, as it is often underdiagnosed or misdiagnosed as hemorrhoids or other conditions [2]. However, some studies have estimated that IRP affects about 2–27% of the population with constipation [3], and that it is more common in women, older adults and people with chronic straining or pelvic floor dysfunction. Rectal prolapse is a condition in which the rectal mucosa protrudes through the anal sphincter, causing discomfort, bleeding, and fecal incontinence. Although rare, it is more prevalent in children than in adults, especially in those younger than 4 years of age. The etiology and pathophysiology of rectal prolapse in children are not fully understood, but several factors have been associated with its occurrence, such as constipation, cystic fibrosis, malnutrition, parasitic infections, and psychosocial stress. The management of rectal prolapse in children varies depending on the severity and frequency of the episodes, ranging from conservative measures to surgical interventions.

Constipation caused by internal rectal prolapse is due to mucosal folds that occur in the distal rectum, which is a type of obstructive constipation and resistant to laxatives. Due to its radiological appearance like Hirschsprung's disease, some radiologists and pediatric surgeons mistake it and subject it to colostomy and pull-through surgeries. If left undiagnosed and untreated, in addition to persistent and distressing constipation, it leads to rectal dilatation and impaction of fecal masses, and ultimately fecal incontinence. In a research project, 153 children with clinical symptoms and radiological evidence of internal rectal prolapse who were treated were compared with 150 other children as the control group, who were undergoing surgery for hernia, undescended testicle, circumcision, cleft lip, and palate, and did not have clinical symptoms of internal rectal prolapse, with the consent of their parents. The control group had negative anal manometry. Since there is less information on the diagnosis and treatment of this disease in the literature, this section will discuss these topics in detail regarding the above-mentioned information.

2. Clinical symptoms

The most important sign of internal rectal prolapse is difficulty in defecation accompanied by constipation. Unlike what is seen in idiopathic constipation, the patient's constipation is not long-lasting, and more defecation attempts are observed than in other internal constipation and surgeries. The duration of constipation in these patients has been reported to be from 6 to 12 years. However, pain and facial flushing, sweating, and stiffening of the back during defecation are specific features of internal rectal prolapse [4].

Due to the severity of pain, most children cry during defecation. The crying of children leads to the emotional state of the mother and family members who cry with the child. The child is not ready to sit on the toilet and in some way tries to escape from the toilet and tries to do his/her defecation by holding his/her back in the corner of the room, behind the door, or by clinging to the edges of the table. In some children, this condition is accompanied by embarrassment and shame from family members, and they ask them not to be next to them. Unsuccessful attempts to defecate or incomplete emptying sensation are other symptoms of the disease in some patients. The presence of stool masses is another feature of this constipation. The family's analogy of stool to animal shapes during the explanation of defecation means relatively rounded stool masses. Of course, every 15 days, a large volume of fecal matter is expelled from the rectum, which is mostly the result of small stool masses sticking to each other.

Due to the accumulation of fecal masses throughout the large intestine, a type of bowel obstruction occurs that results in loss of appetite, insufficient growth in children, and soiling under oneself. This incontinence is not functional but rather a result of fecal accumulation and overflow, and in fact, is a type of false fecal incontinence. Other symptoms of the disease include abdominal pain caused by the buildup of fecal masses in the large intestine, which can be reduced or eliminated by enema and defecation. For this reason, the onset of nausea can lead some physicians to mistakenly diagnose acute abdominal conditions.

Observation of rectal prolapse in some cases is due to the abrasion of the rectal mucosa during the passage of hard fecal masses. In some cases, due to the obstruction caused by the accumulation of fecal matter throughout the colon and the inability to expel gas, bloating is observed in the small intestines. In advanced cases, such as intussusception, mucous secretions are seen from the rectum, which varies from colorless to blood-stained secretions. Internal rectal prolapse in older children, like adults, can lead to anal fissure, and a burning sensation and itching in the anal area are other symptoms of this condition.

In some patients, a feeling of heaviness in the pelvic floor has been observed. In research conducted, the prevalence of disease symptoms in boys and girls is shown in Table 1. All of these patients have been resistant to drug therapy. Laxatives can relieve constipation for a short period but do not alleviate pain during defecation or other symptoms. Patients are referred to various groups of physicians, including pediatric specialists, pediatric gastroenterologists, and pediatric surgeons. After not receiving a response from drug therapy, they turn to herbal medicine practitioners. Due to the radiological similarity of barium enema, patients with advanced internal rectal prolapse (Grade IV) with intussusception are recommended to undergo bowel resection surgery by pediatric surgeons. Some believe that internal rectal prolapse ultimately leads to external prolapse [5]. With the advancement of technology and the introduction of advanced diagnostic devices such as defecography, etc., it took many years to distinguish the gender and prevalence of these two diseases in children by experts [6].

The prevalence and incidence of internal rectal prolapse are not clear. In this study, out of 153 cases, 66 pediatric patients (43%) were female and 78 pediatric patients (57%) were male. The age of patients was 10–15 years in 14 cases (9%), 5–9 years in 52 cases (34%), 1–4 years in 86 cases (56%), and less than one year in 10 female cases (1). The average age of female patients was 4.28 years, the average age of male patients was 5.10 years, and the overall average age of patients was 4.7 years.

3. Physiopathology

The most important factor in the development of internal rectal prolapse in children is the weakness of the connective tissue between the rectal mucosa and muscle in the submucosal layer, which leads to the invagination of the rectal mucosa towards the

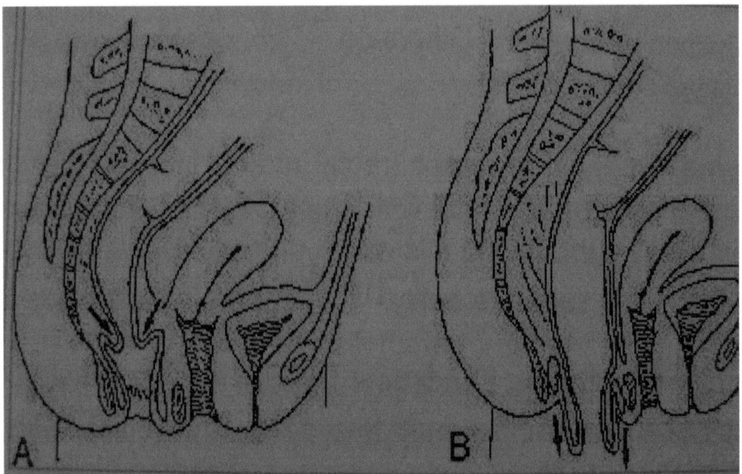

A. Internal rectal intussusception. B. External (complete) recta
prolapse

Figure 1.
Differentiated between internal prolapse.

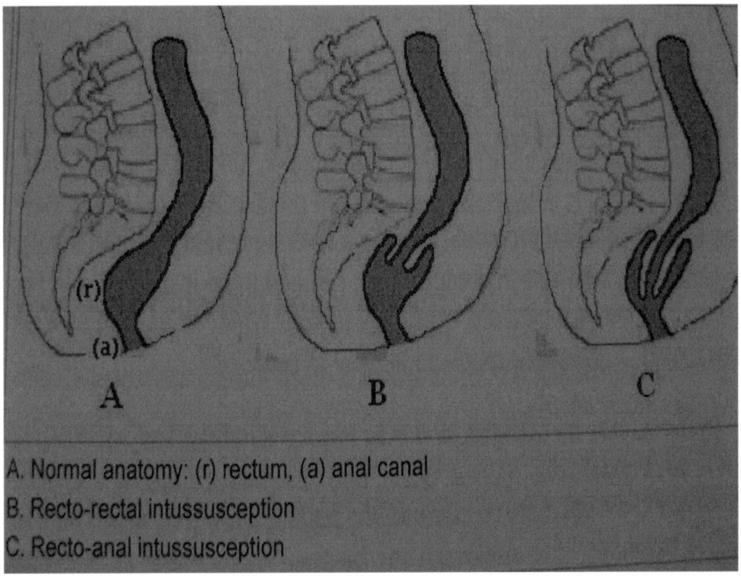

A. Normal anatomy: (r) rectum, (a) anal canal
B. Recto-rectal intussusception
C. Recto-anal intussusception

Figure 2.
Entrapment of the rectal prolapsed mucosal layer between the fecal mass and the anal sphincter muscle.

distal end and the creation of a fold (intussusception) (**Figure 1**). This event causes relative obstruction of the rectal lumen during defecation. Entrapment of the prolapsed mucosal layer between the fecal mass and the anal sphincter muscle leads to severe pain during defecation (**Figures 1** and **2**). The fecal mass, when faced with obstruction, moves proximally through antiperistalsis and returns distally again. This

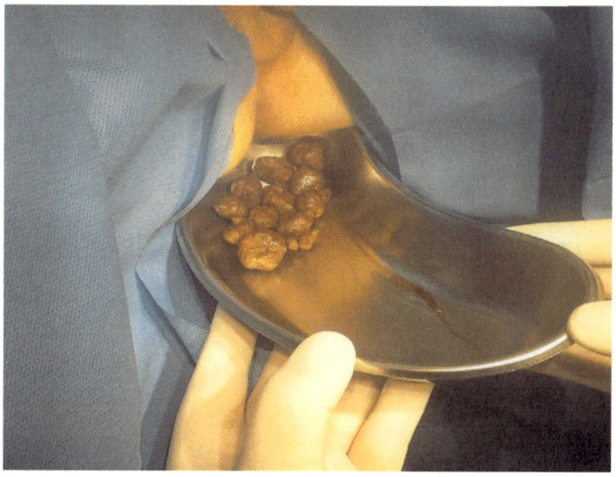

Figure 3.
Patchy stools caused by intestinal obstruction.

invagination causes the fecal matter to be compacted and firmer due to the absorption of water. The patient unconsciously and based on previous experiences, tightens their back muscles, which results in the pulling of the rectal mucosa and leads to the partial opening of the intestinal obstruction, allowing the fecal matter to be expelled in small pieces (**Figure 3**) [7].

4. Differential diagnosis

Internal rectal prolapse in children is often mistaken for idiopathic constipation and Hirschsprung [8, 9]. Pediatric specialists and pediatric gastroenterologists prescribe various types of laxatives for these children. In subsequent visits, they try other types of laxatives that are usually ineffective. Pediatric surgeons, when they suspect Hirschsprung, request a barium enema and observe a narrow painful area in the distal rectum, especially if the bowel mass does not pass after 24 h (**Figures 4** and **5**). With a probable diagnosis of Hirschsprung, the pediatric surgeon recommends the patient undergo a pull-through and colostomy surgery, but during the operation, when the pathologist's biopsy report shows the presence of ganglion, they are surprised. It has been observed that a pull-through operation has also been performed, but the pathologist did not find an aganglionic area in the bowel.

5. Radiological findings

In barium enema images, the observation of mucosal defects in the distal rectum with barium-filled lines along the mucosal folds is indicative of the severity and progression of the disease, and the size of rectal mucosal defects increases (**Figures 4** and **6–8**). Failure to pass fecal masses over time and their accumulation in the rectosigmoid and colon pathway, transforming them into hard, non-expellable masses, in the delayed image (24 h later), fecal mass accumulation mixed with barium is like Hirschsprung's disease and the radiology specialist mistakenly writes the

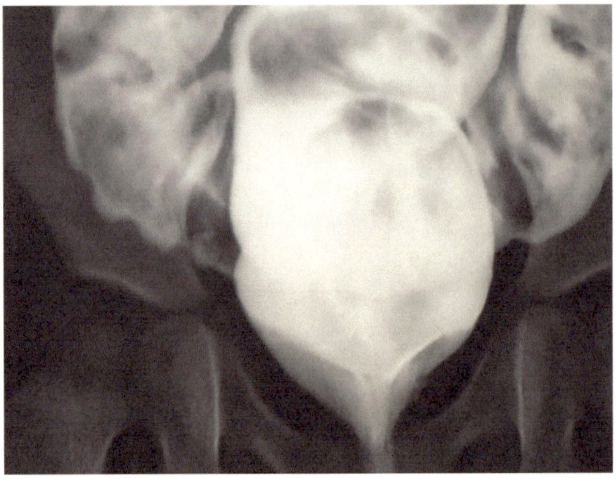

Figure 4.
Narrow region of the distal rectum like Hirschsprung's syndrome.

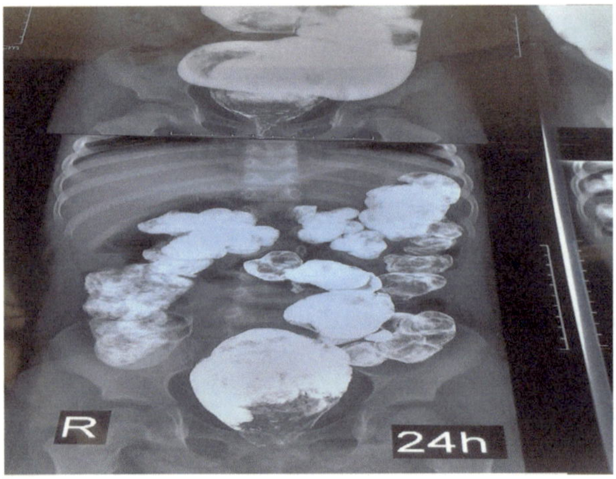

Figure 5.
Narrow region of the distal rectum like Hirschsprung's syndrome.

diagnosis of Hirschsprung's disease in their report (**Figure 6**) [10]. Therefore, the treating physician needs to correlate radiological findings with clinical signs to avoid misdiagnosis. The clinical signs mentioned in this topic should be considered as they are entirely different from constipation symptoms in Hirschsprung's disease.

5.1 Final diagnosis with the Mesh test

Clinical symptoms in the patient's history, along with radiological imaging, confirm the possibility of rectal prolapse. However, the Meah test must be performed under anesthesia for a definitive diagnosis. The "Delshad Mesh" test is performed by

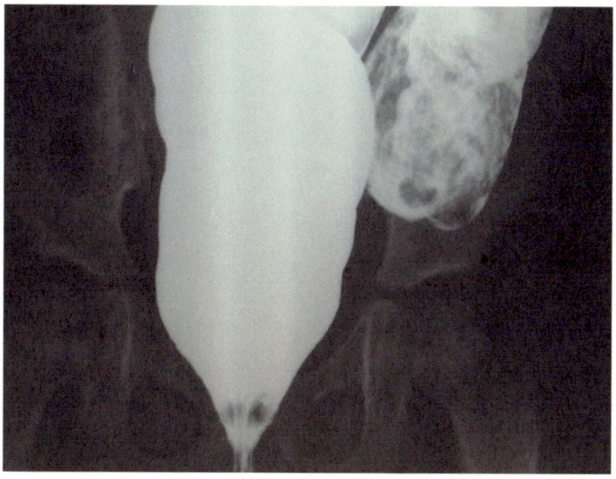

Figure 6.
Increasing the size of rectal mucosa defects due to the severity and progression of the disease.

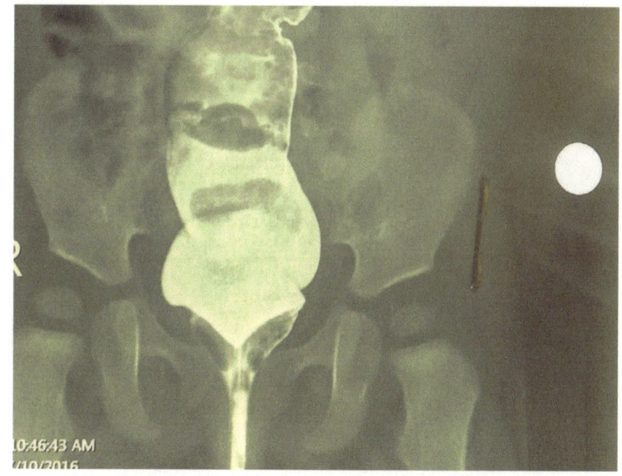

Figure 7.
Increasing the size of rectal mucosa defects due to the severity and progression of the disease.

inserting a gas infused with iodine into the rectum using a balloon. It is then pulled out, mimicking the passage of stool. In patients with rectal prolapse, the pulling of the balloon causes the rectal mucosa to fold, which can be observed (**Figures 9** and **10**). The observation of mucosal folds confirms the diagnosis. It is noteworthy that as the severity of the disease increases, the thickness of the rectal mucosa becomes more apparent (**Figures 11** and **12**). With parental consent, this test was performed on a control group of children who did not have symptoms of rectal prolapses, such as hernia, undescended testicles, circumcision, cleft lip, and palate. However, rectal mucosal discharge was not observed. A positive test result paves the way for the treating physician to perform appropriate treatment with complete confidence, to relieve the suffering of the child.

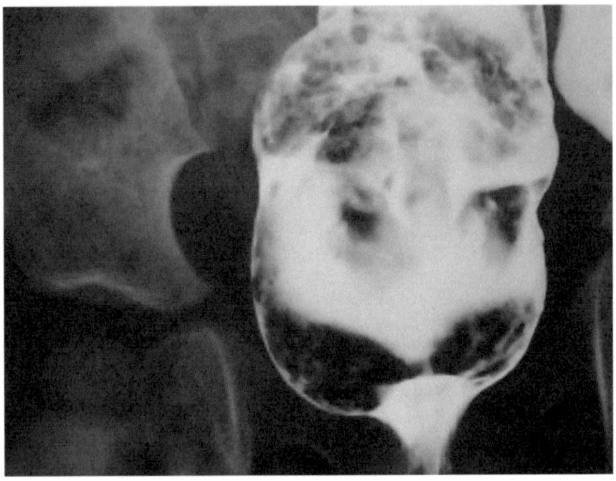

Figure 8.
Increasing the size of rectal mucosa defects due to the severity and progression of the disease.

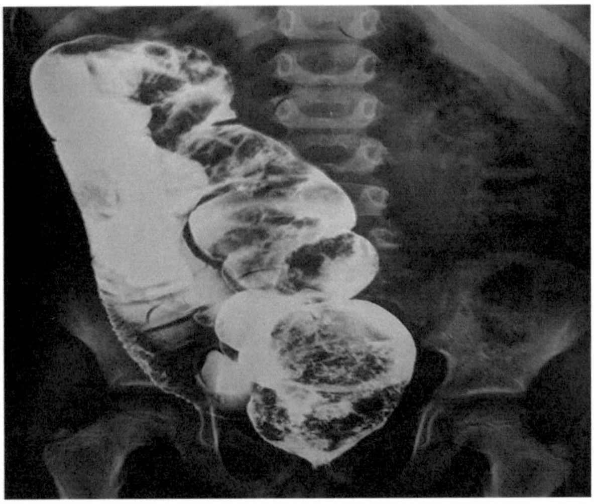

Figure 9.
Creation of rectal mucosal folds due to stretching of the Delshad's mesh.

6. Classification

Internal rectal prolapse is classified based on the thickness of the prolapsed mucosa measured by the Delshad mesh test. It has been observed that as the severity of the disease increases, the thickness of the prolapsed mucosa also increases. The treatment approach also varies according to the severity of the disease. In this study, internal rectal prolapse is classified into 4 categories based on the Delshad mesh test [11, 12].

Grade I: The thickness of the prolapsed mucosa is up to 3 millimeters (**Figure 9**). Usually, the prolapsed mucosa does not protrude from the anal orifice during mucus discharge and is visible, but not palpable. It is a type of recto-rectal prolapse.

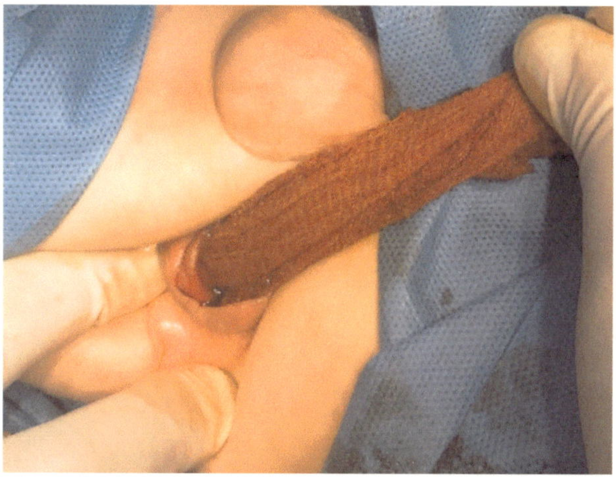

Figure 10.
Creation of rectal mucosal folds due to stretching of the Delshad's mesh.

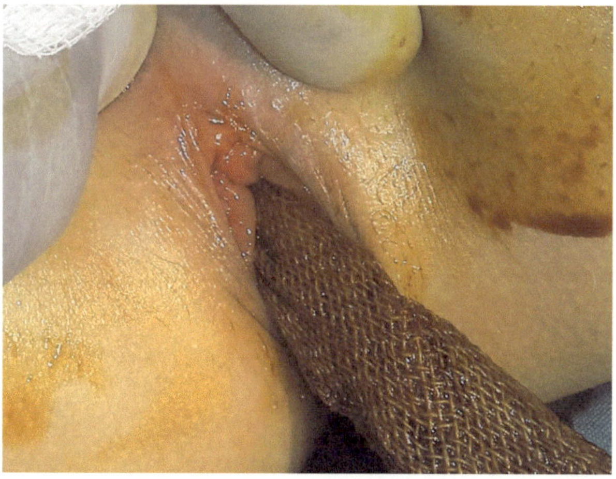

Figure 11.
Grade 4 thickness of mucous membrane prolapse.

Grade II: The thickness of the prolapsed mucosa is up to 5 millimeters (**Figure 10**). In normal conditions, the prolapse is not visible or palpable during defecation. Degrees II and I can be seen as small mucosal defects in barium enema (**Figure 6**).

Grade III: The thickness of the prolapsed mucosa is up to 10 mm (**Figures 13** and **14**). During defecation, the edge of the prolapsed mucosa may protrude from the anal canal and be palpable with a finger. A larger rectum is observed compared to Grades II and I (**Figure 7**).

Grade IV: The thickness of the prolapsed mucosa is more than 10 millimeters (**Figures 11, 12** and **15**). In many cases, the edge of the prolapsed mucosa is visible and palpable outside the anus during defecation (recto-anal). In the barium enema images, the extent of the rectal mucosal defect is greater than what was seen in grade III (**Figure 8**). In advanced cases of grade IV, severe pain during defecation may be present, and fecal incontinence and soiling may occur.

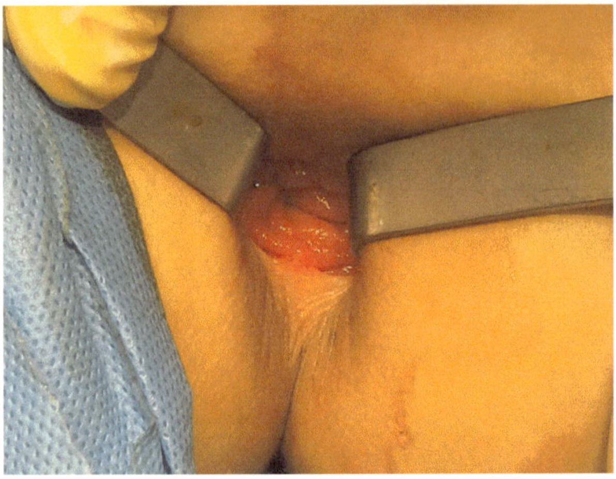

Figure 12.
Grade 4 thickness of mucous membrane prolapse.

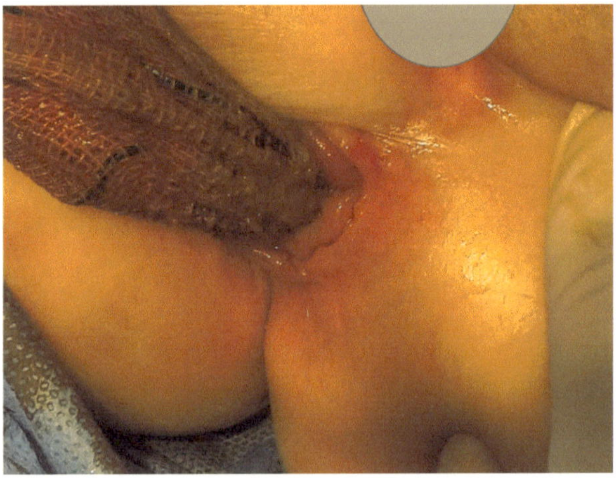

Figure 13.
Grading of rectal internal prolapse based on Delshad's mesh test.

7. Treatment

The treatment varies according to the degree and severity of the disease. In degrees I and II, injecting a sclerosing solution between the mucosa and the rectal muscle, which leads to adhesion of these two layers and prevents the development of mucosal fissures during defecation, can treat the disease. Alcohol 90°, 20% saline solution, 50% dextrose, and Glycerin phenique are used for sclerotherapy. Due to the side effects of the first three solutions, the author prefers to use Glycerin phenique. If this solution is injected properly, no side effects are observed. In children over 2 years old up to 10 years old, 2 ccs of Glycerin phenique solution is injected at 4 points at 12, 3, 6, and 9 o'clock, every 2 centimeters above the Dentate Line, between the mucosa and the rectal muscle.

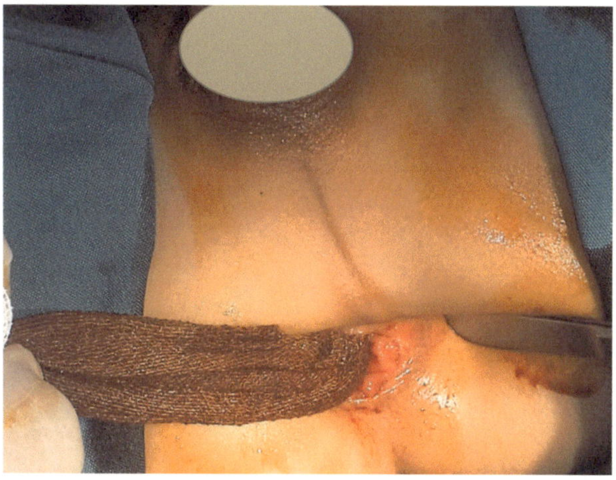

Figure 14
Grade 3 thickness of mucous membrane prolapse.

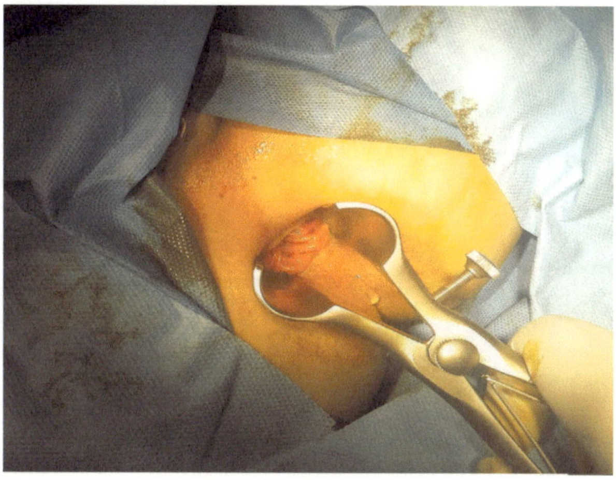

Figure 15.
Grade 4 thickness of mucous membrane prolapse.

This procedure is performed under anesthesia, and the patient is placed in a lithotomy position. It is better to use a purple angiocath. The needle tip, along with the mandrel, is inserted into the wall of the rectum from the skin around the anus (**Figures 16** and **17**), with the aid of a finger guide inserted into the rectum. The needle entry point is touched under the mucosa and prevented from moving into the muscle or out of the mucosa (**Figure 18**). Before injection, it is better to perform an anorectoscopy to visualize the rectal mucosal duplications (**Figure 19**). If there are fecal masses present, they should be evacuated (**Figures 20** and **21**). In patients with long-standing constipation and fecal impaction in the rectosigmoid and colon, it is recommended to prepare them for admission one day before treatment with oral mannitol and ring solutions.

In patients who suffer from long-term constipation and fecal impaction in the rectosigmoid and colon, it is recommended to prepare the bowel with oral solutions of

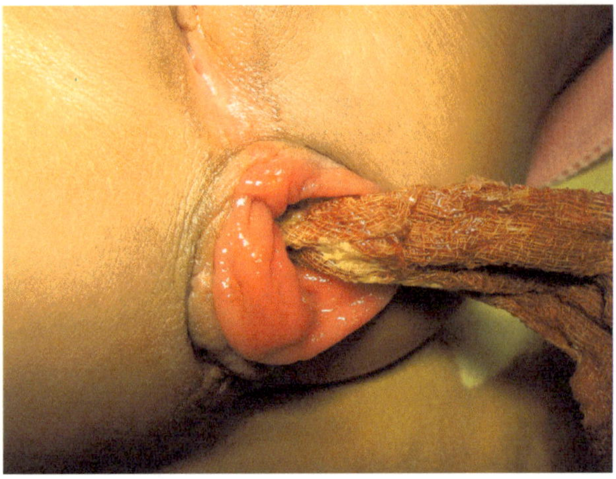

Figure 16.
Mucous prolapse treatment according to the degree and severity of the disease.

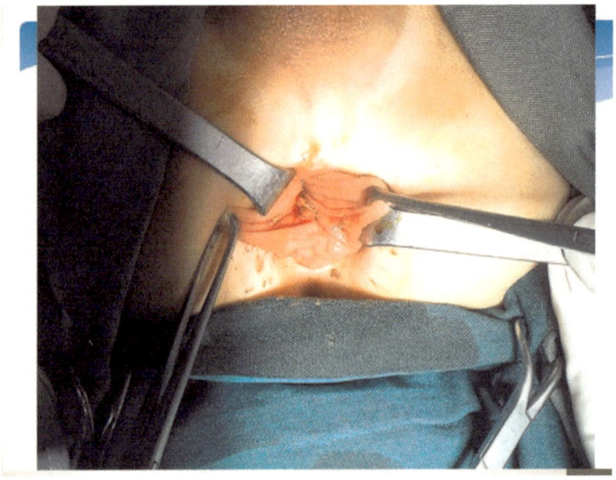

Figure 17.
Mucous prolapse treatment according to the degree and severity of the disease.

mannitol and ringers one day before hospitalization and treatment. Mannitol solution of 10% concentration should be given in two doses with a 5-hour interval, calculated based on the patient's weight at 10 ccs per kilogram. This solution causes rapid bowel evacuation. To compensate for electrolyte loss, twice the amount of the mannitol solution, Ringer's solution, should be consumed half an hour after each mannitol dose. Normal saline enema is also recommended after mannitol evacuation to complete bowel preparation. Despite all these measures, due to long-term fecal impaction in the colon, fecal masses may still be seen during the examination under anesthesia and injection of sclerosing solution. These masses need to be evacuated.

In grade III treatment, injection of a sclerosing solution (Glycerin phenique) is used, but in most cases, a second injection is required 3 months after the first injection. About 8% of grade III cases require excision of prolapsed mucosa after the second injection. In grade IV prolapse treatment, surgery is performed, and the

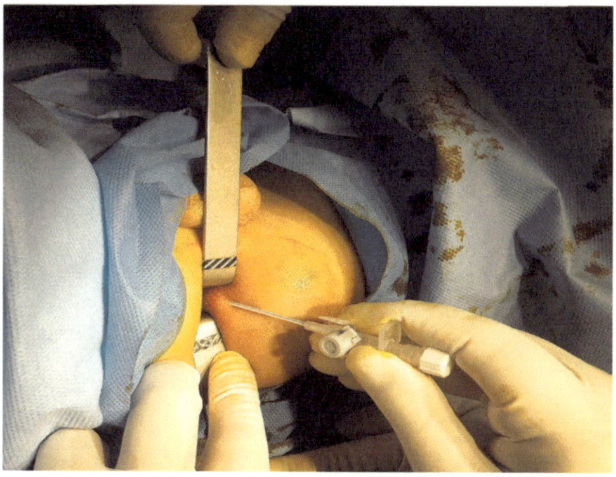

Figure 18.
Mucous prolapse treatment according to the degree and severity of the disease.

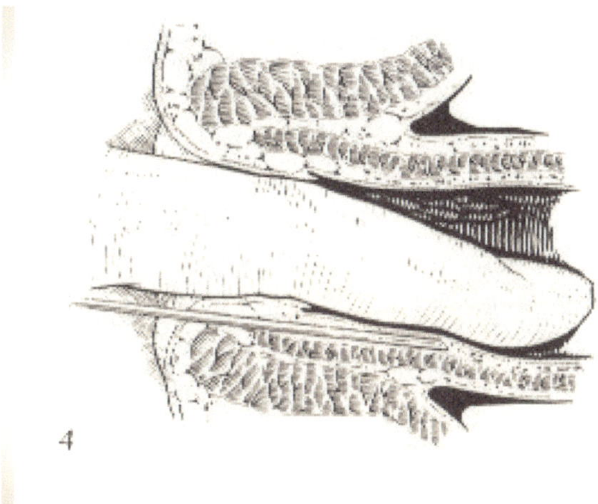

Figure 19.
Mucous prolapse treatment according to the degree and severity of the disease.

prolapsed mucosa is excised through the anus, and the edges of the rectal mucosa are anastomosed with another suture (**Figures 21–23**).

For excision and anastomosis of the rectal mucosa, a stapler device can also be used, which has a significant effect on reducing bleeding and anastomotic leakage. Fortunately, the side effects reported with sclerosing solutions other than glycerin phenylbutyrate, such as local tissue necrosis, have not been observed with the use of this solution, and the adhesion resulting from this injection has remained stable. Glycerin phenylbutyrate solution is easily accessible and does not require pre-use disinfection. It should be attempted to use a 10-ml syringe in all cases and the appropriate amount of glycerin phenylbutyrate solution should be drawn into it based on the need (**Figures 24** and **25**).

The maximum dosage for children is also 10 milliliters. It is always recommended to use the purple-colored angiocath. When injecting, after placing the Farabeuf

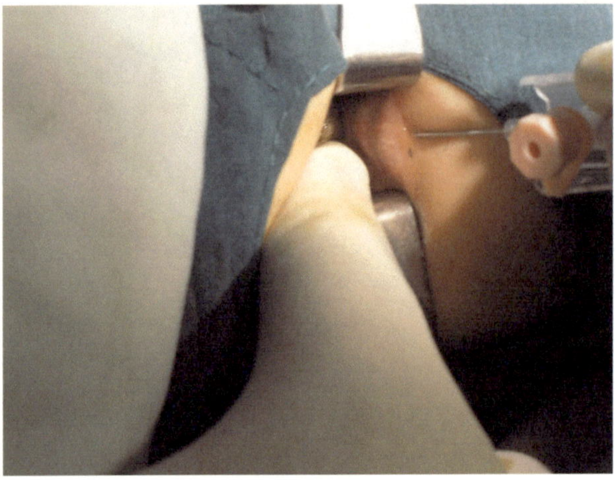

Figure 20.
Mucous prolapse treatment according to the degree and severity of the disease.

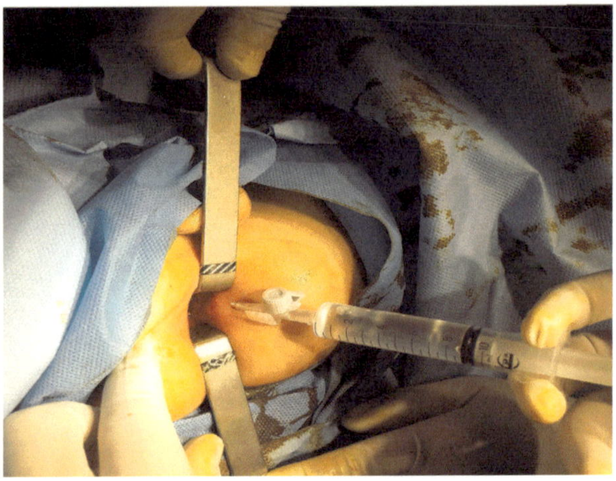

Figure 21.
Mucous prolapse treatment according to the degree and severity of the disease.

Retractor at 12 and 6 o'clock, the injection sites at 3 and 9 o'clock are prepared. First, the angiocath needle with its mandrel is inserted through the anal verge into the rectal wall, and, as mentioned, with the finger touching the shaft, the needle is directed under the mucosa. Then the mandrel is pulled out, and a syringe containing glycerin phenique is connected to it. The injection is slowly and carefully performed under the mucosa and at a distance higher than the dentate line to both sides and beyond as needed. After that, the retractors are placed at 3 and 9 o'clock, and the injection under the rectal mucosa is performed at 12 and 6 o'clock. After the injections are finished, and it is ensured that there is homeostasis and that the mesh inside the rectum is removed, the patient can be discharged. If the internal rectal prolapse is high and requires excision, the patient remains NPO for 24 hours and can be discharged on the fourth day after receiving and tolerating fluids and food.

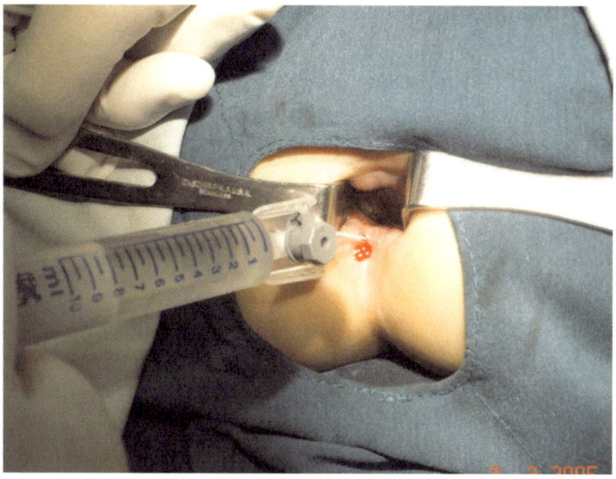

Figure 22.
In grade IV prolapse, the treatment is surgery, and the prolapsed mucosa is excised through the anus, and the edges of the rectal mucosa are anastomosed with another thread.

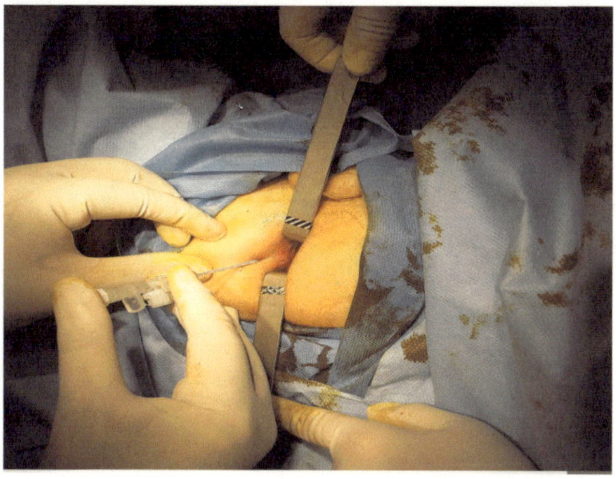

Figure 23.
In grade IV prolapse, the treatment is surgery, and the prolapsed mucosa is excised through the anus, and the edges of the rectal mucosa are anastomosed with another thread.

8. Postoperative care

Since patients with long-standing constipation have accumulated stool in their entire large intestine, it seems necessary to evacuate fecal matter in the postoperative period (**Figure 26**). In cases where relative obstruction is caused by prolapsing folds in the distal rectum, the peristaltic movement decreases due to rectosigmoid expansion. Therefore, in such cases, prescribing laxatives and a dietary regimen to prevent re-constipation is necessary. In cases where the symptoms of the disease persist for a long time, it takes time to adapt the patient to new conditions, and with the help of family or a psychologist, the patient should be continuously

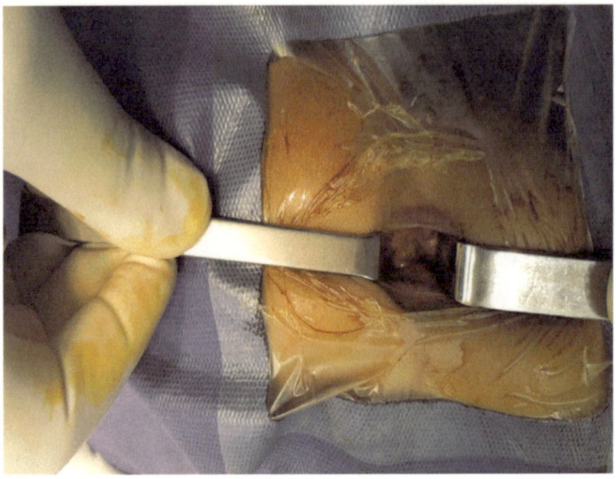

Figure 24.
Complications of prolapse treatment in children.

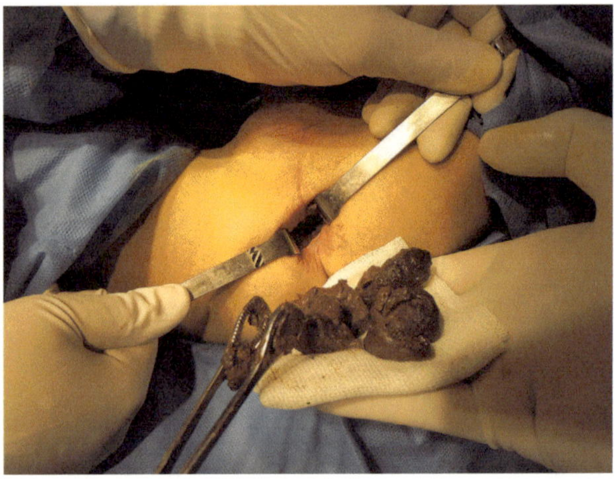

Figure 25.
Complications of prolapse treatment in children.

encouraged to adapt to the new conditions. In addition to efforts to defecate and eliminate the fear of defecation, it is necessary to encourage the patient to sit on the toilet.

9. Adverse effects

9.1 Temporary immobility of the anal sphincter muscle

Injection of sclerosing solution beside the anal sphincter muscle may create fibrotic tissues and temporarily cause incontinence or soiling. Therefore, it is emphasized that the injection site of sclerosing solution be placed 2 cm above the Dentate Line.

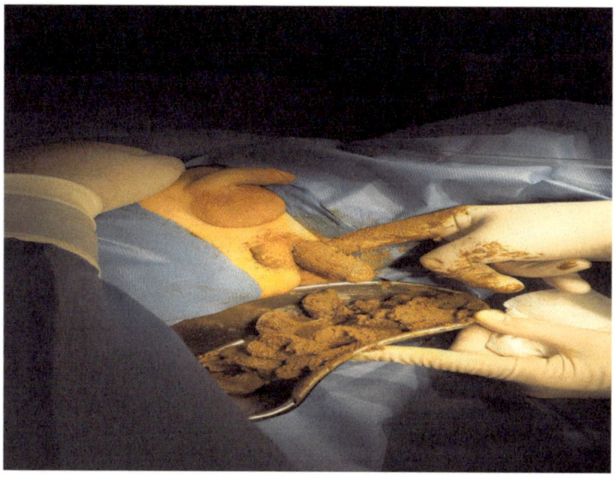

Figure 26.
Complications of prolapse treatment in children.

9.2 Relative obstruction of the rectal lumen due to severe mucosal swelling

In cases where more than the standard amount of sclerosing solution is injected, it may cause mucosal swelling and result in relative obstruction of the rectal lumen temporarily. The injection volume should be proportional to the age and volume of the rectum, ranging from 1 ml to 2.5 ml at each point, and should not exceed this amount. In children under 12 months of age, a maximum of 1 ml should be injected at each point. In children over 12 months, the injection volume at each point should not exceed 2.5 ml.

9.3 Phenol-glycerin solution toxicity

Due to the possibility of phenol-glycerin solution toxicity, it should be used with caution to prevent it from entering the bloodstream during injection. Therefore, before injecting the sclerosing solution, the syringe plunger should be pulled back when inserting the angiocath needle under the rectal mucosa, and it should be ensured that the needle does not enter the veins. If the needle tip has entered a vein, it should be removed from the skin and inserted through another route, and checked again to ensure that it is not inside the vein.

9.4 Leakage of sclerotherapy solution into vagina

As there is a small distance between the rectal wall and the vaginal wall in children, if the needle is not carefully inserted at 12 o'clock position, it may enter the lumen of the vagina and the sclerotherapy solution will spill inside the vagina without any therapeutic effect at the intended site. Therefore, after removing the needle, it should be reinserted at a different point close to the previous one with more precision.

9.5 Temporary urinary retention

In boys, during injection at 12 o'clock, in case of insufficient accuracy and spreading of sclerosing solution around the urinary sphincter, there is a possibility of

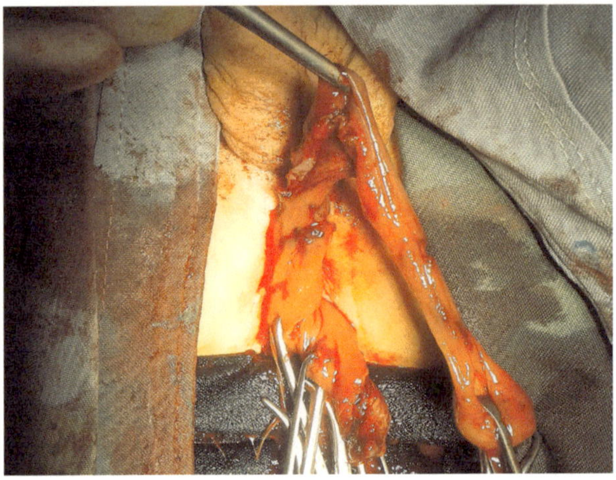

Figure 27.
Complications of prolapse treatment in children.

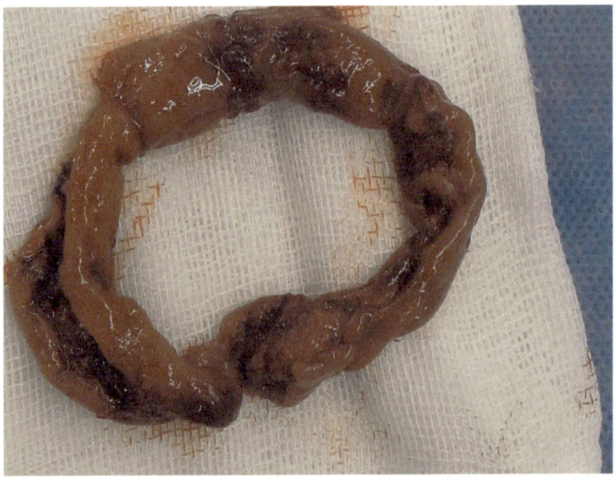

Figure 28.
Complications of prolapse treatment in children.

temporary urinary retention, and the physician may need to use a Nelaton catheter for urine evacuation. This condition may last for 2–3 days but returns to normal afterward (**Figures 27–29**).

10. Results

The results of treating internal rectal prolapse with both injection and mucosal excision of the rectum are very satisfactory. Out of 113 cases with grade I and II prolapses, complete improvement was achieved with one injection of a sclerosing solution under the rectal mucosa in 101 patients, and all symptoms before treatment, including constipation, difficulty in defecation, pain during defecation, standing and defecation by tightening the back, passing stool in pieces and running away from the toilet were resolved. In 4 cases, fear of using the toilet lasted for up to 3 months and

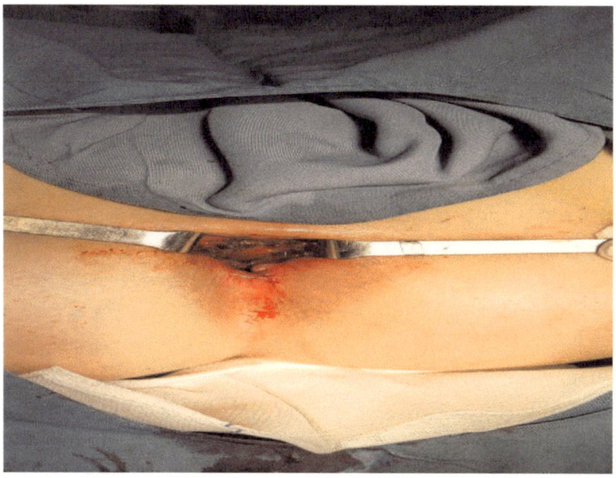

Figure 29.
Complications of prolapse treatment in children.

then disappeared. In 12 cases (including the 4 previous cases), some symptoms persisted for up to 2 months, after which improvement was achieved.

Due to the accumulation of fecal masses throughout the colon and insufficient evacuation before surgery, the re-accumulation of feces in the rectosigmoid causes constipation and the recurrence of previous symptoms. In such cases, the patient needs to be treated with bowel evacuation agents such as normal saline. In resistant cases with rectosigmoid dilation, they can be hospitalized for one day under bowel preparation with mannitol and Ringer's solution. If despite the improvement of all symptoms, the fear of using the toilet persists, psychotherapeutic treatment methods can be used to combat this phenomenon. Family cooperation and encouraging their child, even by giving gifts, will play an effective role in correcting this situation.

Families must try to treat their children with love, compassion, and understanding and avoid threatening, intimidating, and bad behavior. Since the spirit of such children has been greatly damaged over the years of suffering from this disease and they feel inferior compared to other children, efforts should be made to improve this spirit as soon as possible. Of the 29 cases in the Grade III group, complete recovery was achieved, and in 2 cases, the need for mucous prolapse excision and anastomotic stenosis was found, after which symptoms were completely resolved. In 9 cases of the Grade IV group, after complete excision of the prolapsed mucosa and anastomotic stenosis of the edges, complete recovery was achieved. Stapler device was not used in any of the cases. The use of 3.5 Vicryl thread is recommended for anastomosis. In advanced cases that led to fecal incontinence, bowel control was established after this treatment.

11. Discussion

Our study on internal rectal prolapse (IRP) in children sheds light on a commonly misdiagnosed condition that is often overlooked as a cause of constipation. The findings we have presented contribute valuable insights into the evaluation and treatment of IRP in pediatric patients.

One of the most significant findings of our study is the high prevalence of IRP in children with persistent constipation. We have demonstrated that a significant number of children with chronic constipation actually suffer from IRP. This finding underscores the importance of considering IRP as a potential underlying cause when evaluating children with constipation, particularly in cases where conventional treatments have proven ineffective. Our findings align with previous studies that have also reported a high incidence of IRP in children with refractory constipation [2].

Our study also highlights the crucial role of a comprehensive evaluation for children suspected of having IRP. We emphasize the need for a thorough medical history, physical examination, and diagnostic tests such as anorectal manometry and defecography. These investigations play a vital role in identifying and differentiating IRP from other causes of constipation, leading to a more accurate diagnosis and targeted treatment. It is important to note that our approach aligns with several guidelines and reviews on the management of rectal prolapse in children [13].

Furthermore, our study explores various treatment approaches for IRP in children. We discuss the efficacy of non-surgical interventions, including dietary modifications, behavioral changes, and pelvic floor exercises. These conservative measures often provide relief and improve bowel function in children with IRP. However, we also acknowledge that some cases may require surgical intervention, especially in those with severe or refractory symptoms. We describe different surgical techniques for IRP, such as Thiersch wire placement, Delorme's procedure, and laparoscopic rectopexy. Importantly, we report favorable outcomes and low complication rates associated with these procedures.

The implications of our study's findings are significant for both clinicians and pediatric patients. By raising awareness about IRP, we emphasize the need for healthcare providers to consider this condition in the differential diagnosis of constipation in children. Early recognition and appropriate treatment of IRP can help prevent complications such as fecal incontinence and rectal dilation.

Moreover, our study underscores the importance of a multidisciplinary approach to managing IRP in children. Collaboration between pediatric gastroenterologists, colorectal surgeons, and other healthcare professionals is crucial for optimizing patient outcomes. This collaborative effort allows for the selection of the most appropriate treatment strategies tailored to the specific needs of each patient.

While our study provides valuable insights into IRP in children, it is important to acknowledge certain limitations. The retrospective design of our study and the relatively small sample size may restrict the generalizability of our findings. Additionally, obtaining long-term follow-up data on the outcomes of different treatment modalities would enhance our understanding of the efficacy and durability of these interventions.

12. Conclusion

Constipation and resistant stool in internal rectal prolapse disease can be easily diagnosed and treated with medical therapy. Treatment with sclerosing solution injection in grade IV rectal prolapse can save the child from the severe complications of this disease.

Funding

None.

Contributors' statement

Dr. Salahedin Delshad: conceptualized and designed the study, drafted the initial manuscript, and reviewed and revised the manuscript. Designed the data collection instruments, collected data, carried out the initial analyses, and reviewed and revised the manuscript. Coordinated and supervised data collection, and critically reviewed the manuscript for important intellectual content.

Conflict of interest

The authors deny any conflict of interest in any terms or by any means during the study.

Human and animal rights

No animals were used in this research. All human research procedures followed were by the ethical standards of the committee responsible for human experimentation (institutional and national), and with the Helsinki Declaration of 1975, as revised in 2013. This study was approved by the Research Ethics Board of Alborz University of Medical Sciences.

Consent for publication

Informed consent was obtained from each participant.

Availability of data and materials

All relevant data and materials are provided with in manuscript.

Author details

Salahedin Delshad
Maryam Hospital, Karaj, Iran

*Address all correspondence to: dr.salahedindelshad@gmail.com

IntechOpen

© 2023 The Author(s). Licensee IntechOpen. This chapter is distributed under the terms of the Creative Commons Attribution License (http://creativecommons.org/licenses/by/3.0), which permits unrestricted use, distribution, and reproduction in any medium, provided the original work is properly cited.

References

[1] Selection Criteria for Internal Rectal Prolapse repair by Delorme's Transrectal Excision. SpringerLink. Available from: https://link.springer.com/article/10.1007/BF02236355

[2] Cariou de Vergie L, Venara A, Duchalais E, Frampas E, Lehur PA. Internal rectal prolapse: Definition, assessment and management in 2016. Journal of Visceral Surgery. 2017;**154**:21-28. DOI: 10.1016/j.jviscsurg.2016.10.004

[3] The Assessment and Management of Rectal Prolapse, Rectal Intussusception, Rectocoele, and Enterocoele in Adults. The BMJ. Available from: https://www.bmj.com/content/342/bmj.c7099.extract

[4] Salahedin D, Naser P, Zahra M. The most common symptoms of internal rectal prolapse in children referred to Maryam Hospital, Karaj: During 2015 to 2020. AUMJ. 2021;**10**:106-114

[5] Impact of Rising Grades of Internal Rectal Intussusception on Fec...: Ingenta Connect. Available from: https://www.ingentaconnect.com/content/wk/dcr/2016/00000059/00000001/art00014

[6] Laparoscopic Ventral Rectopexy for Internal Rectal Prolapse Using Biological Mesh: Postoperative and Short-Term Functional Results. SpringerLink. Available from: https://link.springer.com/article/10.1007/s11605-011-1793-2

[7] Delshad S, Delshad B, Mogheimi P, Heidari G. Treatment of internal rectal prolapse in children: A cross sectional study. Annals of Medicine and Surgery. 2022;**84**:104886. DOI: 10.1016/j.amsu.2022.104886

[8] Neshatian L, Carrington EV. Rectal intussusception: Medical management and timing of the decision to operate. Seminars in Colon and Rectal Surgery. 2023;**34**:100940. DOI: 10.1016/j.scrs.2022.100940

[9] Rectal Intussusception: Characterization of Symptomatology. SpringerLink. Available from: https://link.springer.com/article/10.1007/s10350-004-0834-2

[10] What are the Symptoms of Internal Rectal Prolapse? - Wijffels - 2013 - Colorectal Disease - Wiley Online Library. Available from: https://onlinelibrary.wiley.com/doi/full/10.1111/j.1463-1318.2012.03183.x?casa_token=o3aTBpJBzrcAAAAA%3AmtcqfuZB2pF_PsmiT9kmTp-b3N3uZBcthiMMTpvZbaFKYZMw6MkCozaWqKGpcmY6-Bq9TJqsVBXaLw

[11] Delshad S, Delshad B, Mogheimi P, Heidari G. Introducing a new grading method for the diagnosis and grading of internal rectal prolapse in children. International Journal of Surgery Open. 1 Dec 2022;**49**:100580

[12] Bloemendaal ALA, Buchs NC, Prapasrivorakul S, Cunningham C, Jones OM, Hompes R, et al. High-grade internal rectal prolapse: Does it explain so-called "idiopathic" faecal incontinence? International Journal of Surgery. 2016;**25**:118-122. DOI: 10.1016/j.ijsu.2015.12.004

[13] Rectal Prolapse in Children: An Update to Causes, Clinical P... : Journal of Pediatric Gastroenterology and Nutrition. Available from: https://journals.lww.com/jpgn/fulltext/2020/02000/rectal_prolapse_in_children__an_update_to_causes,.21.aspx?casa_token=

MOPTQfcHhF4AAAAA:
OITGNMVMPEBmn6rO9SHlIgh
wBq8KXn6r4-GoIJ_VYxItQXad
XKptS7Dd1O9FP0IUuglyIqeTFZpe
MUA1XdoKzAiHrg

Chapter 8

Surgical Treatment of Rectal Prolapse: Preoperative Evaluation and Surgical Options

Tommaso Cipolat Mis, Béatrice Vinson-Bonnet, Antonio d'Alessandro, Valeria Basso and Andrea Pierre Luzzi

Abstract

Rectal prolapse is a debilitating medical condition known to significantly compromise an individual's quality of life. Optimal management typically entails trans-abdominal minimally invasive surgical interventions, particularly when performed with stringent adherence to appropriate indications. Such surgical interventions hold the potential to ameliorate patients' symptoms and enhance their overall quality of life. A prerequisite for the successful execution of these surgical procedures is a comprehensive preoperative assessment, encompassing a thorough analysis of rectal and anal functionality. This essential evaluation serves as a crucial determinant in achieving optimal surgical outcomes. Moreover, due to the frequent concurrence of anterior prolapse with urinary and gynaecologic dysfunctions, a multidisciplinary assessment becomes imperative. A multidisciplinary discussion involving various medical specialties is pivotal in guiding treatment decisions. In conclusion, a meticulous preoperative assessment is paramount in selecting the most suitable surgical approach, thereby facilitating an enhancement in the patient's quality of life.

Keywords: rectal prolapse, rectocele, ventral rectopexy, perineal surgical approach, complication rate

1. Introduction

Rectal prolapse denotes a pathological condition characterised by the complete or partial invagination of the upper rectum [1]. This phenomenon manifests in two distinct forms: internal and external (**Figure 1**), with the latter being discernible upon perianal examination if reduction cannot be achieved. Following a Valsalva manoeuvre, rectal prolapse may either spontaneously resolve or necessitate manual reduction via digital pressure. In select instances, it may prove non-reducible, thereby inducing symptoms such as pain, ulceration, haemorrhaging, incarceration, and gangrene (**Figure 2**). In such cases, rectal prolapse constitutes a formal surgical indication requiring immediate attention [2]. This surgical intervention typically entails resection and the creation of a stoma.

The incidence rate of rectal prolapse is reported as 2.5 cases per 100,000 inhabitants, with a notably higher prevalence among elderly women, demonstrating a gender

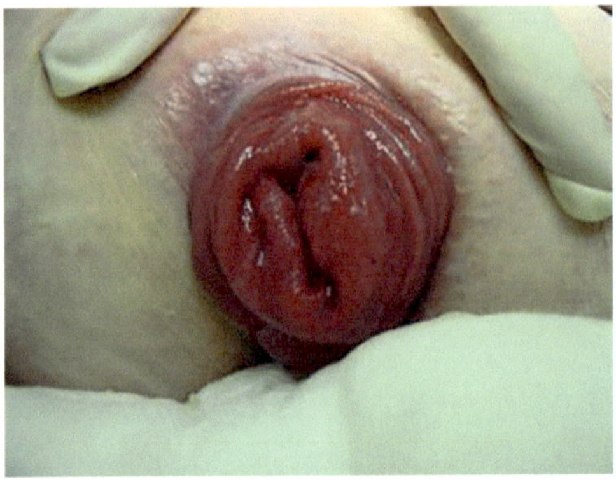

Figure 1.
External rectal prolapse.

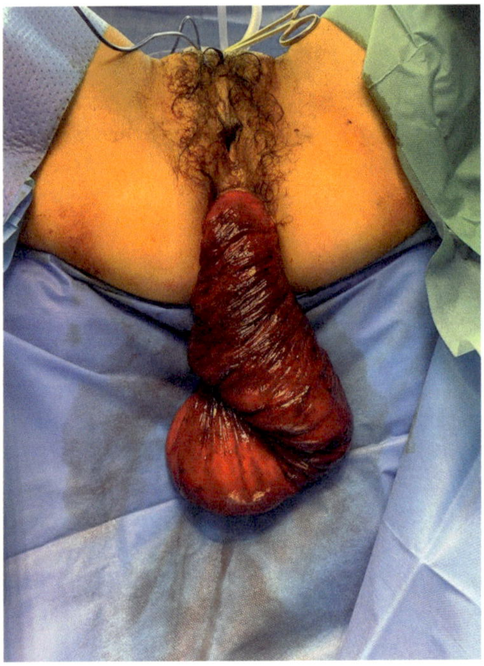

Figure 2.
Complicated large external recto-sigmoid prolapse with mucosal ischemia.

ratio of 9:1 [1, 3]. In a recent work published by El-Dhuwaib et al. [4] including one of the largest databases concerning this pathology including more than 25,000 patients treated between 2001 and 2012, a higher incidence was found that rose to 18.5 cases per 100,000 inhabitants per year. Frequently, this condition is observed in patients with a medical history characterised by chronic constipation, strenuous defecation, pelvic floor dysfunction, or perineal obstetric injuries [1, 2]. Despite ongoing research efforts, the precise pathophysiological mechanisms underpinning rectal prolapse remain inadequately understood [5]. There exists some systemic pathology like the Ehlers-Danlos syndrome and the mucoviscidosis or cystic fibrosis that are found to be risk factors for the development of the rectal prolapse. In a paper published by

Joshi et al. [6] they found an increased quantity of elastic fibres in patients with rectal prolapse compared to the control population.

Another recent paper published by Attaallah et al. [7] demonstrate a possible role of the rectal redundancy in the physiopathology of the rectal prolapse.

Patients with rectal prolapse commonly exhibit various anatomical anomalies, including a rectum with a straight alignment, absence of fascial attachments between the rectum and the sacrum, redundancy of the sigmoid colon, diastasis of the levator ani muscles, abnormal deep Douglas pouch, and a patulous anus [2].

These patients are characterised by a medical history that often includes symptoms such as incontinence and constipation. In cases where external full-thickness prolapse is present, patients may experience passive incontinence, urge incontinence, or soiling as additional symptoms [2].

Constipation is used to describe symptoms that relate to difficulties in defecation; this includes infrequent bowel movements, hard or lumpy stools, excessive staining, a sensation of incomplete evacuation of blockage, and, in some cases, the use of manual manoeuvres to facilitate evacuation. The chronic constipation affects around 10–15% of the population and is one of the prevalent gastroenterological entities. Following the Rome IV criteria, constipation is categorised into four different subtypes [8]:

- Functional constipation
- Irritable bowel syndrome avec constipation
- Opioid-induced constipation
- Functional defecation disorders, including inadequate defecatory propulsion and dyssynergic defecation.

Obstructive defecation syndrome (ODS) is a functional defecation disorder characterised by excessive staining, the sensation of incomplete evacuation, the sensation of anorectal obstruction or blockage, and/or manual assistance to facilitate the evacuation in more than 25% of bowel movements over the last 12 consecutive weeks [9]. From an anatomical perspective, ODS is primarily associated with specific anatomical factors, namely rectocele, internal rectal prolapse, and enterocele.

Rectocele is characterised by the protrusion of the rectum into the vaginal cavity. This occurrence results from damage to the posterior compartment, leading to the weakening of the posterior vaginal wall support [10], or it can involve the herniation of the anterior rectal wall into the posterior vagina [11]. Enterocele, on the other hand, entails the compression of the small intestine against the rectal wall, typically occurring in patients with an abnormal deep Douglas pouch. Enterocele is a type of elitrocele [12], which is defined as a herniation of the Douglas pouch which is interposed between the vagina and the rectum. Based on the content of this deep Douglas pouch, we should talk about:

- Enterocele: the presence of a small bowel in the deep part of the Douglas pouch hernia
- Sigmoidocele: the presence of a sigmoid colon, usually in the case of a dolico-sigmoid

- Epiplooncele: the presence of epiploon in the deepest part of the Douglas cavity

It is worth noting that internal rectal prolapse and rectocele frequently coexist.

Rectocele is diagnosed in more than half of women presenting with pelvic floor disorders [10], although its true incidence and pathogenesis remain subject to controversy [11]. In approximately 80% of cases, rectocele coexists with an internal rectal prolapse, whereas isolated rectocele is found in only 10% of cases [13]. Surgical intervention is recommended when rectocele is symptomatic; however, if a non-symptomatic rectocele is discovered, surgical intervention is not advised. The primary objective of surgical treatment for this type of functional pathological finding is symptom resolution [10].

Some authors have identified significant correlations between pelvic floor disorders and certain factors, including a younger age at first delivery, a higher body mass index, forceps delivery, and a history of previous gynaecologic surgery [2, 10].

On occasion, rectifying the underlying anatomical disorder may not necessarily correspond to an amelioration of symptoms. This observation raises the possibility of a common tendency to underestimate other potential contributing factors in this intricate syndrome [14]. Such factors can exert a significant influence on individuals' quality of life and carry substantial social and economic implications, particularly within the context of an ageing population [15]. It's so important in this type of situation to tailor the preoperative management and the surgical indication based on the individual patient's characteristics.

2. Clinical findings and diagnosis

Patients with rectal prolapse typically present with several common complaints, including the sensation of a protruding mass following defecation or the need to manually reduce this protrusion [1]. Additionally, they may experience mucous discharge during defecation, and in some cases, bleeding can occur due to a solitary ulcer. In elderly patients, incontinence can be reported in up to 88% of cases, while constipation may affect as many as 70% of individuals with rectal prolapse [1].

The preoperative assessment of symptom severity holds paramount importance [3]. It enables a more objective evaluation of the post-operative course and facilitates the assessment of functional outcomes during follow-up. Various scoring systems are available for this purpose, such as the Wexner, FISI, GIQL (general Quality of Life), and Vaizey scores.

Clinical examination, which can be conducted under general anaesthesia and includes both anorectal and vaginal assessments, plays a pivotal role in diagnosing internal rectal prolapse. If it's performed under general anaesthesia, the gynaecological position is preferred, differently the lateral decubitus or four-legged position it's possible with a combined vaginal and rectal evaluation performed in dorsal decubitus. The classification of rectal prolapse is based on the Oxford classification, which comprises five grades (**Table 1**) [16].

Notably, rectocele is a common finding, even in asymptomatic individuals undergoing radiological examinations. It is observed in approximately 80% of women [11] with half of these cases involving rectoceles exceeding 1 cm in size. Larger complex rectoceles, typically measuring more than 3–4 cm [3, 17], are associated with a variety of symptoms, including obstructive defecation syndrome, constipation, rectal pain, and bleeding. Patients often describe the sensation of a vaginal mass during

			Definition	Radiological definition
Internal rectal prolapse (IRP)	Recto-rectal intussusception	Grade I	High recto-rectal prolapse	Descends no lower than proximal limit of rectocele
		Grade II	Low recto-rectal prolapse	Descends into the level of rectocele but not onto anal canal
	Recto-anal intussusception	Grade III	High recto-anal prolapse	Descends onto anal canal
		Grade IV	Low recto-anal prolapse	Descends into anal canal
External rectal prolapse (ERP)		Grade V	External prolapse	Protrude from anus

Table 1.
Oxford classification of the rectal prolapses.

defecation, and manual assistance through vaginal compression of the rectocele is reported in 20–75% of cases.

A multidisciplinary preoperative assessment that includes thorough radiological and instrumental evaluations assumes paramount importance in the management of rectal prolapse. Equally crucial is the multidisciplinary discussion of cases, involving collaboration with gynaecologists, urologists, proctological specialists, and pelvic surgeons [3].

When urological or gynaecological symptoms are present, a focused evaluation becomes imperative, potentially leading to the consideration of combined surgical interventions, particularly in cases involving anterior uro-vaginal prolapse.

The preoperative instrumental evaluation comprises several key components [3, 18, 19]:

- Colonoscopy: this procedure is essential to rule out other potential causes of rectal bleeding, such as polyps or tumours, particularly when a recent and negative endoscopy report is not available.

- Defecography or Dynamic-MRI: defecography stands as the preferred radiological test due to its ability to capture the natural positioning during the examination. However, radiological imaging is unnecessary when dealing with external prolapse. The dynamic-MRI, if performed by an expert radiologist in pelvic floor imaging, is the best imaging for the evaluation of the elitrocele, enterocele, sigmoidocele, epiplooncele, and rectocele. For the internal rectal prolapse, the dynamic defecography, if performed by an expert radiologist, is, in our experience, the best radiological evaluation.

- Manometry: manometric assessment proves valuable in cases of reducible prolapse. It enables a functional evaluation of the sphincters and the identification of any alterations in the coordination between the rectal and sphincter muscles, such as anismus. In cases where anismus is detected, preoperative biofeedback rehabilitation is recommended, with resolution sought before proceeding with surgery [14].

- Transanal Echography: this evaluation is employed to assess the integrity of the anal sphincter if there exists any suspicion of a possible sphincter lesion or an abnormal sphincter hypotonia at the anorectal manometry was found.

- Colic Transit Time: in situations involving severe constipation that could not be referred to as obstructive defecation syndrome, colic transit time assessment is performed to facilitate a differential diagnosis from obstructive defecation syndrome [1] or a combined situation of colic constipation and obstructive defecation syndrome; in the case of presence of colic constipation, a medical treatment is mandatory. A gastroenterological follow-up is usually performed to allow an improvement of the colic constipation. A new patient assessment will be performed to evaluate the persistence of obstructive defecation syndrome caused by a pelvic floor disorder.

- Peripheral neurological disease may necessitate the inclusion of pudendal nerve motor latency testing and other relevant neurophysiological assessments in patient evaluations.

Several absolute contraindications, particularly for the abdominal surgical approach, merit careful consideration [3]:

- Pregnancy: surgical intervention during pregnancy is not advisable.

- Absence of Anatomical Abnormality: in cases where there is no identifiable anatomical abnormality, surgery should be avoided.

- Severe Intrabdominal Adhesions: the presence of extensive intrabdominal adhesions poses a significant contraindication.

- Active Proctitis: surgical intervention is not recommended in the presence of active proctitis.

- Psychological Instability: patients with significant psychological instability, as indicated in the literature [20], may not be suitable candidates for surgery.

For some conditions, there are relative contraindications that warrant consideration, including:

- High-Grade Endometriosis: high-grade endometriosis should be evaluated carefully, and the decision for surgery should be made judiciously.

- Previous Pelvic Radiotherapy: patients with a history of previous pelvic radiotherapy should be assessed individually to determine the appropriateness of surgical intervention.

- Previous Complicated Sigmoid Diverticulitis: a history of complicated sigmoid diverticulitis should also be taken into account when considering surgery.

To resume, in our experience the preoperative patient assessment is based on several key points steps (**Table 2**).

	When
Personal medical history with particular attention to past gynaecological history and pelvic-floor surgical history Evaluation of the patient's medical treatment	Always
Carful clinical examination that includes the abdominal and pelvic examination of the perineal region, the anorectal, and vaginal examination. Rigid anoscope or rectoscopy.	Always The diagnosis of rectal prolapse is fundamentally clinical
Clinical examination under general anaesthesia	If the standard clinical evaluation does not allow a complete evaluation
Colonoscopy	If we do not have a recent endoscopic evaluation or in the presence of newly appeared rectorragia In presence of solitary rectal ulcer
Defecography performed by an expert radiologist	To diagnose internal rectal, prolapse, and rectocele
Dynamic-MRI performed by an expert radiologist	Better in case of elitrocel, sigmoldocel, enterocel, epiplooncel, rectocele, and major rectal prolapse
Manometry	Useful in case of internal prolapse with ODS and/or rectocele at elitroclele
Trans anal echography	If a sphincteric lesion is suspected, in case of incontinence with a past medical history of gynaecological surgery and suspicion of an obstetrical lesion
Colic transit time	If a colic constipation is suspected
Pudendal nerve motor latency	In the case of concomitant neurologic pathology
Discussion of the case in a multidisciplinary setting	Always
Urodynamic evaluation	In case of concomitant urological symptoms

Table 2.
Key steps of the preoperative evaluation.

3. Surgical treatment options

The definitive treatment for rectal prolapse is exclusively surgical. However, the absence of robust results from large prospective randomised controlled trials has led to a lack of international consensus regarding the gold-standard surgical intervention for both internal and external rectal prolapse [12, 13]. Currently, the ventral mesh rectopexy, as described by D'Hoore, is considered a leading approach in the field [9].

Two primary surgical approaches are commonly employed: the abdominal approach and the perineal approach [21]. While the literature documents over a hundred surgical techniques, we will focus our attention on those that are most widely practiced both in everyday surgical procedures and in published literature. In **Table 3** there is a list of the most discussed surgical approaches in international literature. We will focus our attention on the three most performed procedures as you should see later.

Non-operative management is typically reserved for individuals who are not suitable candidates for surgery. This approach relies on interventions such as a high-fibre diet, laxative therapy, enemas, and biofeedback rehabilitation [1, 21].

Abdominal approach	Perineal approach
Ventral mesh rectopexy D'Hoore	Perineal recto-sigmoidectomy – Altemeier technique
Posterior mesh rectopexy	Rectal mucosal sleeve resection – Delorme technique
Orr-Loygue rectopexy	Anal encirclement Thiersch
Resection rectopexy	Perineal suspension fixation – Wyatt
Anterior suture rectopexy	

Table 3.
The most common surgical procedures ordered based on the surgical approach.

The selection of the optimal surgical approach hinges on achieving the best functional outcomes, minimising recurrence rates, and reducing post-operative comorbidities. Regrettably, the existing literature lacks prospective randomised studies capable of conclusively identifying the superior approach [1, 3, 5]. In the randomised studies published within the last decade [3, 5], the perineal approach exhibited a non-significantly higher recurrence rate. Furthermore, in terms of functional results and improvements in quality of life post-surgery, both randomised studies conducted by Senapati et al. [5] and Smedberg et al. [3] failed to detect any significant differences. A prospective trial by Emile et al. [22] showed a non-statistically significant increase in recurrence rates and longer post-operative hospital stays following Delorm's procedure.

In conclusion, no single procedure demonstrates clear superiority in functional outcomes and post-operative morbidity. However, data suggests that the abdominal approach may be more suitable for young, healthy patients with a lower risk of general anaesthesia-related complications. The perineal approach, on the other hand, may be reserved for elderly and more frail patients who can undergo spinal or epidural anaesthesia [1, 21].

The perineal surgical approach principally encompasses two procedures: full-thickness rectal resection with colo-anal anastomosis (Altmeier procedure) and circumferential mucosal resection (Delorm's procedure).

Various abdominal procedures involve rectal mobilisation with rectopexy [1], with or without sigmoid resection [23]. Some authors have proposed rectal mobilisation without pexy, but a multicentre randomised controlled trial by Karkas et al. [24] demonstrated a significantly higher recurrence rate at 5 years after non-rectopexy versus rectopexy (8.65 vs. 1.5%, $p = 0.003$).

A subset of surgeons suggests concomitant sigmoid resection (Frykman-Goldberg procedure) during rectopexy to reduce post-operative constipation compared to preoperative and non-resection rectopexy; this procedure is more commonly performed in the United States clinical practice [1]. In Europe, resection rectopexy is not commonly performed due to an increased risk of colorectal anastomotic fistula and the availability of less risky surgical options with similar outcomes. We do not have experience in resection rectopexy that we decide not to perform considering the higher risk of complications.

Rectal mobilisation can be performed anteriorly or posteriorly. A study by Aitola et al. [25] demonstrated that posterior mobilisation worsens constipation or leads to de novo constipation. Other publications suggest that anterior mobilisation is associated with less constipation [3]. Consequently, posterior rectopexy is considered an obsolete and abandoned technique [1].

The anterior rectopexy, or Ripstein technique, and its subsequent variants were first described in 1959 [1]. The physiological and anatomical objective is to restore the rectum's anatomical position and correct pelvic floor descent [1, 26].

Rectopexy can be executed using non-absorbable sutures or a mesh. However, a meta-analysis by Lobb et al. [26] failed to establish that mesh rectopexy significantly reduces recurrence rates. The lack of robust results in this regard can be attributed to the heterogeneity of the studies included in the analysis.

During rectal mobilisation in rectopexy, the lateral ligaments should either be preserved or divided. The division may lead to denervation and damage to the parasympathetic component of the inferior hypogastric plexus, potentially resulting in a higher rate of post-operative constipation [1].

Regarding abdominal procedures, the minimally invasive laparoscopic approach has gained popularity since the introduction and standardisation of the ventral rectopexy procedure by D'Hoore [27].

In conclusion, the most widely favoured surgical procedure for rectal prolapse treatment is minimally invasive ventral mesh rectopexy [1]. Within the perineal approach, Delorm's and Altmeier's procedures are the most frequently performed [1].

3.1 Altmeier's procedure

The rectosigmoid resection with colo-anal anastomosis, performed via a perineal approach, was initially described by Mikulicz in 1889 [28]. This surgical procedure can be conducted under locoregional anaesthesia, which carries a relatively low surgical risk.

The patient is positioned in a modified lithotomic position with splayed arms. At the time of incision, a broad-spectrum antibiotic regimen (comprising Cefazolin and Metronidazole) is administered, along with a low-dose heparin treatment [3, 29].

A urinary catheter is inserted and left in place for a duration of 48 hours. The use of a Lone-Star divaricator is essential as it allows for optimal exposure of the anal region, facilitating the coloanal manual anastomosis.

The procedure commences with an incision made in the rectal wall, positioned approximately 15 mm above the dentate line in the lower rectum. This incision is full-thickness and extends to the opening of the Douglas space. Subsequently, both the rectum and sigmoid colon are mobilised through this incision. In the posterior aspect, the mesorectum and mesosigmoid are ligated and subsequently sectioned. The peritoneum layer is closed using absorbable sutures, while the posterior muscular plane is sutured using non-absorbable sutures.

The anastomosis is executed via separate full-thickness sutures, typically employing Vicryl 2 or 4/0 sutures. We recommend the placement of four cardinal points, which are carefully tensioned with the assistance of the Lone-Star divaricator, followed by the positioning of additional sutures to ensure the creation of an optimal anastomosis.

Furthermore, the anastomosis should be of a mechanical nature. In such cases, the rectal wall is incised 3 cm above the dentate line to avoid anastomosis directly on the dentate line, as this could potentially lead to chronic pain.

3.2 Delorm's procedure

The Delorme's procedure involves the mucosectomy of the prolapsed rectum, followed by a muscular layer plication and a muco-mucosal anastomosis. Delorme first described this technique [28].

The patient's positioning and perioperative measures are the same as those employed for the Altmaier procedure.

The procedure begins with a circumferential incision made approximately 15 mm above the dentate line. Subsequently, the mucosa is separated from the circular muscular layer, corresponding to the internal sphincter. Typically, this detachment of the mucosa is achieved through electrocoagulation. An instrument is used to grasp the mucosa, and traction is applied with a finger within the prolapsed lumen. Once adequate mucosal dissection is achieved, the muscular layer is repositioned and sutured, typically using separate stitches. The muco-mucosal anastomosis commences with four cardinal stitches and is then completed with additional stitches to ensure a comprehensive anastomosis.

3.3 Ventral mesh rectopexy

The ventral mesh rectopexy is currently the most frequently performed surgical technique for rectal prolapse and was initially described in 2005 by D'Hoore et al. [27]. This minimally invasive surgical approach is widely accepted. The original description of ventral rectopexy, known as the Orr-Loygue technique, involved full rectal mobilisation and suturing of two meshes onto the antero-lateral wall [19]. However, full rectal mobilisation has been largely abandoned due to its negative impact on functional outcomes.

The patient is positioned in a modified lithotomic decubitus with arms placed alongside the body. A urinary catheter is inserted, which can be removed post-surgery.

At the time of incision, a broad-spectrum antibiotic is administered, and a low-dose heparin is given [3].

The laparoscopic column is placed on the left side of the patient, while the second surgeon may be positioned on the right side or the opposite side [28].

A periumbilical optic trocar placement is carried out, and pneumoperitoneum is induced either through an open technique or by inserting a Verres needle at the Palmer point in the left hypochondrium. Three or four operative 5 mm trocars are placed, with specific trocar placement varying based on surgeon preference (**Figure 3**). A 30° scope is recommended, although some authors have used a 0° scope as well [28]. A three trocars procedure is also possible with the suspension of the uterus, but a suboptimal exposure will be achieved with this operative setting.

The sigmoid colon descends into the pelvis and should be secured with an omental flap attached to the left abdominal wall [28]. In non-hysterectomized women, trans-parietal fixation of the uterus is performed to free up the pelvis. A malleable valve of a laparoscopic pence is used to expose the rectovaginal space.

The patient is placed in a Trendelenburg position at 20° or 25°, with a 10° tilt. The rectosigmoid junction is retracted to the left, and an inverted-J incision is made on the right side of the rectum, over the deepest part of the Douglas pouch. Care must be taken to avoid damage to the hypogastric nerve. Dissection proceeds along the anterior rectal wall in the rectovaginal septum, with special attention to avoiding vaginal or rectal injury. No lateral or posterior dissection is performed. The anterior dissection is continued right to the elevator muscular plain; this step is useful to perform an intraoperative rectal or/and vaginal exploration to evaluate the completeness of the dissection. A non-absorbable polypropylene 3 × 17 cm mesh is secured to the anterior wall of the distal rectum with 3 up to 6 separate non-absorbable sutures.

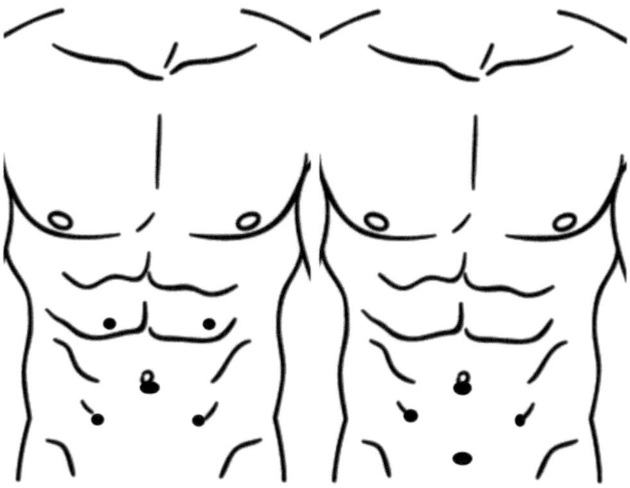

Figure 3.
Trocar placement.

Some authors as Maggiori et al. [9] use a quite bigger mesh 4 × 20 cm. The mesh is also fixed to the sacral promontory using non-absorbable sutures or non-absorbable tacks [30]. Proper suspension of the rectum is crucial to avoid excessive tension and potential functional complications [3]. The posterior vaginal wall is sutured to the anterior aspect of the mesh, allowing for the closure of the rectovaginal septum and correction of vaginal prolapse; this is not a mandatory aspect in our experience and it can be avoided.

Closure of the peritoneal flap is performed using running sutures or separate stitches. This step is essential to prevent adhesions, obstructions, and reduce the risk of recurrence and symptomatic elitrocel [3]. In our experience, we use a 3–0 barbed V-Loc™ reabsorbable suture.

This technique, as reported by D'Hoore et al. [27], achieves a recurrence rate of 5% with a median follow-up of 5 years. The median recurrence rate for anterior mesh rectopexy varies in the literature from 0 to 16% (**Figure 4**) [26].

Studies have evaluated the efficacy of biological mesh versus non-absorbable synthetic mesh. While no randomised trials directly compare the two options, some meta-analyses suggest no significant difference in post-operative complications and recurrence rates [2]. However, biological mesh tends to be more expensive. Conversely, a review conducted in 2008 by the National Institute for Health and Care Excellence (NICE) reported a higher failure rate with biological mesh (23 vs. 9%) compared to synthetic mesh [30]. Relative indications introduced in 2013 by a panel of experts [3] recommend the use of biological mesh in specific situations, such as young adolescents or patients of reproductive age, diabetics, smokers, or those with a history of pelvic irradiation, or in cases of intra-operative injury to the rectum or vagina.

Regarding synthetic mesh, two primary mesh materials have been tested: polyester and polypropylene. Polyester mesh was associated with a significantly higher rate of erosion [31]. Moreover, synthetic mesh erosion rates were 1.87% for polypropylene compared to 0.22% for biological mesh. In our experience, we prefer a polypropene mesh. We do not have experience in this field with biological mesh; considering the

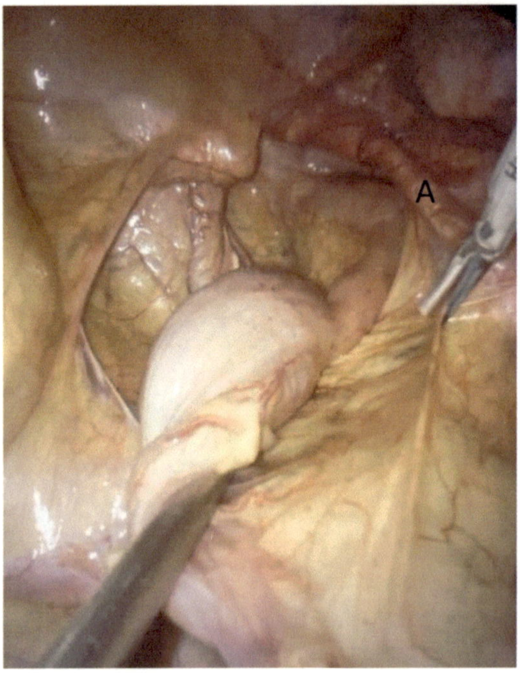

Figure 4.
Case of recurrent internal rectal prolapse with symptomatic rectocele in hysterectomised patient. Beginning of the J incision of the peritoneum at the right side of the rectum. At right side, we can remark the presence of the previous mesh.

experience with this type of mesh in some abdominal wall procedures, we find the manipulation of this mesh in a minimally invasive setting not easy.

In the initial description of the surgical technique, a synthetic suture was used to secure the mesh to the rectum [32]. However, it was found that a polydioxanone sulphate (PDS) 2–0 suture had a 0% erosion rate, whereas a polyester suture (Ethibond) had a 3.7% erosion rate [31]. Some authors have also explored the use of tissue glue (cyanoacrylate or synthetic hydrogel) to secure the mesh to the rectum, showing promising results, but further analysis is required. In our experience, we use a 2–0 PDS suture.

In cases of abdominal adhesions, the same surgical procedure can be performed via laparotomy.

The minimally invasive robotic approach has been evaluated in recent years. A retrospective study by Dumas et al. [33] found a longer operative time but significantly shorter hospital stays, higher patient satisfaction, and lower recurrence rates. Another meta-analysis published in 2021 showed no difference in post-operative outcomes but a shorter hospital stays [34]. Although a longer operative time is often reported, this finding was not confirmed by Flynn et al. [34]. Conversely, a meta-analysis conducted by Albayati et al. [35] comparing the two minimally invasive approaches found no difference in outcomes, but the robotic approach did require a longer operative time.

A technical variation of the ventral rectopexy that we start performing recently is the ventral mesh rectopexy with the retroperitoneal tunnelization of the mesh; this technique allow to avoid the complete lateral opening of the peritoneum with the J incision preserving both lateral and utero-sacral ligaments. Two separate incisions of the peritoneum are performed: the first at the sacral promontory and the second at the Douglas to open the recto-vaginal plain. A laparoscopic instrument is passed in the retroperitoneal space between the two incisions to create a retroperitoneal tunnel to allow the passage of the mesh. In the retrospective analysis performed by Campenni et al. [36], comparing the tunnelization technique with the classic ventral rectopexy, the modified tunnelization technique seems to be safe and faisable.

4. Outcomes and complications

Surgical complications associated with rectal prolapse repair can be categorised into inadequate technique-related issues, procedure-specific complications, and general medical complications that may occur during hospitalisation. Addressing the first two categories, the treatment could require a laparoscopic revision surgery or a conservative treatment. Technical errors identified in revision surgery, as reported by some authors [30], include insufficient evidence of ventral dissection or inadequate fixation of the mesh to the rectum or promontory.

Mesh-related complications can arise, such as mesh erosion into the rectal, vaginal, or bladder walls, particularly in patients who have undergone hysterectomy. This erosion may result in the palpable presence of mesh during rectal or vaginal examinations. The incidence of erosion can reach up to 7% with synthetic mesh but remains at 0% with biological mesh [30].

Another mesh-related complication is rectal stricture [30], which manifests as obstructive defecation syndrome and/or pelvic pain. The study by Badrek-Al Amoudi [30] attributed this complication to inadequate mesh fixation at the mid-sacrum rather than at the promontory.

Chronic pelvic pain is a rare complication that may be linked to pudendal nerve irritation. Establishing the exact cause can be challenging, but it may be associated with chronic inflammation.

Recurrence rates reported in the literature range from 0 to 16% [26], with most recurrences occurring within the first 2–3 years. The duration of follow-up is a key consideration in interpreting these rates. In a study conducted by D'Hoore et al. [27] the recurrence rate was 5% at 5 years, consistent with published literature. Maggiori et al. [9] reported a similar range, with a recurrence rate of 6% and a median follow-up of 42 ± 7 months.

A structured training program to ensure proper technical execution of the surgery is essential. The learning curve, as recognised by the Association of Coloproctology of Great Britain and Ireland, typically comprises around 25–30 procedures [31]. As discussed by Badrek-Al Amoudi [30], the learning curve may influence both functional outcomes and complication rates. However, Trompetto et al. [29] reported a prolapse rate exceeding 40% after 4 years of follow-up following Altmeier's procedure.

In a meta-analysis comparing abdominal ventral rectopexy with the perineal approach (Delorme and Altmaier techniques) published in 2022 by Pellino et al. [37] a higher recurrence rate was observed with the perineal approach, particularly in studies with longer follow-up periods. This difference was statistically significant in non-randomised trials but not in randomised trials. The study also found that the rate of post-operative incontinence was higher with the perineal approach, while the rate of constipation was higher with the abdominal approach.

5. Conclusions

Rectal prolapse presents a complex anatomical condition that frequently leads to debilitating symptoms and a decline in overall quality of life. Internal rectal prolapse is commonly accompanied by the presence of a rectocele. The typical clinical syndrome that leads the patient to a specialistic evaluation can include more frequently an incontinence in case of external prolapse and the obstructive defecation syndrome in case of internal rectal prolapse. When these symptoms are evident, a surgical intervention is the most viable solution. A preoperative tailored evaluation is mandatory to achieve a good post-operative functional outcome; a multidisciplinary discussion of each case is the most appropriate way to achieve the best patient selection. In case of suspicion of anisme, a preoperative well-performed rehabilitation by biofeedback is essential to achieve a favourable functional outcome.

Currently, the most effective technique and the ones that we suggest in terms of recurrence rate and the enhancement of functional aspects and quality of life is ventral mesh rectopexy, a procedure that can be safely carried out through minimally invasive settings by laparoscopic or robotic approach [9]. In case of contraindication for medical or anaesthesiologic reasons or in case of adhesions or any difficult and too risky intrabdominal surgical condition, a perineal procedure can be preferred. In this case, according to our experience, the Altmeier is preferred in case of major external prolapse and a Delorme procedure in case of minor external rectal prolapse but there a no study in literature that demonstrates the superiority of one of two techniques.

Author details

Tommaso Cipolat Mis[1*], Béatrice Vinson-Bonnet[1], Antonio d'Alessandro[1], Valeria Basso[1] and Andrea Pierre Luzzi[2]

1 Service de Chirurgie Digestive, Proctologique et Viscérale, CHI Poissy – Saint Germain-en-Laye, France

2 Beaujon Hospital, Clichy, France – University of Genoa, Genoa, Italy

*Address all correspondence to: tommaso.cipolat@gmail.com

IntechOpen

© 2024 The Author(s). Licensee IntechOpen. This chapter is distributed under the terms of the Creative Commons Attribution License (http://creativecommons.org/licenses/by/3.0), which permits unrestricted use, distribution, and reproduction in any medium, provided the original work is properly cited.

References

[1] Gallo G et al. Consensus statement of the Italian Society of Colorectal Surgery (SICCR): Management and treatment of complete rectal prolapse. Techniques in Coloproctology. 2018;**22**(12):919-927. DOI: 10.1007/s10151-018-1908-9

[2] Faucheron JL, Trilling B, Girard E, Sage PY, Barbois S, Reche F. Anterior rectopexy for full-thickness rectal prolapse: Technical and functional results. World Journal of Gastroenterology. 2015;**21**(16):5051-5053. DOI: 10.3748/wjg.v21.i16.5049

[3] Mercer-Jones MA et al. Consensus on ventral rectopexy: Report of a panel of experts. Colorectal Disease. 2014;**16**(2):1431-1433. DOI: 10.1111/codi.12415

[4] El-Dhuwaib Y, Pandyan A, Knowles CH. Epidemiological trends in surgery for rectal prolapse in England 2001-2012: An adult hospital population-based study. Colorectal Disease. 2020;**22**(10):1359-1366. DOI: 10.1111/codi.15094

[5] Senapati A et al. PROSPER: A randomised comparison of surgical treatments for rectal prolapse. Colorectal Disease. 2013;**15**(7):858, 861, 865-867. DOI: 10.1111/codi.12177

[6] Joshi HM et al. Histological and mechanical differences in the skin of patients with rectal prolapse. International Journal of Colorectal Disease. 2015;**30**(8):1117-1122. DOI: 10.1007/s00384-015-2222-x

[7] Attaallah W, Akmercan A, Feratoglu H. The role of rectal redundancy in the pathophysiology of rectal prolapse: A pilot study. Annals of Surgical Treatment and Research. 2022;**102**(5):289. DOI: 10.4174/astr.2022.102.5.289

[8] Aziz I, Whitehead WE, Palsson OS, Törnblom H, Simrén M. An approach to the diagnosis and management of Rome IV functional disorders of chronic constipation. Expert Review of Gastroenterology & Hepatology. 2020;**14**(1):39-46. DOI: 10.1080/17474124.2020.1708718

[9] Maggiori L, Bretagnol F, Ferron M, Panis Y. Laparoscopic ventral rectopexy: A prospective long-term evaluation of functional results and quality of life. Techniques in Coloproctology. 2013;**17**(4):431-436. DOI: 10.1007/s10151-013-0973-3

[10] Gluck O, Matani D, Rosen A, Barber E, Weiner E, Ginath S. Surgical treatment for rectocele by posterior colporrhaphy compared to stapled transanal rectal resection. Journal of Clinical Medicine. 2023;**12**(2):1-3. DOI: 10.3390/jcm12020678

[11] Zbar AP, Lienemann A, Fritsch H, Beer-Gabel M, Pescatori M. Rectocele: Pathogenesis and surgical management. International Journal of Colorectal Disease. 2003;**18**(5):369-384. DOI: 10.1007/s00384-003-0478-z

[12] Agnès Sénéjoux. Rectocèle, entérocèle et élytrocèle : diagnostic et prise en charge. POST'U. 2023:300-302

[13] Van Iersel JJ, Paulides TJC, Verheijen PM, Lumley JW, Broeders IAMJ, Consten ECJ. Current status of laparoscopic and robotic ventral mesh rectopexy for external and internal rectal prolapsed. World Journal of Gastroenterology. 2016;**22**(21):4978-4984. DOI: 10.3748/wjg.v22.i21.4977

[14] Picciariello A et al. Obstructed defaecation syndrome: European consensus guidelines on the surgical management. British Journal of Surgery. 2021;**108**(10):1150-1152. DOI: 10.1093/bjs/znab123

[15] Formisano G et al. Update on robotic rectal prolapse treatment. Journal of Personalized Medicine. 2021;**11**(8):706. DOI: 10.3390/jpm11080706

[16] Tsunoda A, Takahashi T, Yagi Y, Kusanagi H. Rectal intussusception and external rectal prolapse are common at proctography in patients with mucus discharge. Journal of the Anus, Rectum and Colon. 2018;**2**(4):139-144. DOI: 10.23922/jarc.2018-003

[17] Wong MTC, Abet E, Rigaud J, Frampas E, Lehur PA, Meurette G. Minimally invasive ventral mesh rectopexy for complex rectocoele: Impact on anorectal and sexual function. Colorectal Disease. 2011;**13**(10):e320-e326. DOI: 10.1111/j.1463-1318.2011.02688.x

[18] Fu CWP, Stevenson ARL. Risk factors for recurrence after laparoscopic ventral rectopexy. Diseases of the Colon and Rectum. 2017:179. DOI: 10.1097/DCR.0000000000000710

[19] Smedberg J, Graf W, Pekkari K, Hjern F. Comparison of four surgical approaches for rectal prolapse: Multicentre randomized clinical trial. BJS Open. 2022;**6**(1):1-3, 10-11. DOI: 10.1093/bjsopen/zrab140

[20] Marceau C, Parc Y, Debroux E, Tiret E, Parc R. Complete rectal prolapse in young patients: Psychiatric disease a risk factor of poor outcome. Colorectal Disease. 2005;**7**(4):360-365. DOI: 10.1111/j.1463-1318.2005.00762.x

[21] Formijne Jonkers HA et al. Evaluation and surgical treatment of rectal prolapse: An international survey. Colorectal Disease. 2013;**15**(1):115, 118-119. DOI: 10.1111/j.1463-1318.2012.03135.x

[22] Emile SH et al. Laparoscopic ventral mesh rectopexy vs Delorme's operation in management of complete rectal prolapse: A prospective randomized study. Colorectal Disease. 2017;**19**(1):50-53. DOI: 10.1111/codi.13399

[23] Tou S, Brown SR, Nelson RL. Surgery for complete (full-thickness) rectal prolapse in adults. Cochrane Database of Systematic Reviews. 2015;**2015**(11):5. DOI: 10.1002/14651858.CD001758.pub3

[24] Karas JR et al. No Rectopexy versus Rectopexy following rectal mobilization for full-thickness rectal prolapse: A randomized controlled trial. Diseases of the Colon and Rectum. 2011;**54**(1):29-34. DOI: 10.1007/DCR.0b013e3181fb3de3

[25] Aitola PT, Hiltunen K-M, Matikainen MJ. Functional results of operative treatment of rectal prolapse over an 11-year period. Diseases of the Colon and Rectum. 1999;**42**(5):655-660. DOI: 10.1007/BF02234145

[26] Lobb HS, Kearsey CC, Ahmed S, Rajaganeshan R. Suture rectopexy versus ventral mesh rectopexy for complete full-thickness rectal prolapse and intussusception: Systematic review and meta-analysis. BJS Open. 2021;**5**(1):1-3. DOI: 10.1093/bjsopen/zraa037

[27] D'Hoore A, Cadoni R, Penninckx F. Long-term outcome of laparoscopic ventral rectopexy for total rectal prolapse. British Journal of Surgery. 2004;**91**(11):1500-1505. DOI: 10.1002/bjs.4779

[28] Lechaux D, Lechaux J-P. Trattamento chirurgico del prolasso rettale completo dell'adulto. EMC – Tecniche Chirurgiche

Addominale. 2014;**20**(3):1-16. DOI: 10.1016/S1283-0798(14)68235-8

[29] Trompetto M, Tutino R, Realis Luc A, Novelli E, Gallo G, Clerico G. Altemeier's procedure for complete rectal prolapse; outcome and function in 43 consecutive female patients. BMC Surgery. 2019;**19**(1):1. DOI: 10.1186/s12893-018-0463-7

[30] Badrek-Al Amoudi AH, Greenslade GL, Dixon AR. How to deal with complications after laparoscopic ventral mesh rectopexy: Lessons learnt from a tertiary referral Centre. Colorectal Disease. 2013;**15**(6):707-712. DOI: 10.1111/codi.12164

[31] Mercer-Jones MA, Brown SR, Knowles CH, Williams AB. Position statement by the pelvic floor society on behalf of the Association of Coloproctology of Great Britain and Ireland on the use of mesh in ventral mesh rectopexy. Colorectal Disease. 2020;**22**(10):1429-1435. DOI: 10.1111/codi.13893

[32] Collinson R, Wijffels N, Cunningham C, Lindsey I. Laparoscopic ventral rectopexy for internal rectal prolapse: Short-term functional results. Colorectal Disease. 2010;**12**(2):97-104. DOI: 10.1111/j.1463-1318.2009.02049.x

[33] Dumas C et al. Is robotic ventral mesh rectopexy for pelvic floor disorders better than laparoscopic approach at the beginning of the experience? A retrospective single-center study. International Journal of Colorectal Disease. 2023;**38**(1):216. DOI: 10.1007/s00384-023-04511-9

[34] Flynn J, Larach JT, Kong JCH, Warrier SK, Heriot A. Robotic versus laparoscopic ventral mesh rectopexy: A systematic review and meta-analysis. International Journal of Colorectal Disease. 2021;**36**(8):1621-1631. DOI: 10.1007/s00384-021-03904-y

[35] Albayati S, Chen P, Morgan MJ, Toh JWT. Robotic vs. laparoscopic ventral mesh rectopexy for external rectal prolapse and rectal intussusception: A systematic review. Techniques in Coloproctology. 2019;**23**(6):529-535. DOI: 10.1007/s10151-019-02014-w

[36] Campennì P, Marra AA, De Simone V, Litta F, Parello A, Ratto C. Tunneling of mesh during ventral rectopexy: Technical aspects and long-term functional results. Journal of Clinical Medicine. 2023;**12**:294. DOI: 10.3390/jcm12010294

[37] Pellino G et al. Abdominal versus perineal approach for external rectal prolapse: Systematic review with meta-analysis. BJS Open. 2022;**6**(2):1-3, 5, 7. DOI: 10.1093/bjsopen/zrac018

Section 4

Rectal Disorders

Chapter 9

Haemorrhoids: Aetiology to Management

Ajit Naniksingh Kukreja

Abstract

The definition of "haemorrhoids" and the epidemiology of these conditions have long been contentious. Unfortunately, we still do not understand the full scope of this phenomenon despite years of studies, discussions, and pathogenetic theories. The ancient Greek words "haema," which means blood, and "rhoos," which means flow, are where the name "haemorrhoid" is derived from. The word "piles," which is derived from the Latin word "pila," which means anal swelling (round mass), is another term for haemorrhoids. Since the birth of English physician John of Arderne (1307 AD), when haemorrhoids were typically referred to as piles, the term "piles" has become widely used. Haemorrhoids are still used to refer to piles with mass rather than haemorrhagic (bleeding) piles. One of the most common disorders affecting adults in industrialized nations is haemorrhoids. According to published statistics, 60–70% of those over the age of 40 experience haemorrhoid symptoms. In the hierarchy of coloproctological illnesses, haemorrhoids make up roughly 40%. Coloproctologists have already firmly incorporated minimally invasive treatments for haemorrhoids into their routine care in recent years. These treatments have a variety of benefits over surgical approaches, including the capacity to be used as outpatient procedures without causing any impairment, high efficacy in the early stages of the disease, and few complications. Internal and external haemorrhoids are two different types of haemorrhoids. Haemorrhoids may be caused by a low-fibre diet, constipation, prolonged pushing, pregnancy, and obesity. The diagnosis of haemorrhoids must be made after a thorough review of the patient's medical history, physical examination, and further evaluation. The treatment for haemorrhoids, which includes both medication and surgical options, is dependent on how severe the condition is. In this chapter, we attempt to cover everything from aetiology to the management of haemorrhoids.

Keywords: haemorrhoids, IRC, DGHAL-RAR, Milligan-Morgan, MIPH, laser hemorrhoidoplasty

1. Introduction

Since the dawn of time and ever since humans learned to walk, haemorrhoids have plagued mankind, and we have yet to discover a permanent cure [1]. It was the same as what we see today and had been haunting humanity for millennia, but it was unclearly comprehended, and names were probably hard to decipher. Even though most illnesses experienced by our ancestors are not explicitly stated in the literature, haemorrhoids and anorectal problems are one set of illnesses that are referenced in the earliest literature. Convincing references can be discovered in both Buddhist and Old Testament literature. Some known mentions of this condition include the existence of physicians attending to haemorrhoids in Egyptian palaces as early as 2500 BC; the treatment records are found in the Edwin Smith and Ebbers Papyri (both 1700 and 1500 BC), as well as in records from India, China, Greece, and Rome [2].

2. Epidemiology

Numerous epidemiological studies over the years have shown how environmental factors might affect the development of haemorrhoidal illness [3].

The prevalence of haemorrhoids varies according to sociocultural factors. For instance, haemorrhoids are extremely uncommon in native Africans, but they are more common in Africans or African Americans exposed to Westernized dietary practices. Both sexes and people of all ages can develop haemorrhoids.

More than a million Americans, or 4.4% of the population, are estimated to experience haemorrhoids yearly in the United States. In addition, haemorrhoids have been reported to cause symptoms in 50% of people over 50.

Race-related differences also exist, with Caucasians being more prevalent. It is challenging to determine the precise prevalence of haemorrhoids because there are far more cases of people who self-diagnose than those with a medical diagnosis.

Just a few years before Burkitt's theory, Hyams and Philpot were among the pioneers of the contemporary era to investigate the occurrence of haemorrhoids [4]. Age, sex, socioeconomic level, race, religion, bowel habits, and pregnancy were used to categorize the patients. The most significant finding was that haemorrhoidal illness affected one in four people over 30 years of age.

Women may undoubtedly experience haemorrhoids during or after pregnancy, childbirth, or menstruation. Although haemorrhoid tissues include oestrogen receptors, physical rather than hormonal variables, such as increased pelvic pressure, have a bigger impact on the development of haemorrhoids.

The influence of family history is significant, but there is insufficient evidence to conclusively link haemorrhoids to genetics, similar food patterns, or similar lifestyle choices.

Patients presenting with haemorrhoidal disease are more frequently white, from higher socioeconomic status, and in urban areas.

There is no known sex predilection, although men are more likely to seek treatment.

However, pregnancy causes physiologic changes that predispose women to develop symptomatic haemorrhoids. As the gravid uterus expands, it compresses the inferior vena cava, causing decreased venous return and distal engorgement.

External haemorrhoids occur more commonly in young and middle-aged adults than in older adults.

The prevalence of haemorrhoids increases with age, with a peak in persons aged 45–65 years.

3. Anatomy, pathophysiology

The most common anorectal illness is a haemorrhoidal disease (HD) [3, 5–9], which is characterized by the symptomatic enlargement and/or distal displacement of the typical anal cushions known as haemorrhoids. Haemorrhoids are normal vascular cushions underlying the distal rectal mucosa and they contribute approximately 15–20% of the resting anal pressure and ensure complete closure of the anal canal. External haemorrhoids develop from the external haemorrhoidal plexus, whereas internal haemorrhoids develop from the internal haemorrhoidal plexus. The dentate line is the anatomical line that separates the internal haemorrhoidal plexus from the exterior haemorrhoidal plexus. Three soft engorgements known as anal cushions or "haemorrhoids" make up the normal internal haemorrhoidal plexus. Therefore, if the phrase "internal haemorrhoids" is taken in its precise literal definition, it does not denote a disease state. However, in clinical practice, the term "internal haemorrhoids" is only used to refer to the illness brought on by the abnormal enlargement of anal cushions, or, more specifically, by their metamorphosis into anal nodules. This term is more specifically limited to haemorrhoidal symptoms, i.e., anal cushions are called "haemorrhoids" when they bleed and/or prolapse.

The surgical procedure and haemorrhoid therapies are equally as crucial as having a thorough understanding of pathophysiology. Varicose vein theory, vascular hyperplasia theory, anal lining (cushion) sliding theory, and hyperactivity of the internal sphincter hypothesis are the top established hypotheses up until recently. Although the cushion tissue of haemorrhoids should technically be referred to as "pathologic haemorrhoids" because it is normal tissue, for the sake of simplicity, this chapter will simply refer to them as haemorrhoids.

Thomson [10] compared the varicose vein theory, the vascular hyperplasia theory, and the sliding anal lining theory, the three primary hypotheses for the cause of haemorrhoids, and concluded that the sliding anal lining theory was accurate.

4. Anal cushion

4.1 Vascular part

In the typical surgical anal canal, three primary anal cushions are primarily identifiable. Anal cushions contain a significant component of non-vascular tissue despite being tissues that are mostly of vascular origin. Arterioles, venules, and their functional anastomoses (arteriolar-venular anastomoses) make up the internal haemorrhoidal plexus. The surgical anal canal's scarlet colour is a result of the presence of veins inside cushions.

The superior (SRA) and middle (MRA) rectal arteries supply blood to the internal haemorrhoidal plexus. Most frequently, a plexus of these arteries develops behind the rectum. This plexus, which is entirely different from the internal haemorrhoidal plexus, typically offers three main terminal branches that penetrate the rectal wall and ultimately terminate submucosally in the anus above the dentate line in three different locations: the left lateral, the right anterior, and the right posterior positions.

The predominant venous branches of the internal haemorrhoid cushions are commonly the superior (SRV) and medium (MRV) rectal veins. While the MRV and the inferior rectal veins are tributaries of the systemic circulation, the SRV drains blood to the inferior mesenteric vein, which is a part of the portal venous circulation [11]. As a result, both portal and systemic circulations drain blood from anal cushions.

Blood flows straight from arterioles to venules inside cushions via numerous arteriolar-venular anastomoses. Since most arteriolar-venular anastomoses lack a muscle wall, they are classified as sinusoids. In an idealized three-way intersection, sinusoidal haemorrhoidal tissue receives arterial blood from the SRA and MRA, oxygenates the cushion's non-vascular region, and then emits venous blood to the SRV and MRV's minuscule root venules. The sinusoids are thus filled with a mixture of blood from the arterial, systemic, and portal venous circulations [11].

The development of sinusoidal plexus occurs nearly exclusively in specific locations of the upper anus because of the preferred artery supply to those regions. The anal cushions are situated where the submucosal tissue's left lateral (3 o'clock), right anterior (11 o'clock), and right posterior (7 o'clock) terminal major artery branches are located (**Figure 1**) (when looked at with the patient in the lithotomy position, i.e. anterior is 12 o'clock).

4.2 Non-vascular part

Transitional epithelium, elastic, and collagenous connective tissue, and Treitz muscle make up the cushion's non-vascular portion. Treitz's muscle is thought to be one of the most significant pathogenetic elements in the development of haemorrhoids since it tightly holds the cushions in their natural position. The anal submucosal muscle, whose fibres subside submucosally between the sinusoids, fixes the cushions to the "floor" of the haemorrhoids (i.e., to the internal anal sphincter), while the mucosal suspensory ligament (Park's ligament), which penetrates the internal sphincter, fixes the sinusoids to the conjoined longitudinal muscle.

Despite not being anatomically a part of the anal cushion, the conjoined longitudinal muscle is just as crucial to preventing haemorrhoidal illness as Treitz's muscle. It appears to work like a backbone that holds the internal and external sphincters in place and secures the anorectum to the pelvis.

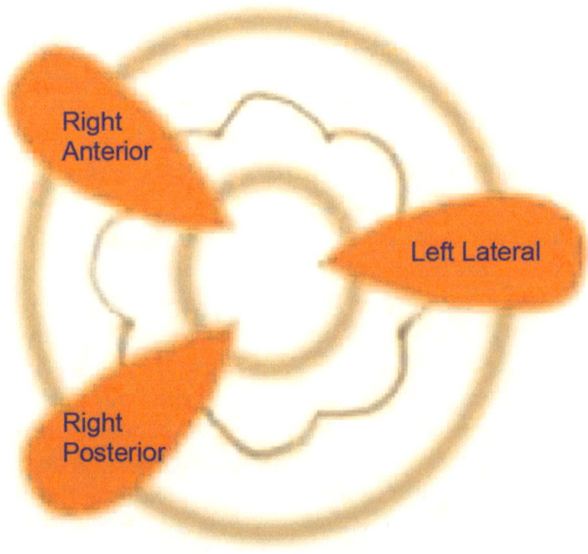

Figure 1.
Position of normal anal cushions.

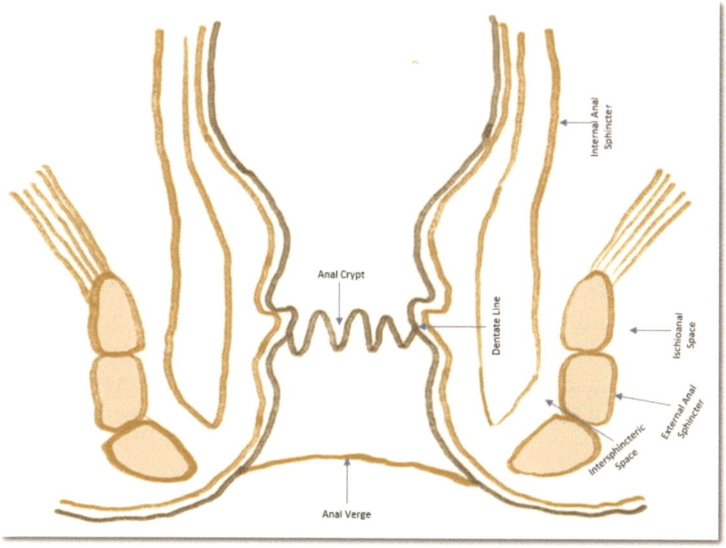

Figure 2.
Anatomy of the Anal canal.

Four anatomical safety elements guarantee the firm anchoring of normal anal cushions above the dentate line, the maintenance of their regular size, and the avoidance of their prolapse:

1. the integrity of the accompanying connective tissue, which supports the sinusoids and holds them to the internal sphincter.

2. the Treitz's muscle and the conjoined longitudinal muscle in their whole anatomically.

3. the structure resembling a sphincter that is seen in the terminal arterioles; and

4. the terminal branches of the supplying arteries are small in diameter.

The reduction in anal cushion size is caused by two additional mechanisms: During defecation, the internal anal sphincter and haemorrhoids work together. The decreasing pressure of the relaxed internal anal sphincter allows blood to flow from the anal cushions to the SRV and MRV, thereby reducing the size of the anal cushions; the submucosal ligament of Treitz's muscle contracts the anal cushions while the descending stool directly widens the anal canal. Simultaneously, the anal cushions descend, forming anal lips that shield the internal anal sphincter beneath. After faeces, the anal cushions rise to their normal posture, rapidly filling with blood until they are full; thus, faecal soiling is avoided (**Figure 2**).

5. The theory of varicose veins

From the time of Hippocrates and Galen until recently, the varicose vein theory was thought to be the most significant among the pathophysiology of haemorrhoids since distended vessels were frequently seen in cases of anal tissue or excised haemorrhoidal tissues during surgery. Haemorrhoidal procedures with extensive excision that are based on this hypothesis are being performed, even though it is no longer widely acknowledged. Through resected samples of haemorrhoids, John Hunter et al. were able to see prolonged veins, and they surmised that these veins were pathologic outcomes that are uncommon in healthy individuals.

Although the precise pathophysiology of haemorrhoids is still unknown, it is generally accepted that unusually clogged and descending anal cushions are the primary cause of haemorrhoids [12]. It was believed that several types of anorectal varices included haemorrhoids. However, there is solid proof that anorectal varices and haemorrhoids are two different conditions. Patients with varices and portal hypertension do not experience more haemorrhoids than healthy people do. Due to the multifactorial nature of haemorrhoids, several risk factors, including pregnancy, ageing, constipation, chronic diarrhoea, and internal rectal prolapse, have been linked to their development.

5.1 The theory of sliding anal cushions

According to Thomson [10], the concept of sliding anal cushions or sliding anal canal lining is now widely acknowledged. It suggests that haemorrhoids form when the anal cushion's supporting tissues break down or degenerate.

This hypothesis was first proposed by Thomson [10], and it has since been expanded upon by Gass, Adams, Hughes, Patey, and Parks. They also believed that haemorrhoids could form from the deterioration of loose and coarse connective tissue.

Elastic fibre, collagen, and subepithelial smooth muscle (also known as the mucosal suspensory ligament or Treitz's muscle) are the basic components of supporting tissue.

The anal cushions' elasticity is provided by elastic fibres, and their tensile strength is a result of collagen and smooth muscle.

Anal cushions move downhill due to the tearing of muscle fibres and connective tissue within them because of the shearing force of faecal material, especially hard and bulky stools.

Anal cushions positioned improperly may interfere with venous drainage, causing haemorrhoidal plexus venodilatation.

The cushions are more likely to be forced out of the canal and have their venous return further impeded by increased intraabdominal pressure and strain.

A higher expression of enzymes related to the deterioration of supporting tissues was seen in haemorrhoid specimens, in addition to the direct harm caused by stool passing through anal cushions.

The protrusion of anal cushions and the development of haemorrhoids may be partially caused by anomalies in the composition and metabolism of collagen. Researchers have looked at the kind and quantity of collagen fibres in haemorrhoid sufferers.

5.2 The theory of vascular abnormality

Based on the histologic findings of marked venodilatation in haemorrhoid specimens and the bleeding symptoms of prolapsing and "non-prolapsing" haemorrhoids, vascular abnormality, and the dysregulation of blood supply to, from, and within anal cushions may be linked to the development of haemorrhoids. The anorectal blood flow is regulated by several mechanisms. Some processes, such as intrinsic vascular tone and endothelial factors, come from within blood vessels, while others, like cytokines and hormones, come from the surrounding tissue. Dysregulation of vascular tone is brought on by an imbalance between vasoconstrictor and vasodilator chemicals.

Haemorrhoids showed a rise in powerful vasodilatory chemicals including nitric oxide. Haemorrhoid tissue exhibited an upregulation of inducible nitric oxide synthase.

When compared to healthy controls, patients with haemorrhoids had significantly greater peak velocities and acceleration velocities of afferent arteries, according to a trans perineal colour Doppler ultrasound examination of the anorectal vascular plexus as demonstrated by Aigner. Patients with haemorrhoids also had significantly increased arterial blood flow. Patients with haemorrhoids had terminal branches of the superior rectal artery that supplied the anal cushion that was noticeably larger than those in healthy individuals. The severity of haemorrhoids was oddly well linked with an increase in artery calibre and flow.

5.3 The theory of rectal redundancy

Haemorrhoids may have a pathogenesis that extends beyond the anal cushions. Many medical professionals say internal rectal prolapse or rectal redundancy is linked to circumferential prolapsing haemorrhoids. The correct anchoring of supporting tissue within anal cushions to the rectal wall may be hampered by rectal redundancy. Straining and frequent stool passing, which result in clogged and prolapsed haemorrhoids, are two signs of blocked defecation that are frequently caused by high-graded internal rectal prolapse. Using a trans anal circular stapler, the stapled haemorrhoidopexy or procedure for prolapse and haemorrhoids (PPH) repositions prolapsing haemorrhoids back up into the anal canal by removing a ring of redundant anorectal mucosa just above the haemorrhoids. The blood flow to haemorrhoid tissue is also decreased with stapled haemorrhoidopexy, leading to the shrinkage of haemorrhoids.

5.4 The theory of increased pressure on the anorectal vascular plexus

According to Palit et al., defecation requires the integration and coordination of the sensorimotor functions of the colon, rectum, anal canal, pelvic floor muscle, and its associated nerve supply. In real life, a reflex expulsion will happen if intrarectal pressure is over 50 mmHg, such as when faeces are present in the rectal ampule. The voluntary contraction of the abdominal muscles and the adoption of the squatting position have an impact on the efficacy of defecation as well. Both movements raise the intraabdominal pressure, which then raises the intrarectal pressure. According to Morio et al., people with functional constipation or blocked defecation condition have noticeably high intrarectal pressure. Anal cushion venous engorgement & haemorrhoids are caused by abnormally high intraabdominal and intrarectal pressures that interfere with the venous drainage of the anorectal vascular plexus. Haemorrhoids are thought to be caused by several conditions that raise intraabdominal pressure, or they may aggravate acute haemorrhoid symptoms. Pregnancy, persistent cough, abdominal obesity, constipation, straining, vigorous activity, and weightlifting are some of these conditions.

6. The causes of haemorrhoids

- Low-fibre diet and constipation.
- Prolonged Straining with defecation.
- Diarrhoea.
- Hereditary predisposition.
- Pregnancy.
- Occupation.
- Sports.
- Leisure activities.
- Psychological disorders.
- Spinal Paralysis.

6.1 Classification of haemorrhoids

A disease classification system helps compare the numerous treatment choices that are available as well as select the best course of action for a certain class. Haemorrhoids are often classified according to where they are located and how much prolapsed they are. However, none of the classification systems for haemorrhoids is complete enough to provide a detailed clinicopathological description of haemorrhoids in a specific patient.

1. Goligher's classification of haemorrhoids is the one that is most frequently used. Internal haemorrhoids are further rated according to the degree of prolapse in Goligher's classification.

    - Grade I: haemorrhoids do not prolapse even though they bleed.
    - Grade II: haemorrhoids prolapse when the patient strains, but they reduce spontaneously.
    - Grade III: haemorrhoids prolapse but need to be repositioned manually; and
    - Grade IV: haemorrhoids prolapse and are not reducible (**Figure 3**).

    Drawbacks of Goligher's classification: the inadequacy of not considering the related symptoms and extension (dynamic evolution) of this classification to the complete haemorrhoidal system (internal and external), to get around the basic differentiation between internal and external haemorrhoids.

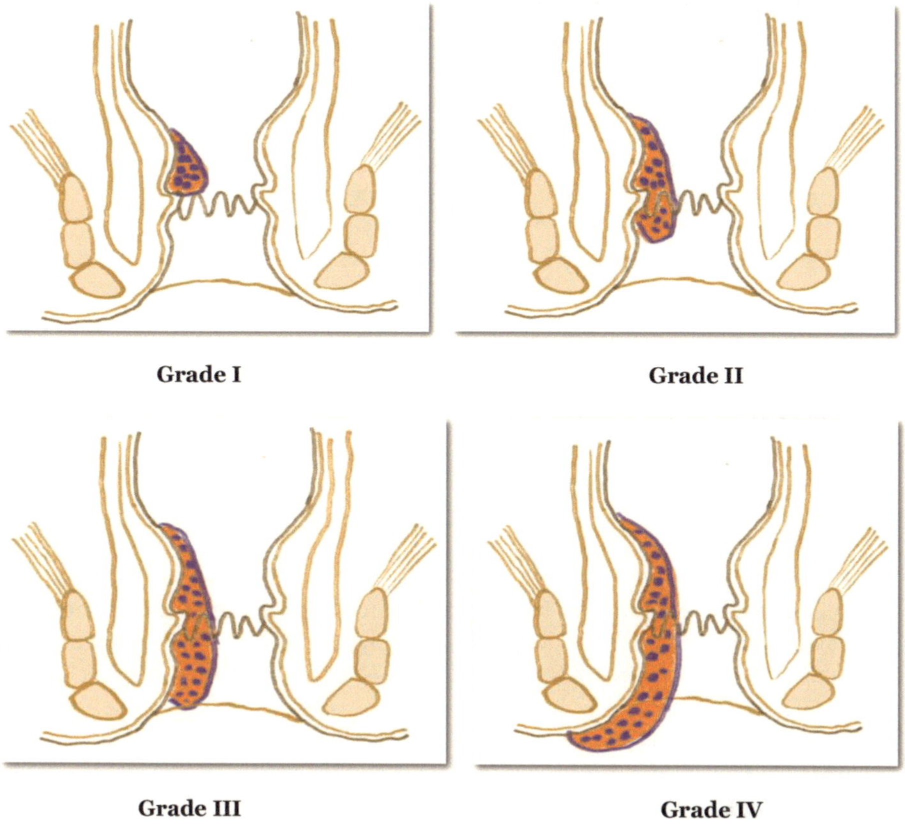

Figure 3.
Grades of Haemorrhoids.

- Basic irreducible haemorrhoids and acutely thrombosed, incarcerated internal haemorrhoids are both classified as fourth-degree haemorrhoids.
- This classification does not specify:
    - the number of haemorrhoidal columns involved,
    - the size of the haemorrhoids, or
    - whether they are circumferential or isolated.

2. Depending on the relation to the dentate line,
    - Internal – the internal haemorrhoids are covered by mucosa (columnar or cuboidal epithelium) and originate above the dentate line.
    - External – the external haemorrhoids arise below the dentate line and are covered by anoderm (squamous epithelium).

- Mixed – Mixed (interno-external) haemorrhoids arise both above and below the dentate line.

3. Based on the anatomical locations of haemorrhoids,

    - Primary – Primary haemorrhoids occur at the three primary positions of the anal cushions, which have been classically described,

    - Secondary – Secondary haemorrhoids arise in between the primary anal cushions, and

    - Circumferential.

4. Based on symptoms,

    - Prolapsing, and (**Figure 4**)

    - Non-prolapsing.

5. Depending on the number of haemorrhoids and the presence of circumferential haemorrhoids or thrombosis, each primary Goligher grade (I to IV) of haemorrhoids is further categorized by using the suffixes (a to d), as mentioned below [13].

    a. Single pile mass

    b. Two piles but with <50% circumference

    c. Circumferential piles occupying >50% circumference of the anal canal.

    d. Thrombosed or gangrenous piles (complicated)

6.2 Symptoms

- Bleeding – Fresh red blood during or after defecation, the level of haemoglobin may fall with long-term bleeding, dark red blood along with stool points to colonic disease, and tar-like dark-coloured blood suggests bleeding from the upper GI Tract.

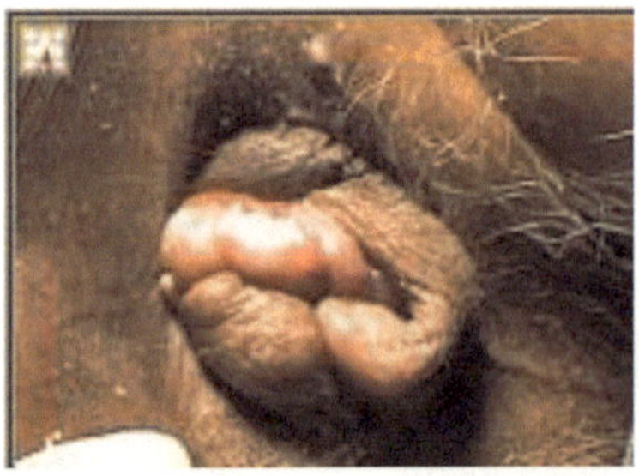

Figure 4.
Prolapsing Grade IV haemorrhoids.

- Prolapse – Apart from bleeding, prolapse is the second most important symptom of haemorrhoids. Goligher classification is based on the degree of prolapse. Patients with third-or fourth-degree haemorrhoids frequently complain of something coming out of their anus, as well as inflamed tissue in the perianal region.

- Pain – Internal haemorrhoids are not painful except for the ones that have been forcibly reduced or are incarcerated. Anal conditions such as thrombosed external haemorrhoids or anal fissures, which are distal to the dentate line of the anal canal, usually cause pain.

- Itching – Itching around the anus is a common complaint among patients with internal haemorrhoids. Mucosal prolapse causes an increase in perianal discharge, which irritates the perianal skin and causes itching. Pruritus ani may also be brought on by mycosis, allergic dermatitis, contact dermatitis, psoriasis, benign tumours, malignancies, oxyuriasis, and diabetes, among other conditions.

- Discharge – Typically, the mucosa proximal to the dentate line is where the mucoid secretion occurs. Prolapsed haemorrhoids may also cause mucoid discharge. Apart from prolapsed haemorrhoids, mucoid discharge is a symptom of several illnesses, including rectal polyps, anal fistulas, ulcerative colitis, Crohn's disease, and irritable bowel syndrome.

- Soiling – Some individuals with third and fourth-degree haemorrhoids have soil in the form of mucus discharge due to an impairment of the fine regulation of continence.

6.3 Differential diagnosis

Because most patients who complain of haemorrhoids have a variety of anorectal symptoms, it is crucial to rule out alternative causes of haemorrhoid symptomatology.

All aspects of the differential diagnosis are based on the patient's symptoms.

The causes of discomfort, such as fissures, abscesses, fistulas, external haemorrhoid thrombosis, or prolapsed thrombosed internal haemorrhoids, are nearly often detected in pathologies distal to the dentate line when anal pain is the patient's primary complaint.

6.4 Acute pain

- Anorectal abscess

- Acute anal fissure

- Anorectal fistula

- Impaction

- Rectal trauma

- Thrombosed haemorrhoid.

6.5 Chronic pain

- Anorectal abscess
- Anal fissure
- Anorectal fistula
- Anal stenosis
- Crohn's disease affecting the anal canal
- Thrombosed haemorrhoid.

6.6 Bleeding per rectum

- Fissure in ano
- Inflammatory bowel disease
- Malignancy
- Polyps
- Proctitis
- Ruptured thrombosed haemorrhoids
- Pruritus Ani
- Anogenital warts (condyloma acuminata)
- Anal incontinence
- Eczema
- Fistula
- Fungal infection
- Infections (sexually transmitted diseases — STDs)
- Rectal prolapse

6.7 Swelling or lump

- Abscess
- Anal tumour
- Rectal tumour

- Rectal polyp
- Rectal prolapse
- Thrombosed haemorrhoids.

6.8 Haemorrhoids, portal hypertension and rectal varices

Anorectal varices must be distinguished from bleeding haemorrhoids since they require very distinct treatments. Magnetic resonance imaging and endoscopic ultrasonography are non-invasive techniques for diagnostic and post-treatment control.

The trans anal suture technique, transhepatic inferior mesenteric venography and embolization, or any of the portal-systemic shunting and decompression techniques can all be used to treat bleeding from varices.

6.9 Examination, workup, and diagnosis

Patients with haemorrhoid complaints should undergo the following examinations: [once you have assured the patient and thoroughly explained what you are going to accomplish.]

Inspection: Gently spread the buttocks to facilitate a thorough examination of the following areas: – The squamous section of the anal canal - The perianal, Genital, Perineal, and Sacrococcygeal regions.

Palpation: The key to diagnosis is palpation, which helps to localize symptoms, including pain, soreness, induration, swelling, lumps, and growths.

Digital rectal examination: This is the fundamental assessment for each patient with anorectal pathology.

Anoscopy/Proctoscopy: The simplest tool for visualizing the interior haemorrhoidal cushions and anoderm. Proctoscopy or flexible sigmoidoscopy must be carried out when symptoms indicate a need to check for neoplasms and inflammatory bowel disease in the rectum and lower colon.

It is usually recommended that all individuals who have anorectal symptoms undergo an anoscopy, rigid proctosigmoidoscopy, and/or flexible sigmoidoscopy.

Additional evaluation and workup may be scheduled based on the results of the physical examination, the patient's age, and his or her medical history.

In the following circumstances, a colonoscopy or barium enema to examine the colon is advised:

- The anorectal examination is inconclusive.
- The bleeding does not indicate haemorrhoids.
- Anaemia is present.
- There is positive occult blood in stool; and
- There are significant risk factors for colonic neoplasia present (family history, personal joint pathology, pulmonary disease, significant abdominal symptoms, weight loss, change in bowel habits, age older than 50 years, or other risk factors for colonic malignancy).

Describe anatomically where each anal pathology is located (e.g., anterior, posterior, left, right, etc.) or by the numbers that go around a clock's face in a clockwise direction.

6.10 Laboratory investigations

A CBC could be a helpful indicator of anaemia & infection.

Haemorrhoidal bleeding can sometimes cause anaemia, and on rare occasions, the presence of such anaemia should suggest a different diagnosis.

6.11 Imaging studies and manometry

Rectal prolapse may require a defecography. The sphincter complex and its mechanism of action can be assessed using endoanal ultrasonography and anorectal manometry. This is crucial in the evaluation before haemorrhoid intervention since it could affect the type of intervention the surgeon chooses based on the possibility of developing incontinence following surgery.

6.12 Treatment and management

An old saying about haemorrhoids asserts that if you take care of your bowels, your haemorrhoids will take care of themselves. A simple and frequent defecation of soft stool can help to prevent, or at least limit, anal mucosal prolapse; thus, it is important to consider all medical and hygienic suggestions for the control of haemorrhoid symptoms.

The management of haemorrhoids has undergone a facelift with better and safer modalities available for different grades of haemorrhoids, with less postoperative complaints. These modalities range from reassurance to surgical hemorrhoidectomy to newer minimally invasive modalities [14].

6.12.1 Lifestyle modifications

Every patient should get lifestyle recommendations for both initial therapy and to lower the likelihood of recurrence in those who need additional intervention. These recommendations include improving anal hygiene; increasing dietary fibre and fluid intake; avoiding foods and beverages like nuts, coffee, spicy foods, and alcohol; avoiding straining during defecation; avoiding delaying the urge to urinate; avoiding spending too much time on the toilet seat; and avoiding constipation or diarrhoea.

The use of sitz baths and refraining from straining when using the toilet may also be advised, albeit there is scant scientific evidence to support this.

In a small number of situations, the symptoms can be alleviated by changing the patient's defecatory behaviours, such as advising them to refrain from reading on the toilet and sitting in a particular position on the toilet. Symptoms are anticipated to improve to some extent with conservative treatment for all types of haemorrhoids, whether they are in an early stage or an advanced stage.

Therefore, regardless of the severity, conservative treatment should be advised as a first line of management. Early internal or external haemorrhoids may be treated using the following conservative measures:

- A warm sitz bath
- Medicine
- Diet
- Defecation advice

6.12.2 Conservative treatment

a. Sitz Bath: It is essential for the conservative treatment of benign anal disorders such as haemorrhoids and anal fissures, postoperative management, and prevention. Sitz baths reduce pain by lowering anal pressure, assisting in keeping the anus clean and enhancing anal blood circulation, which reduces congestion and oedema.

b. Timed Toilet Training: If possible, patients should be advised to initiate their defecation after breakfast and to finish their bowel movement within 3 minutes, even if they feel like they need to defecate more. If someone has a propensity to go to the toilet shortly after waking up, they should be told to drink one to two cups of water to trigger the gastrocolic reflex. Teach people to rinse with water rather than using tissue after defecating. If a tissue is required, tell people to use it only after soaking it in water.

c. Medical Therapy: To maintain soft stools and prevent straining, medical therapy may involve the use of laxatives, which are typically fibre-based.

Although there are several topical medications in the form of creams, ointments, and suppositories in the market, there is no strong proof that they work.

These include various combinations of corticosteroids, vasoconstrictors, local anaesthetics, antiseptics, and astringents. They might offer some symptomatic relief in the short term, but prolonged usage is not advised, especially with corticosteroid-containing treatments, because it may lead to ulceration and skin thinning. Again, there is scant support for these agents.

The role of oral medicines in the treatment of haemorrhoids is either as a preventative measure for early stages where prolapse is not significant or as a crucial means of controlling severe bleeding until definite office procedures or surgery can be performed. Despite the lack of clear data, phlebotonics (such as oral flavonoids) [15] may have some role in the management of acute symptoms and may help ease symptoms following surgical therapy.

A heterogeneous group of medications known as phlebotonics are made utilizing -plant-derived substances like calcium dobesilate or flavonoids, which can be either manufactured or taken from plants like Euphorbia prostrata, Gingko Biloba, etc. Because of their abilities to strengthen blood vessel walls, increase venous tone, promote lymphatic drainage, normalize capillary permeability, and their antagonistic effects on the molecular mediators of inflammation, they treat acute and chronic haemorrhoidal diseases. Their precise mode of action, however, is not completely understood. These medications are nevertheless routinely utilized in patients with symptomatic haemorrhoidal illness despite concerns about their efficacy due to methodological study limitations, heterogeneity, and potential publication bias.

Diosmin was isolated in 1925 from the plant *Scrophularia nodosa* and was first introduced as a therapeutic agent in 1969. Micronized Purified Flavonoid Fraction, which contains 10% hesperidin and 90% diosmin, has shown promise in the treatment of haemorrhoids.

Patients with grade I and II haemorrhoids who received MPFF-based treatment prior to irreversible degenerative changes in the ligaments of the haemorrhoidal plexuses experienced the best results. It also helped promote ideal conditions during the postoperative phase and avoid symptom relapse in patients with more severe haemorrhoidal disease [16].

Symptomatic haemorrhoids appear to respond favourably to therapy with flavonoids. Flavonoids reduce the risk of not getting well or having persistent symptoms by 60%, and they also appear to considerably reduce the risks of bleeding, chronic discomfort, and itching. However, each of these outcomes exhibits significant variation. With conflicting outcomes in multiple trials, it is still unclear whether supplementing treatment with fibre with a flavonoid is advantageous. Flavonoids are sometimes taken at doses that are higher than those that are generally recommended.

In conclusion, medical therapies can alleviate symptoms of haemorrhoids at any stage; those who do not respond, however, should receive additional care.

6.12.3 Office procedures

a. Sclerotherapy: Haemorrhoids were successfully treated with sclerosing agent injections 200 years ago. Molgan published the first account of the injection-based use of iron sulphate in England in 1869. Michael utilized a mixture of olive oil and phenol (2:1) in 1871 and reported positive results. Inflammation and fibrosis, which result in vascular compression, hemostasis, and fixation of prolapsed haemorrhoid tissues in the anal canal, are the fundamental principles of sclerotherapy.

    Indications and Contraindications – Indicated in first andd second-degree non-prolapsing haemorrhoids. Contraindicated for thrombosed external haemorrhoids, concomitant anal diseases such as fistulas, tumours, anal fissures, and skin tags.
    Procedure: Sclerotherapy is commonly performed without anaesthesia; however, with the availability of topical local anaesthetic sprays, the patient's anxiety can be decreased by their use.
    Depending on the surgeon's preference, the procedure can be readily carried out with the patient in a lithotomy or prone jackknife position.
    The rectal ampulla is reached by inserting the anoscope or proctoscope through the anal canal. The scope is then slowly dragged out until the mucosa "prolapses" over its opening. Once the haemorrhoidal tissue has been located, inject 5 ml of your selected sclerosant into the submucosa at the haemorrhoid's base.
    Complications: Injecting the sclerosant solution can result in momentary, acute precordial and upper abdominal pain. Other known complications are sloughing, thrombosis and necrosis, burning, local abscess and paraffinoma, bacteraemia and sepsis.

b. Rubber band ligation: The most often used non-invasive treatment for haemorrhoids is rubber band ligation. Using a rubber band to stop the blood flow, promotes ischaemic necrosis to remove the haemorrhoidal tissue. This procedure can be done in an outpatient clinic without the need for anaesthesia, and it can also be used to remove relatively minor piles that are left behind after the primary, larger pile has been removed.

    Indications and Contraindications: Indicated in early second and third-degree haemorrhoids, haemorrhoids in patients with comorbidities of heart, liver, and lung where corrective surgery is not possible, residual piles after hemorrhoidectomy, removal of a rectal polyp. Contraindicated in patients on anticoagulants.
    Procedure: The patient should normally be positioned in the left lateral decubitus posture to facilitate the procedure. Equipment that is suited for the procedure and has adequate lighting is also necessary. Few medical professionals recommend placing the band on the redundant mucosa above the haemorrhoid. Thus, the benefits of maintaining the anal cushions and ensuring that the ligations are well above the dentate line, thereby reducing the possibility of post-ligation pain, are provided. Some experts recommend placing two bands on the same column in one sitting. Although ligating three columns in one sitting has been documented, it is better to only ligate one to two columns at a time to save the patient the unpleasant experience of severe discomfort and pain.
    Complications: Delayed bleeding, External haemorrhoidal thrombosis, Ulceration Slippage of the ligature, severe pain, nagging abdominal pain, urinary retention, sepsis and rarely death.

c. Infrared Coagulation: An effective therapy option for internal haemorrhoids that are low-grade and symptomatic is infrared coagulation. It can be performed with a specialized device and the probe inserted through an anoscope. Infrared coagulation involves the direct application of infrared light at the haemorrhoid's base, where it is converted to heat. This causes tissue destruction to a depth of 3

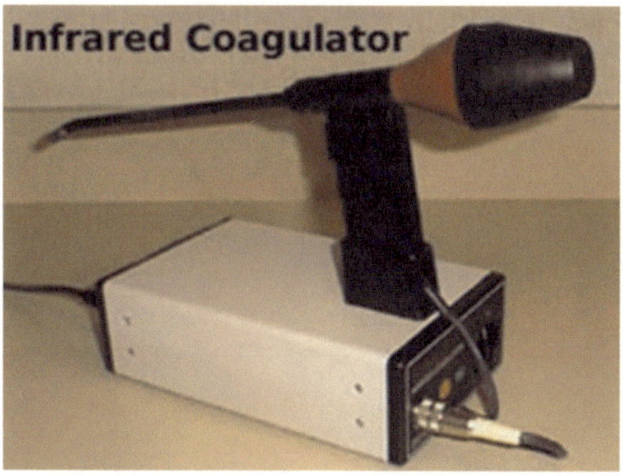

Figure 5.
Infrared coagulator.

mm, protein denaturation, and inflammation, resulting in fibrosis and subsequent scarring, shrinkage, and fixation of the redundant haemorrhoid tissue to the muscular layer beneath (**Figure 5**).

Advantages: Modern, user-friendly technology that is quick and painless to use, instantaneous coagulation without smoke or odour, works even in wet fields, less painful and less complicated than rubber band ligation, and cross-contamination elimination without the need for disinfection.
Complications: The postoperative recovery is excellent, except for tolerable pain. Occasionally, a patient may complain of severe pain if the coagulation is performed at the mucocutaneous junction. Some patients may bleed during the first week. This bleeding does not require treatment other than assurance.

d. Radiofrequency coagulation and excision: What Is the Basic? The basic principle behind radiosurgery is to deliver radio waves between 5.0 and 6.0 MHz through a radiofrequency electrode while keeping the temperature low. Radiofrequency coagulation can be used for first and second-degree haemorrhoids and radiofrequency excision for grade III and grade IV haemorrhoids (**Figure 6**).

Advantages: Advantages of the procedure include: No postoperative stay is necessary; Easy learning curve; Patient can return to work the following morning; It can be done as an outpatient treatment; It can be done under local anaesthesia, regional anaesthesia, or short general anaesthesia.

e. **Embolization** [17]: In response to the hypothesis that haemorrhoids become arterially vascularized, a novel approach has recently been introduced. The idea is to permanently restrict blood flow to the haemorrhoids by embolizing the main feeding arteries of the piles. The treatment involves pushing 2–3 mm fibre coils with a microcatheter through a right femoral route to the distal branches of the superior rectal arteries while under local anaesthesia. The primary indication appears to be a patient who has a haemorrhoidal illness with disabling chronic bleeding, a medical contraindication to surgery, or who has not responded to instrumental or surgical treatment.

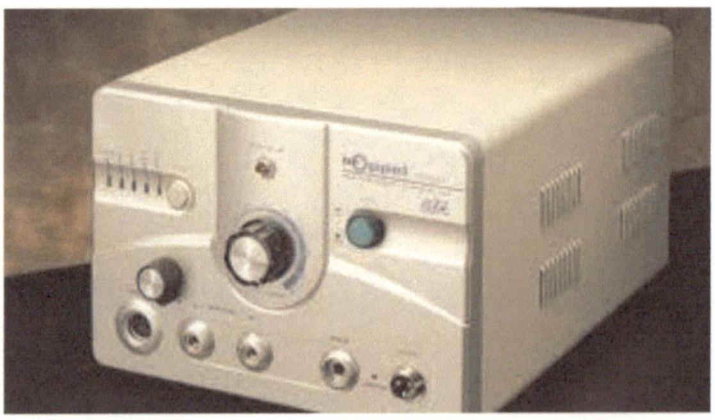

Figure 6.
Radiofrequency.

DOI: http://dx.doi.org/10.5772/intechopen.1002689

6.12.4 Surgical procedures

a. Conventional hemorrhoidectomy [18, 19]: Hemorrhoidectomy is one of the most frequently performed anorectal operations, with two well-established methods, the "open" Milligan-Morgan excision and the "closed" Ferguson technique, being used by most colorectal surgeons. Hemorrhoidectomies have historically served as the gold standard for surgical care and are taught as such. Both procedures carry the risk of postoperative bleeding, urinary retention, and late anal stenosis, and the convalescence is similarly long and challenging after both operations. The complication rate must be kept in mind, and modern management asks for diverse approaches. When patients are asked to consent, it is appropriate to inform them that hemorrhoidectomy delivers the best long-term efficacy with the worst pain control in the first two weeks following surgery, meaning a longer recovery period before returning to work. Modern energy sealing devices that are employed for dissection during hemorrhoidectomy contribute to better outcomes for pain management. A partial list of possible complications from surgical hemorrhoidectomy includes the following: Pain, haemorrhage, urinary retention, urinary tract infection, constipation, faecal impaction, anal tags, mucosal prolapse, mucosal ectropion, rectal stricture, anal stenosis, anal fissure, pseudo polyps, epidermal cysts, anal fistula, pruritus ani, faecal incontinence, and recurrent haemorrhoids.

b. Stapled hemorrhoidectomy: Prof. Longo first discussed this in 1998 [20]. The upper anal canal's mucosa and submucosal tissue were removed and anastomosed using a circular stapler. Even though the haemorrhoidal piles are not removed, the haemorrhoids are successfully treated. It was once believed that blocking the blood supply to haemorrhoids was the mode of this treatment, but it now appears to be due to the lifting of the anal canal caused by the removal and suturing of redundant mucosa and submucosal tissue. This procedure was designed to manage pain and discomfort following a haemorrhoid operation, and it conceptually altered how surgical treatment was done. While not addressing

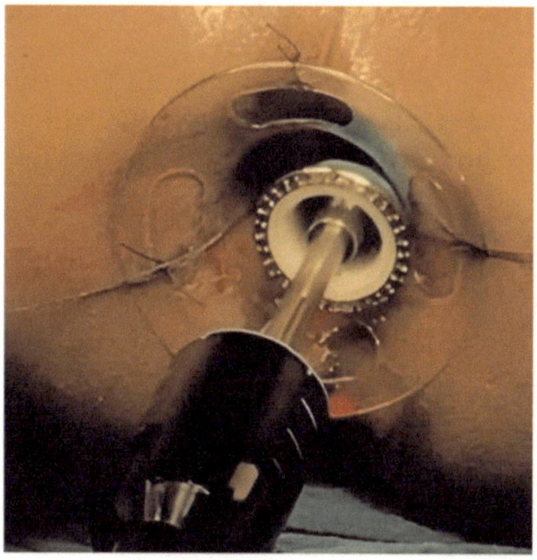

Figure 7.
Stappled haemorrhoidectomy.

any exterior components, a circumferential mucosectomy performed well above the dentate line helps reduce haemorrhoidal cushion prolapse by restoring anatomy to the anorectal junction (**Figure 7**).

With the main advantage of being less painful, haemorrhoidopexy has been advocated as an alternative to traditional hemorrhoidectomy. The most specific indication would be circumferential prolapsed haemorrhoids, always maintaining that any exterior components would need extra operations either concurrently or during a second operation. Stapled haemorrhoidopexy is contraindicated in cases of infection, preoperative stenosis, any degree of incontinence, or sphincter injury. Concerns and Issues Other than in Conventional Hemorrhoidectomy:

Anal intercourse (male or female); Anal fissure; Anal fistula; Skin tags; Hypertrophied anal papillae; Thrombosis; Preexisting sphincter injury or loss; Excessive rectal mucosal prolapse.

c. Doppler-guided haemorrhoidal artery ligation & recto anal repair [21]: In 1995, a Japanese surgeon named Kazumasa Morinaga developed a novel method of treating haemorrhoids. Using a Doppler (ultrasound) approach, he identified the haemorrhoidal arteries. He created a special device with a Doppler transducer and a window that allowed the surgeon to identify the haemorrhoidal arteries and ligate them by ligating a suture (stitch) around them. This is a straightforward method that quickly alleviated the majority of haemorrhoidal symptoms, including bleeding and protrusion. When dealing with prolapse, a mucopexy is added to the artery ligation, and this approach, which is extremely respectful of the anorectal architecture, is genuinely non-excisional. It is ideal for individuals with grades II to III who need surgery because of bleeding [22]. If there is no fibrosis preventing cushions from being lowered to their anatomical place, grade IV haemorrhoids can also be treated in this manner. Sclerotherapy recipients may not be good candidates for mucopexy in that regard. Emergency bleeding management in high-risk patients taking antiplatelet medication has also been effective. A specific characteristic of this operation is the possibility to adapt it to the specific symptoms of each patient (**Figure 8**).

   Adding mucopexy to more or fewer locations is tailored to individual clinical presentations. The cost issue also compares favourably to other operations. The need for Doppler to guide the location of arteries has been questioned and could

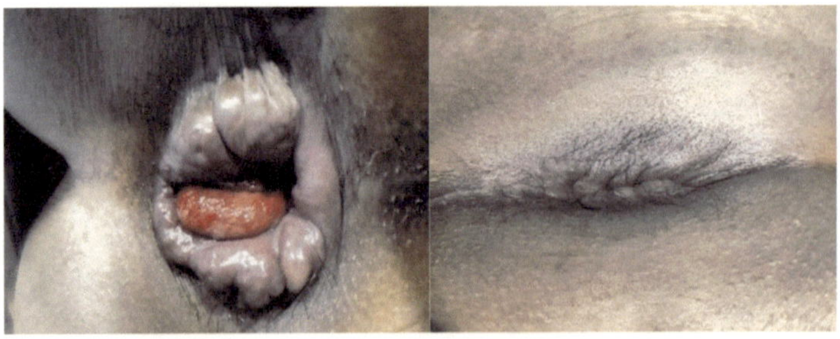

Figure 8.
Preoperative Image – Immediate Post DGHAL-RAR.

also have cost implications. Lower postoperative pain and complications as well as comparatively reduced costs even with a higher rate of recurrence are criteria to propose arterial ligation and mucopexy as a possible first step before considering more aggressive treatments.

d. Laser haemorrhoidoplasty: Laser Hemorrhoidoplasty (LHP) is a novel therapeutic option for haemorrhoids. Lasers were first described for use in haemorrhoid disease over 30 years ago but have only been utilized recently. There are two main laser approaches to haemorrhoidal disease. Laser haemorrhoidoplasty (LH) involves an incision at the base of haemorrhoid, via which the haemorrhoidal tissue is coagulated using the laser probe [23]. A haemorrhoidal laser procedure utilizes a Doppler ultrasound probe to identify the terminal branches of the superior rectal artery, which are first ligated, and then the haemorrhoidal tissue is coagulated using the laser probe. Some authors use finger-guided haemorrhoidal artery ligation of the superior haemorrhoidal arteries followed by coagulation of haemorrhoidal tissue using a laser probe. Although LHP is an effective treatment for grade II to grade IV haemorrhoids, individuals with grade IV haemorrhoids run a substantial risk of bleeding and re-intervention (**Figure 9**).

   Laser haemorrhoidoplasty offers significantly lower pain scores, defecation pain scores, and opioid analgesia use in the early postoperative period, there is statistically significant symptom resolution and improvement in symptom-related patient QoL on long-term follow-up. Laser therapy for haemorrhoids results in less tissue damage and good hemostasis, as well as shorter surgical times and shorter hospital stays. Despite all the advantages, using lasers in therapy necessitates specialized training and safety precautions. Further head-to-head studies comparing LH to other haemorrhoid therapies with larger sample sizes and the utilization of objective postoperative symptom scores are required to determine the most efficacious therapeutic approach for this common condition. Complications include pain, bleeding at the site of entry of fibre, burning pain and itching, postoperative oedema, thrombosis, infection, bleeding, sloughing of mucosa in inexperienced hands, and abscess.

e. Transanal suture rectopexy [24]: Introduced by Dr Chivte from India in 2012. Indicated for grade II to grade IV haemorrhoids, The theory is based on dearterialization, whereby vessels are blocked at two locations, 2 and 4 cm above the dentate line, hence preventing the creation of collaterals and their subsequent recurrence. The learning curve is quite low for trans anal suture

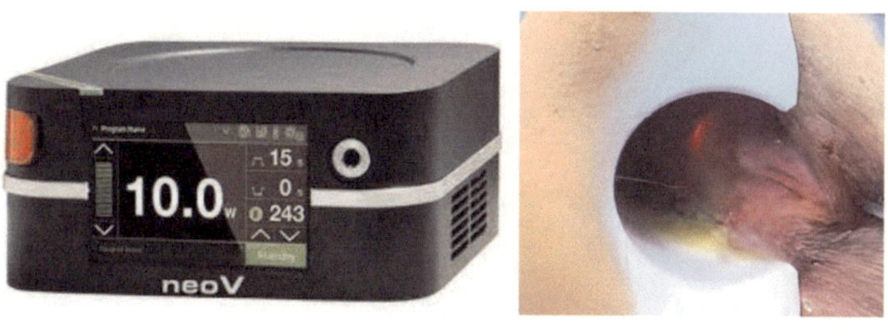

Figure 9.
1470 nm diode laser - the glow of the laser in the submucous plane.

rectopexy for haemorrhoids. All grades of haemorrhoids have an identical rate of success, and different surgeons have demonstrated comparable outcomes. Haemorrhoids' mass, prolapse, and recurrence can be successfully managed by the operation. To be acknowledged as an acceptable painless treatment for haemorrhoids, the novel approach still needs extensive follow-up.

7. Management in specific situations

a. Thrombosed external haemorrhoids [25, 26]: Hematoma from venous rupture and clotting caused by excessive squeezing during defecation are thrombosed haemorrhoids. Commonly occurring on external haemorrhoids, it may occur on internal haemorrhoids also. A painful palpable lump around the anus is the commonest symptom. The size of the lump may vary, the smaller size of the lump, the more easily the pain subsides. Pain itself should be differentiated from the perianal abscess and anal fissure. Anal ultrasound is often used for differential diagnosis.

The treatment is divided into conservative and surgical treatment [27]. If the lump is less than the size of a pea, it can be treated conservatively. Sitz baths, laxatives, anti-inflammatory drugs, and ointments are used for conservative treatment. Usually, the pain settles down within 3–4 days, and the hematoma sometimes ruptures spontaneously; in some cases, it can last for more than 1 month to dissolve completely. The leftovers from the hematoma's complete dissolution frequently manifest as a skin tag (**Figure 10**).

A hematoma that covers more than 30% of the anal circumference is better treated surgically. Even with a lesser thrombosed haemorrhoid, if it frequently reoccurs and is typically accompanied by increasing anal pressure or an anal fissure, then, surgical removal of blood clots is advised together with lateral internal sphincterotomy to lower anal pressure.

b. Thrombosed internal haemorrhoids: Internal haemorrhoids that are acutely thrombosed or strangulated typically manifest in patients as extremely painful, untreatable haemorrhoids. Haemorrhoids that are confined may necrotize and

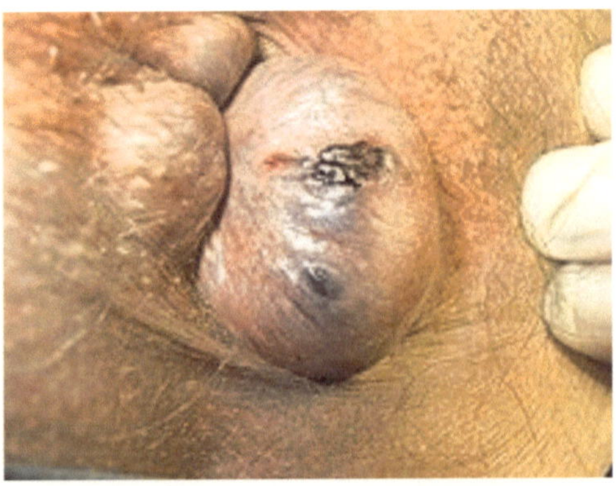

Figure 10.
Thrombosed external haemorrhoids

drain. Treatment for this condition can be challenging, especially if there has been significant strangling, thrombosis, or if there is an underlying circumferential prolapse of high-grade haemorrhoids. Pain and tissue congestion may be lessened by manually decreasing the haemorrhoid masses, either with or without intravenous analgesics or anaesthesia. In these cases, an urgent hemorrhoidectomy is frequently necessary. Mucosa and anoderm should be preserved as much as possible to avoid postoperative anal stricture unless the tissues are necrotic. In skilled hands, the surgical results of an urgent hemorrhoidectomy were on par with those of an elective procedure.

c. Haemorrhoids in pregnancy: Haemorrhoidal issues are frequently an issue for women in the latter stages of pregnancy. Under the effect of progesterone, haemorrhoids and constipation are likely to occur often throughout pregnancy. Drugs should be avoided as much as possible in the early stages of pregnancy. Haemorrhoids are uncommon throughout the middle stages of pregnancy, but during the latter stages, increased abdominal pressure and hunched posture make them prolapse easily. Most of these issues can be effectively managed with sitz baths and bowel control (such as laxatives and stool softeners). Thrombosed haemorrhoids can be surgically removed as usual. In managing haemorrhoids in pregnant women, MPFF is a safe and efficient medical therapy (use is contraindicated in the first trimester) [15]. Maintaining treatment with MPFF during the prenatal stage decreases the incidence and length of relapses of acute haemorrhoid symptoms. For individuals who do not improve after receiving conservative treatment, surgical or non-surgical techniques may be recommended. Only thrombosed or strangulated haemorrhoids should be treated surgically, and this should be done under local anaesthesia.

d. Haemorrhoids in children: Although they are uncommon, haemorrhoids can occur in infants. Most infant haemorrhoids do not require surgical treatment. Children with haemorrhoids should receive prompt treatment and be closely observed to avoid the spread of infections. Children's haemorrhoids are frequently caused by constipation, prolonged chair use, a low-fibre diet, poor toilet training, and prolonged sitting. The most typical symptom is rectal bleeding. Controlling constipation, consuming more fibre while eating less spicy and fatty food, using haemorrhoidal cream, taking sitz baths, and using anti-pruritic medications are conservative treatments for haemorrhoids in children.

e. Haemorrhoids in patients on anticoagulants [28]: In patients with haemorrhoids, anticoagulant or antiplatelet medications may encourage anorectal bleeding and raise the risk of bleeding after surgery or banding. Because most bleeding episodes are self-limited and end spontaneously, stopping antithrombotic medication may not be essential unless the bleeding is continuous or severe. The mainstay of treatment for these patients is, consequently, a conservative approach. When medical treatment is ineffective for bleeding, low-grade haemorrhoids, injection sclerotherapy is the preferred option. The danger of subsequent bleeding makes rubber band ligation contraindicated in individuals taking anticoagulant or antiplatelet medications at the time. It is advised to stop using anticoagulant or antiplatelet medications 5–7 days before and after haemorrhoid banding or any other type of surgery for haemorrhoids.

f. Haemorrhoids in patients with portal hypertension [29]: The bleeding from an anorectal varicose vein and the bleeding from haemorrhoids should be differentiated in patients with portal hypertension. Haemorrhoids are purple, do not collapse under digital pressure, do not extend proximally to the dentate line, and may prolapse during proctoscopy. Rectal varices, on the other hand, are dark blue, extend more than 4 cm above the anal margin, and collapse on digital pressure but do not prolapse. Varices originate from the rectum, anal canal, and perianal area. These three locations can be managed by suturing continually at three to four points from the upper rectum to the perianal area. RBL is typically not advised for patients with severe cirrhosis due to the possibility of postoperative secondary bleeding. In these cases, conservative therapy and coagulopathy correction should be suggested. Patients with concurrent bleeding haemorrhoids and cirrhosis can be effectively and safely treated with injection sclerotherapy. Suture ligation of the bleeder or hemorrhoidectomy may be suggested in a refractory situation.

g. Haemorrhoids in HIV Patients: Approximately 19.7% of HIV-positive patients also have perianal conditions, such as haemorrhoids. As a result, it is important to carry out an effective and safe procedure on these individuals. Numerous studies have found that patients with HIV infection had poor anorectal wound healing. The primary line of treatment for persons with HIV who have symptomatic haemorrhoids should be conservative. If conservative treatment is unsuccessful, surgical methods should be made available along with good CD4 count maintenance and preventative antibiotics. Particularly for HIV-positive patients, TRSRP – DGD MP are safe procedures with a low complication risk and few technical issues [30]. HIV-positive patients have a high level of satisfaction with these procedures.

h. Haemorrhoids in patients with inflammatory bowel disease: In patients with inflammatory bowel disease, or for that matter with any infectious or non-infectious colitis, an exacerbation of haemorrhoidal problems is not at all uncommon. Treatment of haemorrhoids in these situations should be as conservative as possible [31]. Any procedure done on the anus or perianal skin in inflammatory bowel disease patients should be confined to the very minimum necessary to address the patient's complaint. Such patients may experience delayed healing or non-healing after receiving definitive or intensive surgical therapy for any anorectal issue, leaving them more disabled than they were before the procedure. Hemorrhoidectomy is occasionally a reasonable way to cure bleeding or protrusion of haemorrhoids when the illness is dormant and sepsis, fistula formation, and scarring are absent.

i. Recurrent haemorrhoids: A past excisional hemorrhoidectomy may have a significant impact on how recurrent disease is managed. Reevaluating all the baseline features is necessary, and this includes changing one's lifestyle, losing weight, and reassessing if a colonoscopy is necessary. It is also necessary to receive the initial consultation and operation reports. Before advising the best course of treatment, it is essential to consider any previously acknowledged elements that may be influencing the symptoms of bleeding. These factors might be as straightforward as noncompliance or as complicated as undiagnosed

DOI: http://dx.doi.org/10.5772/intechopen.1002689

bleeding diatheses or initial misdiagnosis. Depending on the severity of the issue, the recurrence may now be treatable with non-invasive hybrid procedures or, in rare circumstances, a guided hemorrhoidectomy, if enough anoderm is preserved to prevent stricture.

When, what, and what not in the management of haemorrhoids

a. There is no "one size fits all" approach to treating haemorrhoids.

b. Although there is an ongoing debate on the optimal surgical technique for treating haemorrhoids, none of the techniques that are currently in use come close to the ideal surgical solution, research is ongoing for a technique that is efficient while being painless and safe.

   In actuality, the less painful the surgery, the higher the likelihood of post-op recurrence.

c. The ideal haemorrhoid surgery should be successful with a low recurrence rate, have minimum postoperative pain to allow for an early return to regular activities, and be safe with minimal morbidity. If recurrence is the primary concern, conventional hemorrhoidectomy (CH) remains the "gold standard." It is, however, accompanied by substantial postoperative pain.

d. Anyone managing patients with colorectal issues will frequently have to deal with people who have haemorrhoidal illnesses. We leave you with a few closing remarks even though it is challenging to summarize all you will run against.

e. Recurrence and other complications following therapy for haemorrhoidal disease are very common, although they are frequently preventable with careful patient selection, preoperative planning, and intervention according to the patient's needs.

f. Technical issues following surgical intervention may have a long-term detrimental effect on patient quality of life. It is crucial that you, as the surgeon, are skilled, knowledgeable about the technical details of the treatments you provide, and familiar with the frequency and treatment of procedural-specific complications.

Author details

Ajit Naniksingh Kukreja
Marengo CIMS Hospital, Ahmedabad, India

*Address all correspondence to: dr.ajit.kukreja@ratandeep.com;
dr.ajit.kukreja@marengoasia.com

IntechOpen

© 2023 The Author(s). Licensee IntechOpen. This chapter is distributed under the terms of the Creative Commons Attribution License (http://creativecommons.org/licenses/by/3.0), which permits unrestricted use, distribution, and reproduction in any medium, provided the original work is properly cited.

References

[1] Kaidar-Person O, Person B, Wexner S. Hemorrhoidal disease: A comprehensive review. Journal of the American College of Surgeons. 2007;**204**(1):102-117. DOI: 10.1016/j.jamcollsurg.2006.08.022

[2] Claus F. Everything you ever wanted to know about the history of hemorrhoids. 2018. Available from: https://sciencenordic.com/denmark-forskerzonen-mens-health/everything-you-ever-wanted-to-know-about-the-history-of-hemorrhoids/1461058

[3] Lohsiriwat V. Hemorrhoids: From basic pathophysiology to clinical management. World Journal of Gastroenterology. 2012;**18**(17):2009-2017. DOI: 10.3748/wjg.v18.i17.2009]

[4] Hyams L, Philpot J. An epidemiological investigation of hemorrhoids. American Journal of Proctology. Jun 1970;**21**(3):177-193. PMID: 5425245

[5] Yang HK. Hemorrhoids. Berlin Heidelberg: Springer-Verlag; 2014. DOI: 10.1007/978-3-642-41798-6_12

[6] Yng HK. The pathophysiology of haemorrhoids. In: Yng HK, editor. Hemorrhoids. Berlin Heidelberg: Springer-Verlag; 2014. pp. 15-24

[7] Lohsiriwat V. Treatment of haemorrhoids: A coloproctologist's view. World Journal of Gastroenterology. 2015;**21**(31):9245-9252. DOI: 10.3748/wjg. v21.i31.9245

[8] Margetis N. Pathophysiology of Internal Hemorrhoids. Annals of Gastroenterology. 2019;**32**(2019):264-272. DOI: 10.20524/aog.2019.0355

[9] Richard S. Clinical Anatomy: An Illustrated Review with Questions and Explanations. 4th ed. Philadelphia, Pennsylvania, USA: Lippincott Williams & Wilkins; 2004

[10] Thomson WH. The nature of haemorrhoids. British Journal of Surgery. Jul 1975;**62**(7):542-552. DOI: 10.1002/bjs.1800620710. PMID: 1174785

[11] Bernstein WC. What are hemorrhoids and what is their relationship to the portal venous system? Diseases of the Colon and Rectum. 1983; **26**:829-834

[12] Burkitt DP. Varicose veins, deep vein thrombosis, and hemorrhoids: Epidemiology and suggested aetiology. British Journal of Medicine. 1972;**2**:556-561. DOI: 10.1136/bmj.2.5813.556

[13] Khana MA, Chowdrib NA, Parrayb FQ, Wanib RA, Mehrajb A, Babab A, et al. PNR-Bleed classification and hemorrhoid severity score—A novel attempt at classifying the hemorrhoids. Journal of Coloproctology;**40**(4):398-403. DOI: 10.1016/j.jcol.2020.05.012

[14] Pata F, Gallo G, Pellino G, Vigorita V, Podda M, Di Saverio S, et al. Evolution of surgical management of hemorrhoidal disease: An historical overview. Frontiers in Surgery. 2021;**8**: 727059. DOI: 10.3389/fsurg.2021.727059

[15] Buckshee K, Takkar D, Aggarwal N. Micronized flavonoid therapy in internal haemorrhoids of pregnancy. International Journal of Gynaecology and Obstetrics. 1997;**57**(2):145-151

[16] Misra MC, Parshad R. Randomized clinical trial of micronized flavonoids in the early control of bleeding from acute internal haemorrhoids. The British Journal of Surgery. 2000;**87**:868-872

[17] Moussa N, Sielezneff I, Sapoval M, Tradi F, Del Giudice C, Fathallah N, et al. Embolization of the superior rectal arteries for chronic bleeding due to haemorrhoidal disease. Colorectal Disease. 2017;**19**:194-199. DOI: 10.1111/codi.13430

[18] Simillis C, Thoukididou SN, Slesser AAP, Rasheed S, Tan E, Tekkis PP. Systematic review and network meta-analysis comparing clinical outcomes and effectiveness of surgical treatments for haemorrhoids. BJS. 2015;**102**:1603-1618. DOI: 10.1002/bjs.9913

[19] Yeo D, Tan KY. Hemorrhoidectomy - making sense of the surgical options. World Journal of Gastroenterology. 2014;**20**(45):16976-16983. DOI: 10.3748/wjg. v20.i45.16976

[20] Longo A. Treatment of hemorrhoidal disease by reduction of mucosa and hemorrhoidal prolapse with a circular suturing device: A new procedure. In: Monduzzi A, editor. Proceedings of the 6th World Congress of Endoscopic Surgery. Bologna; 1998. pp. 777-784

[21] Ratto C, Giordano P, Donisi L, Parello A, Litta F, Doglietto GB. Transanal haemorrhoidal dearterialization (THD) for selected fourth-degree haemorrhoids. Techniques in Coloproctology. 2011; **15**:191-197. DOI: 10.1007/s10151-011-0689-1

[22] Giordano P, Overton J, Madeddu F, Zaman S, Gravante G. Transanal hemorrhoidal dearterialization: A systematic review. Diseases of the Colon and Rectum. 2009;**52**:1665-1671. DOI: 10.1007/DCR.0b013e3181af50f4

[23] Anshini J, Chen L, Gamze A, Richard H, Naseem M. Laser hemorrhoidoplasty in the treatment of symptomatic hemorrhoids: A pilot Australian study. Annals of Coloproctology. 19 May 2022. DOI: 10.3393/ac.2022.00164.0023. Epub ahead of print. PMID: 35584917

[24] Chivate SD, Ladukar L, Ayyar M, Mahajan V, Kavathe S. Transanal suture rectopexy for hemorrhoids: Chivate's painless cure for piles. The Indian Journal of Surgery. 2012;**74**(5):412-417. DOI: 10.1007/s12262-012-0461-4

[25] Kumkumsingh KG, Kukreja AN, Chaudhry T, Gupta S. Hemorrhoids Practice Guidelines 2021. India: Association Colon & Rectal Surgeons of India; 2021

[26] Rivadeneira DE, Steele SR, Ternent C, Chalasani S, Buie WD, Rafferty JL. Standards practice task force of the American society of colon and rectal surgeons: Practice parameters for the management of hemorrhoids [Revised 2010]. Diseases of the Colon and Rectum. 2011;**54**:1059-1064

[27] Pattanaarun J, Wesarachawit W, Tantiphlachiva K, Atithansakul P, Sahakitrungruang C, Rojanasakul A. A comparison of early postoperative results between urgent closed hemorrhoidectomy for prolapsed thrombosed hemorrhoids and elective closed hemorrhoidectomy. Journal of the Medical Association of Thailand. 2009; **92**:1610-1615

[28] Nelson RS, Thorson AG. Risk of bleeding following hemorrhoidal banding in patients on antithrombotic therapy. Gastroentérologie Clinique et Biologique. 2009;**33**(6-7):463-465. DOI: 10.1016/j.gcb.2009.05.007

[29] McNabb-Baltar J, Farag A, Hilzenrat N, Al-Busafi SA. Clinical manifestations of portal hypertension. International Journal of Hepatology. 2012;**2012**:203794

[30] Fan Z, Zhang Y. Treatment of prolapsing hemorrhoids in HIV-infected patients with tissue-selecting technique. Gastroenterology Research and Practice. 2017;**2017**:1970985. DOI: 10.1155/2017/1970985

[31] Jeffery PJ, Ritchie JK, Parks AG. Treatment of haemorrhoids in patients with inflammatory bowel disease. Lancet. 1977;**1**(8021):1084-1085

Chapter 10

Perspective Chapter: The Management of Chronic Anal Fissures

Nathalie Mantilla and Juaquito M. Jorge

Abstract

Chronic anal fissure is a common complaint that is associated with excruciating anal pain and bright red bleeding associated to bowel movements. The classic findings during the physical examination are helpful in differentiating the different types of fissures (acute versus chronic and typical versus atypical). Most cases of chronic anal fissures are successfully treated with conservative measures such as dietary and lifestyle modifications, adequate bowel regimen, and topical muscle relaxants such as nifedipine, diltiazem, or nitroglycerine. Refractory cases are usually managed with botulinum toxins injections or more invasive approaches such as internal lateral sphincterotomy with excellent healing rates at the expense of risk of fecal incontinence. In patients without hypertonicity of the anal sphincter, cutaneous flaps can be used with remarkable results.

Keywords: anal pain, anorectal bleeding, anal fissure, sphincterotomy, botox

1. Introduction

An anal fissure is defined as a linear tear of the superficial lining of the anal canal (from the dentate line to the anal verge). As with many other anorectal conditions, it is often assumed to be hemorrhoids and can go undiagnosed, making it difficult to know its exact incidence. Most patients seeking help from a healthcare professional are those with persistent symptoms, given that many acute anal fissures resolve spontaneously.

Anal fissures classifications are simple and based on the length of symptoms (acute or chronic), and location in the anal canal circumference (typical or atypical). The treatment will depend on the type of fissure and associated patients' conditions.

2. Pathophysiology

The exact pathogenesis of this condition has not been precise; however, different theories have been proposed.

The passage of hard bulky stools through the anal canal, anal intercourse or medical instrumentation are described in the mechanical theory as causing trauma on the mucosa overlying the anal canal, with documented hypertonicity of the anal sphincter [1, 2]. This finding is unclear if it is part of the cause or a consequence of the anal pain [3]. During straining, the anorectal angle (ARA) makes the posterior midline (PML) of the anal canal the most vulnerable location [4]. Nonetheless, loose and multiple liquid bowel movements are known to cause anal fissures as well.

Another theory is the one involving the relative ischemia in the PML of the anal canal, which may be aggravated by hypertonicity of the anal sphincter muscle. The combination of these factors creates a vicious cycle where open wound causes worsening pain, which causes anal muscles spasms and increased tone, consequently aggravating the local ischemia and ultimately precluding healing [5].

3. Clinical presentation

Severe sharp pain is a distinguishing characteristic of anal fissures. It is usually associated with bowel movements and can last minutes to hours. The intensity of the pain causes fear of bowel movements, and it is often described as if glass was passing through the anus. The anorectal pain caused by the fissure is commonly accompanied by bright red blood in the toilet.

Anal fissures are classified based on the duration of symptoms in acute (<6 weeks) and chronic (>6 weeks) and according to the location in typical (posterior/anterior midline) and atypical (lateral quadrants) (**Figure 1**).

In chronic anal fissures, it is characteristic to find a triad of a sentinel skin tag (on the distal apex of the fissure), a hypertrophic anal papilla (on the proximal apex), and exposed hypertrophic internal sphincter muscle (**Figure 2**). **Table 1** summarizes the characteristic symptoms, findings on examination, and associated pathologies depending on the type of fissure (**Figure 3**).

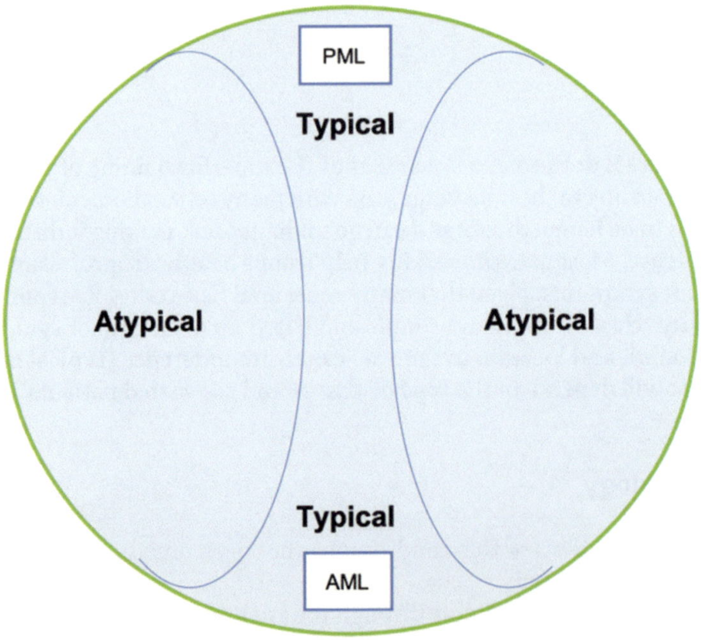

Figure 1.
Anal fissure classification based on location. PML: posterior midline; and AML: anterior midline.

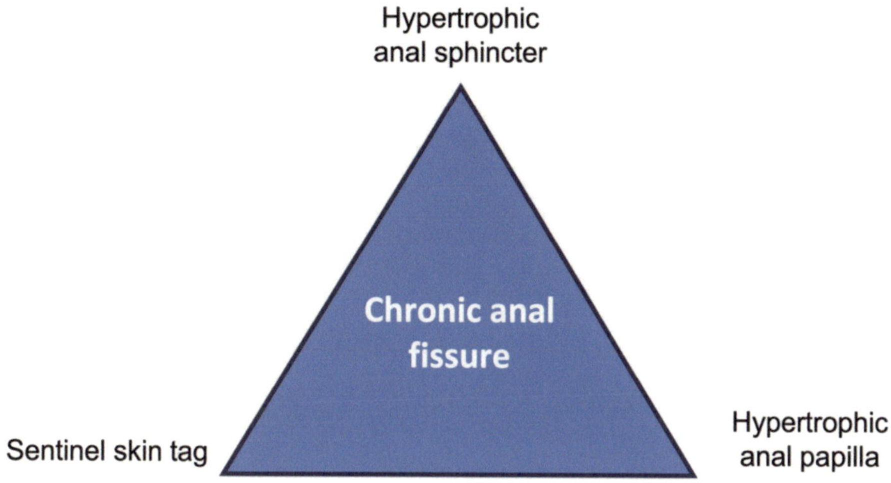

Figure 2.
Chronic anal fissure triad.

Type of fissure	Symptoms	Findings on examination
Acute	• Presentation <6 weeks • Bright red bleeding per rectum (BRBPR) • Sharp pain, and/or burning associated with bowel movements (BM) • Anal spasms after BM	• Linear tear of the anoderm with clean edges • Hypertonic anal sphincter on digital rectal examination (DRE)
Chronic	• Symptoms present beyond 6–8 weeks • Pain and bleeding associated with BM as in acute anal fissures	• Sentinel skin tag at the external apex • Hypertrophic anal papilla at the internal apex • Exposed internal anal sphincter muscle • Thickened raised edges
Type of fissure	**Location and findings on examination**	**Associated pathologies**
Typical	• 73–90% posterior midline (PML) • 10–13% anterior midline (AML) • 3% in both AML and PML • Appearance as described above	• Not associated with other diseases (excluding constipation)
Atypical	• Anywhere in the anal canal, commonly off midline • Deeper ulcerations	• Malignancy • Crohn's disease • Human immunodeficiency virus (HIV) • Syphilis • Tuberculosis

Lu and Herzig [6]; Jobanputra [7].

Table 1.
Characteristic symptoms, findings on examination, and associated pathologies on different types of anal fissures.

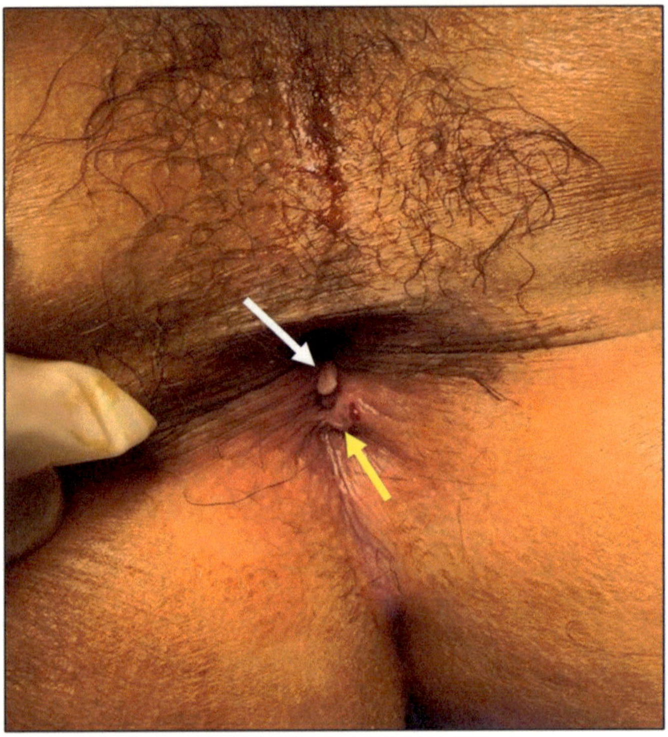

Figure 3.
Chronic AML fissure. White arrow: hypertrophic anal papilla. Yellow arrow: sentinel skin tag.

4. Diagnosis

The cardinal symptom of anal fissures is pain associated with defecation, and that can last several hours. Some patients describe it as "passing broken glass" to describe the sharp and burning nature of the pain. In many cases, pain is associated with bright red bleeding, which is why this condition is often misdiagnosed as symptomatic hemorrhoids (**Figure 4**).

5. Treatment

5.1 Conservative (nonoperative) management

5.1.1 Dietary and lifestyle modifications

Conservative management such as diet and lifestyle modifications should be offered to all patients presenting with acute anal fissures, given the high healing rates (80–90%) and very few side effects associated with these measures [8]. On the contrary, chronic anal fissures only heal with conservative measures in a small group of patients (36%), as reported in a Cochrane review [9]. This is due to the increased anal sphincter tone, the reason why local agents aiming for sphincter muscle relaxation are offered early in the management.

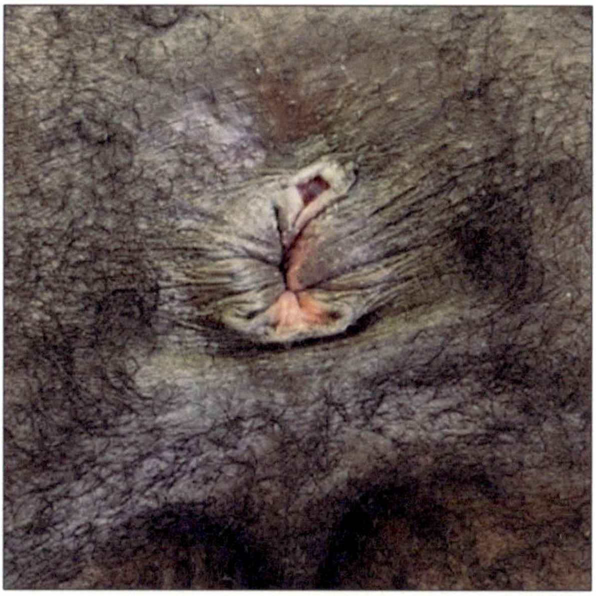

Figure 4.
PML chronic anal fissure with thickened raised edges.

The goal is to preserve an adequate consistency of the stools (formed), avoiding constipation, which helps with healing and preventing recurrences. This can be achieved by pursuing the following recommendations:

- Maintaining a high-fiber diet (20–30 gr per day) or psyllium supplements, with stool softeners as needed.
- Optimization of daily fluid intake to at least 8 glasses of 8 ounces.
- Warm water sitz baths to help relaxing the pelvic muscles.
- Avoid excessive straining and prolong sitting in the toilet (>3–5 minutes).
- Avoid vigorous perianal wiping.

5.1.2 Topical sphincter muscle relaxants

Muscle relaxants are widely used in the management of chronic anal fissures with sphincter hypertonicity. Either through the nitric oxide pathway or by blocking calcium channels in the cell wall, the aim is to relax the anal sphincter muscle to allow blood flow and, consequently, healing of the fissure [1, 2].

5.1.2.1 Glyceryl trinitrate (nitroglycerine)

This agent has been used for decades with healing rates of almost 70% (ranging from 49 to 68%). Recurrence rates have been reported from 51 to 67%. Although most patients report resolution of symptoms with proper use, headache is a well-known side effect experienced in almost 50% of users, leading to discontinuation of treatment in up to 20% of patients. Tachyphylaxis is another undesirable effect of this medication, discouraging further use in some patients.

The initial concentration described and used was 0.2%, prepared as a compound ointment, but several years later, 0.4% became available. Both concentrations can be applied twice a day, perianal or endoanal, for 6–8 weeks. However, the endoanal application of 0.4% ointment specifically has shown healing rates as high as 77%.

When comparing the type of application, perianal versus endoanal, the latter was associated with decreased frequency and severity of headaches. Several studies have investigated the ideal dose by comparing different concentrations from 0.1 to 0.4%, and most results have shown higher healing rates with 0.4% [10, 11].

5.1.2.2 Calcium channel blockers (nifedipine, diltiazem)

This group of topical agents work by blocking the influx of calcium into the cells, allowing relaxation of the anal sphincter muscle. They are considered the first-line treatment for chronic anal fissures due to their good efficacy and lower side effects compared with nitrates. These medications are not available in topical formulation; therefore, they must be prepared as compounds by specialty pharmacies, making availability more limited.

A meta-analysis of randomized controlled trials in the management of chronic anal fissures was published by Nevins and Kanakala, and their results reinforced the outcomes of other publications demonstrating that topical calcium channel blockers and glyceryl trinitrates have comparable healing rates; however, diltiazem 2% and nifedipine produce less often and less severe headaches and have better recurrence rates [12].

5.1.3 Chemical denervation (botulinum toxin)

Botulinum toxin is a protein produced by *Clostridium botulinum*, responsible for muscular relaxation by blocking the release of acetylcholine at the neuromuscular junction. The severity of the muscle relaxation and length of the effect is variable but can last several months (up to 4 months). Botulinum toxin type A is the most widely used, and despite not being specifically approved by the Food and Drug Administration (FDA) for the treatment of chronic anal fissures, it has been shown to significantly improve symptoms when injected directly in the internal anal sphincter muscle. It is relatively well tolerated, with less side effects than muscle relaxants, and despite the need for anesthesia to be applied, it is the second line of treatment for chronic anal fissures and an excellent alternative to surgery, particularly in patients considered high risk for fecal incontinence.

One of the challenges of this treatment is the lack of standardization of application techniques and dosages, including single or multiple injections directly in the internal and external sphincter muscles, in the intersphincteric space, and on the sides of the fissure. Since healing and recurrence rates seem to be similar with low and high doses, it is recommended to use the lowest dose needed to achieve healing to decrease the risk of fecal incontinence.

5.1.4 Topical anesthetic

Topical Lidocaine in gel or ointment is commonly used as an adjuvant in the management of the pain associated with anal fissures. Direct endoanal application is recommended, especially before and after bowel movements. Patients should be educated about its use, intended to help in reducing the pain rather than healing the fissure.

5.2 Operative management

Persistence of the anal fissure after uninterrupted medical treatment for at least 6 to 8 weeks, it is considered a failure of nonoperative management and often requires a surgical intervention.

5.2.1 Anal sphincter dilation

Mechanical stretching of a hypertonic anal sphincter muscle is one of the oldest methods described in the management of chronic anal fissures. Outcomes and details on the technique have shown significant variations in the literature. With the development of more effective treatment options, manual dilation is disfavored, reserving balloon dilation as an option in patients with an increased risk of incontinence.

5.2.2 Lateral internal sphincterotomy (LIS)

The surgical division of the anal sphincter was first described in early 1950s, and despite some variations in the technique, it remains the treatment of choice for hypertonic anal sphincter fissures. The initial description was at the site of the fissure in the posterior midline, which causes fecal soiling in up to 40% of patients due to the anatomic defect of the anal canal ("keyhole deformity"). After the introduction of the lateral sphincterotomy by Notaras in 1969, this procedure became the surgery of choice for patients who failed medical management [13].

5.2.3 Surgical details

As in most outpatient surgeries, our preference is to perform this procedure under spinal anesthesia; however, sedation and local anesthetic is another good option. Pre-operatively, patients receive fleet enemas the night before and the morning of the procedure. After positioning the patient in a prone Jack-knife position with both buttocks taped apart for better exposure of the perianal area and traditional sterile field preparation, a digital rectal examination and a circumferential anoscopy are performed. Antibiotics for surgical prophylaxis are not routinely offered in these cases.

The transection of the sphincter is performed on the right side to avoid bleeding from the left lateral hemorrhoid.

5.2.3.1 Open versus closed

The difference of these techniques is the creation of a radial surgical wound over the intersphincteric groove providing direct visualization of the internal sphincter muscle before transecting it (open approach), as supposed to the insertion of the scalpel in the intersphincteric space with subsequent turning medially and transection of the internal anal sphincter muscle (**Figures 5** and **6**).

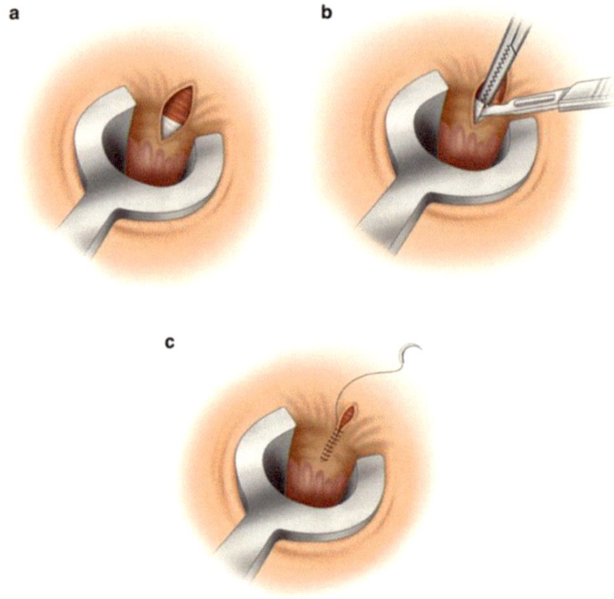

Figure 5.
Open lateral internal sphincterotomy: (a) incision over intersphincteric groove, (b) separation of internal sphincter muscle with a hemostat clamp and division of the muscle using a scalpel, and (c) closure of the wound with absorbable suture (From: Lu and Herzig [6]).

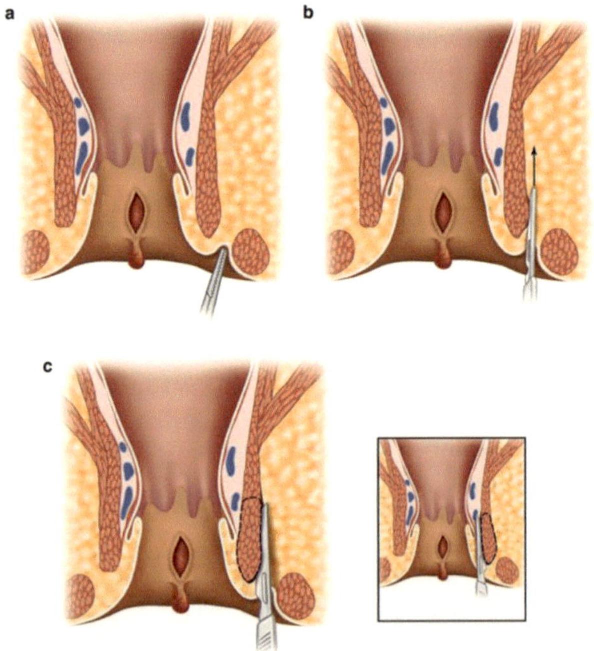

Figure 6.
Closed lateral internal sphincterotomy: (a) identification of the intersphincteric groove, (b) insertion of a scalpel in the sphincteric groove, and (c) medial rotation of the scalpel and transection of the internal sphincter muscle (From: Lu and Herzig [6]).

The results of these two techniques have been studied in multiple opportunities, and in a Cochrane review updated in 2011, similar success and recurrence rates were reported. Fecal incontinence rates are also comparable [14].

5.2.3.2 Conservative versus traditional

The amount of divided muscle, defined by the length of the incision over the internal anal sphincter, differentiates these two approaches. Traditionally, the incision was made to the dentate line (associated with worse incontinence but less recurrence), but more conservative techniques transect the muscle to the level of the apex of the fissure [15].

Individualized care is imperative when deciding the length of the sphincterotomy, to properly balance the risk of incontinence with the healing of the fissure [16, 17]. Some factors to consider include but are not limited to age, gender, history of prior anorectal procedures, prior vaginal deliveries with or without episiotomies or tears, length of the anal canal, prior fissure treatments, consistency of the stools, medications, comorbidities, etc.

5.2.4 Fissurectomy

Fissurectomy has regained attention recently due to its simplicity and virtually no complications associated with the procedure. Whether or not the hypertrophic anal papilla and skin tag are excised, the curettage of the base of the fissure as well as the sharp excision of rolled and epithelialized edges, has been shown to promote healing. The goal is to create a fresh wound and remove fibrosis to facilitate healing by secondary intention. Recurrence rates are higher compared to LIS [18].

5.2.5 Advancement flaps

Patients without hypertonicity of the anal sphincter represent a special challenge, given that topical pharmacologic agents previously discussed aid with healing by relaxing the sphincter muscle. Cutaneous advancement flaps have been reported with excellent results in both types (hypertonic and hypotonic sphincter fissures), with high healing rates and no fecal incontinence [19]. Although this technique requires a certain degree of expertise, it offers a great alternative for patients without sphincter hypertonicity.

5.2.6 Surgical details

Performed as an outpatient procedure under spinal anesthesia is our preferred approach. Pre-operatively, patients receive fleet enemas the night before and the morning of the procedure. Patient are placed in prone Jack-knife position with both buttocks taped apart for a better exposure of the perianal area, and traditional sterile field preparation, a digital rectal examination and a circumferential anoscopy are performed. Antibiotics for surgical prophylaxis are not routinely offered in these cases. Fissurectomy is recommended to create a healthy bed of tissue that supports the cutaneous flap. A wide-base skin and subcutaneous tissue flap is created and advanced toward the anal canal providing full coverage of the fissure. Absorbable interrupted sutures are used to secure the flap in place. In our practice, we often create relaxing superficial incisions on the perianal skin to decrease the tension on the flap (**Figure 7**, **Table 2**).

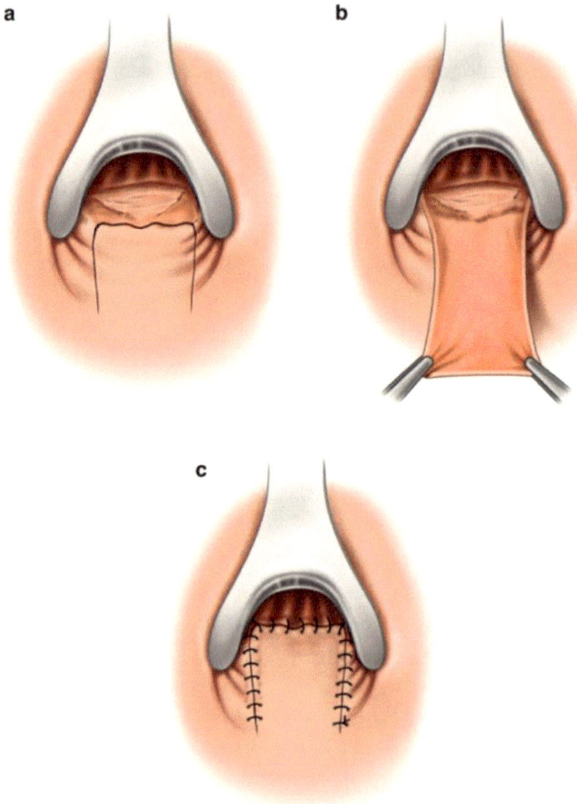

Figure 7.
Dermal advancement flap creation: (a) sharp incision over the skin adjacent to the fissure, (b) dissection of skin and subcutaneous tissue to create a flap, and (c) after advancing the flap over the fissure, it is secure using absorbable sutures (From: Feingold and Lee-Kong [20]).

Type of treatment	Use	Healing rates (%)	Recurrence	Side effects
Nonoperative management	Acute fissures Chronic fissures	80–90 36		
Calcium channel blockers	Chronic hypertonic fissures (first-line treatment)	71–92		Headaches
Nitrates	Chronic hypertonic fissures	49–68	51–67%	Headache 27–50%
Botulinum toxin	Chronic hypertonic fissures (second-line treatment)	45–73	28%	Fecal incontinence
Lateral internal sphincterotomy (LIS)	Chronic hypertonic fissures	93–96		Fecal incontinence 30–40%
Anocutaneous flap	Chronic hypotonic anal fissures	98		

Table 2.
Summary of types of treatments, healing rates and recurrence rates.

6. Special situations

6.1 Crohn's disease

Anal fissures are common in Chron's patients. The atypical location in the lateral quadrants of the anal canal associated with other local (such as fistulas) and systemic symptoms facilitate the diagnosis. These fissures appear as deep ulcerations of the anal area, and adequate treatment involves the management of Crohn's disease with systemic therapy, achieving resolution of symptoms in more than 50% of patients. Surgical intervention is recommended only in cases of complications such as abscesses; however, as a rule for this population of patients, excessive procedures should be avoided. **Figure 8** shows a right anterior anal fissure with an associated posterior midline anal fistula in a Crohn's patient.

6.1.1 Immunosuppressed patients

This subset of patients, particularly those with Human Immunodeficiency Virus (HIV) infection, can develop typical and atypical anal fissures. However, the management can be quite different from non-HIV patients due to comorbidities associated with the disease and its treatment. These include but are not limited to decreased sphincter tone, loose consistency of the stools, impaired wound healing, and increased risk of developing serious infection complications. Therefore, individualized care is strongly advised before determining the best approach.

6.1.2 Anoreceptive patients

Unfortunately, anal fissures are not uncommon in patients with anoreceptive sexual behavior, and this is caused by direct trauma over the anal canal. The management is like those without a history of anal intercourse, ensuring adequate bowel

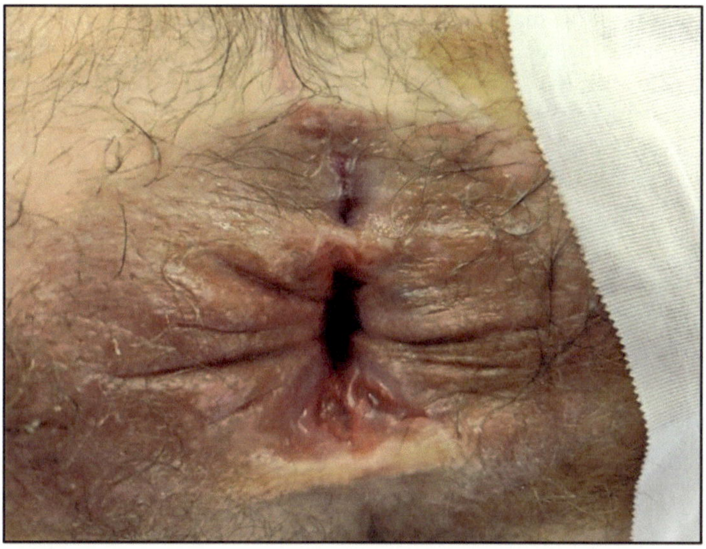

Figure 8.
Right anterior anal fissure with an associated posterior midline anal fistula in a Crohn's patient.

habits and stool consistency. Topical muscle relaxants are also routinely used, and patients are educated to abstain from anal intercourse for the duration of treatment to enable complete healing of the fissures. In cases of failure to nonoperative management, surgical procedures may be necessary; however, caution should be exercised due to the increased risk of fecal incontinence in this population. A thorough discussion of the risks and benefits of any surgical intervention is recommended.

Algorithm of treatment of anal fissure

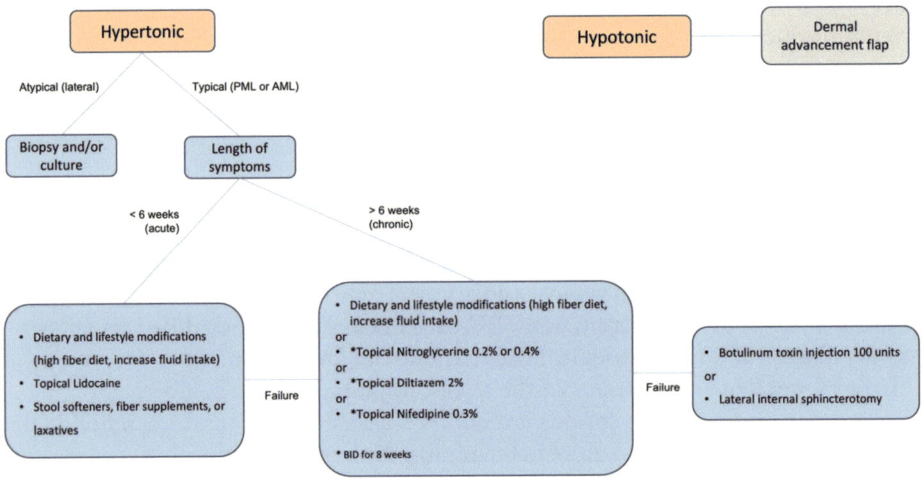

7. Conclusions

Chronic anal fissures are a common reason for colorectal surgery visits, and the diagnosis is usually made with a history of severe anal pain associated with evacuations and bright red bleeding, and physical examination findings of a tear in the anal canal. Nonoperative management with dietary modifications, bowel regimen, and topical muscle relaxants has high rates of achieving resolution of symptoms and healing of the fissures. In cases of failure despite proper medical treatment, a surgical intervention may be warranted. Internal lateral sphincterotomy is an excellent option with high success rates; however, a more conservative approach should be considered in those patients with an increased risk of incontinence. Low-tone fissures are effectively managed with dermal advancement flaps.

Author details

Nathalie Mantilla[1,2]* and Juaquito M. Jorge[3]

1 Cook County Health and Hospitals System, Chicago, IL, USA

2 Rush University, Chicago, IL, USA

3 Tiesenga Surgical Associates, Elmwood Park, IL, USA

*Address all correspondence to: nathaliemantilla@gmail.com

IntechOpen

© 2023 The Author(s). Licensee IntechOpen. This chapter is distributed under the terms of the Creative Commons Attribution License (http://creativecommons.org/licenses/by/3.0), which permits unrestricted use, distribution, and reproduction in any medium, provided the original work is properly cited.

References

[1] Davids JS, Hawkins AT, Bhama AR, Feinberg AE, Grieco MJ, Lightner AL, et al. The American Society of Colon and Rectal Surgeons Clinical Practice guidelines for the Management of Anal Fissures. Diseases of the Colon and Rectum. 2023;**66**(2):190-199. DOI: 10.1097/DCR.0000000000002664

[2] Nelson RL, Manuel D, Gumienny C, Spencer B, Patel K, Schmitt K, et al. A systematic review and meta-analysis of the treatment of anal fissure. Techniques in Coloproctology. 2017;**21**(8):605-625. DOI: 10.1007/s10151-017-1664-2

[3] Farouk R, Duthie GS, MacGregor AB, Bartolo DC. Sustained internal sphincter hypertonia in patients with chronic anal fissure. Diseases of the Colon and Rectum. 1994;**37**(5):424-429. DOI: 10.1007/BF02076185

[4] Nothmann BJ, Schuster MM. Internal anal sphincter derangement with anal fissures. Gastroenterology. 1974;**67**(2):216-220

[5] Gibbons CP, Read NW. Anal hypertonia in fissures: Cause or effect? The British Journal of Surgery. 1986;**73**(6):443-445. DOI: 10.1002/bjs.1800730609

[6] Lu KC, Herzig DO. Anal fissure. In: Steele SR, Hull TL, Read TE, editors. The ASCRS Textbook of Colon and Rectal Surgery. 3rd ed. Springer; 2016. pp. 205-214

[7] Jobanputra SP. Anal fissure. In: Corman ML, editor. Corman's Colon and Rectal Surgery. Lippincott Williams & Wilkins; 2013. pp. 346-366

[8] Jensen SL. Treatment of first episodes of acute anal fissure: Prospective randomised study of lignocaine ointment versus hydrocortisone ointment or warm sitz baths plus bran. British Medical Journal (Clinical Research Ed.). 1986;**292**(6529):1167-1169. DOI: 10.1136/bmj.292.6529.1167

[9] Nelson RL, Thomas K, Morgan J, Jones A. Non-surgical therapy for anal fissure. The Cochrane Database of Systematic Reviews. 2012;**2012**(2):CD003431. DOI: 10.1002/14651858.CD003431.pub3

[10] Bailey HR, Beck DE, Billingham RP, Binderow SR, Gottesman L, Hull TL, et al. A study to determine the nitroglycerin ointment dose and dosing interval that best promote the healing of chronic anal fissures. Diseases of the Colon and Rectum. 2002;**45**(9):1192-1199. DOI: 10.1007/s10350-004-6392-9

[11] Scholefield JH, Bock JU, Marla B, Richter HJ, Athanasiadis S, Pröls M, et al. A dose finding study with 0.1%, 0.2%, and 0.4% glyceryl trinitrate ointment in patients with chronic anal fissures. Gut. 2003;**52**(2):264-269. DOI: 10.1136/gut.52.2.264

[12] Nevins EJ, Kanakala V. Topical diltiazem and glyceryl-trinitrate for chronic anal fissure: A meta-analysis of randomised controlled trials. Turkish Journal of Surgery. 2020;**36**(4):347-352. DOI: 10.47717/turkjsurg.2020.4895

[13] Notaras MJ. Lateral subcutaneous sphincterotomy for anal fissure—A new technique. Proceedings of the Royal Society of Medicine. 1969;**62**(7):713

[14] Nelson RL, Chattopadhyay A, Brooks W, Platt I, Paavana T, Earl S.

Operative procedures for fissure in ano. The Cochrane Database of Systematic Reviews. 2011;**2011**(11):CD002199. DOI: 10.1002/14651858.CD002199.pub4

[15] Menteş BB, Ege B, Leventoglu S, Oguz M, Karadag A. Extent of lateral internal sphincterotomy: Up to the dentate line or up to the fissure apex? Diseases of the Colon and Rectum. 2005;**48**(2):365-370. DOI: 10.1007/s10350-004-0812-8

[16] Elsebae MM. A study of fecal incontinence in patients with chronic anal fissure: Prospective, randomized, controlled trial of the extent of internal anal sphincter division during lateral sphincterotomy. World Journal of Surgery. 2007;**31**(10):2052-2057. DOI: 10.1007/s00268-007-9177-1

[17] Menteş BB, Güner MK, Leventoglu S, Akyürek N. Fine-tuning of the extent of lateral internal sphincterotomy: Spasm-controlled vs. up to the fissure apex. Diseases of the Colon and Rectum. 2008;**51**(1):128-133. DOI: 10.1007/s10350-007-9121-3

[18] Bara BK, Mohanty SK, Behera SN, Sahoo AK, Swain SK. Fissurectomy versus lateral internal Sphincterotomy in the treatment of chronic anal fissure: A randomized control trial. Cureus. 2021;**13**(9):e18363. DOI: 10.7759/cureus.18363

[19] Magdy A, El Nakeeb A, Fouda el Y, Youssef M, Farid M. Comparative study of conventional lateral internal sphincterotomy, V-Y anoplasty, and tailored lateral internal sphincterotomy with V-Y anoplasty in the treatment of chronic anal fissure. Journal of Gastrointestinal Surgery: Official Journal of the Society for Surgery of the Alimentary Tract. 2012;**16**(10):1955-1962. DOI: 10.1007/s11605-012-1984-5

[20] Feingold DL, Lee-Kong SA. Anal fissure and anal stenosis. In: Beck DE, Steele SR, Wexner SD, editors. Fundamentals of Anorectal Surgery. Springer; 2019. pp. 241-255

Chapter 11

Using 3D High-Definition Manometry Evaluating Anal Canal Functions in Children with Congenital Anorectal Malformations: Clinical Studies from China

Weihong Guo, Jiawei Zhao, Yanan Zhang, Yu Xiong and Jinshi Huang

Abstract

Three-dimensional high-definition manometry was used in evaluating anorectal function of 142 post-operative patients with anorectal malformations (ARMs), while 104 non-operative children as controls (CON) who were subdivided into different age groups. Data were collected on the functional length (HPZ-length), resting and squeeze pressure (HPZ-rest, HPZ-sqze), recto-anal inhibitory reflex (RAIR), and strength distribution of the anal canal. The results showed a gradual increase in anal canal function parameters with age in normal infants and children, suggesting that age should be considered as an essential factor when evaluating post-operative anorectal function in ARMs patients. Comparing with CON, a significant decrease in HPZ-rest was observed in all post-operative ARMs groups ($p < 0.05$). The majority of ARMs patients with incontinence had significantly lower HPZ-rest and a higher percentage of asymmetric strength distribution compared to those with continence ($p < 0.05$). The type classification of high and cloaca in ARMs, as well as low HPZ-rest, were identified as two factors affecting post-operative functional outcomes. Manometry is a valuable modality providing distinct details of anal function in the assessment of the underlying functional causes of postoperative defecation disorder, thus helping physicians select the right modality of treatment. Sequential manometry studies are useful for re-evaluating anal function after treatment and biofeedback training.

Keywords: anorectal manometry, anorectal function, anorectal malformation, post-operative anal function, long-term post-operative complication

1. Introduction

Congenital anorectal malformations (ARMs) are developmental malformations of the end digestive tract, with an incidence of 3.17 cases per 10,000 population in China, and 1 case per 5000 live births worldwide [1, 2]. Subsequent surgical interventions in early infancy can be mild, severe, or complex, depending on the type of classification of ARMs. Their post-operative functional outcomes varied, even though they had been treated excellently by the surgery. In other words, ARMs are anatomical or structural abnormalities that need to be repaired, but they are not abnormalities that can simply be corrected by definitive surgery. Whether the reconstructed anus will gain bowel function similar to that of the average person is the most critical concern of both parents and surgeons. Once post-operative complications occur, especially in those with minor abnormalities, parents may be suspicious of surgical management, while surgeons may blame poor development of the anorectum itself.

Constipation and fecal incontinence are common functional complications seen during long-term follow-up. Normally, the post-operative function is assessed using the conventional clinical scoring system based on subjective parameters, such as the number of defecation and the ability to have voluntary bowel movement [3, 4]. Poor scores undoubtedly reflect impaired anorectal function, but they are not a reliable criterion for assessing the outcome of surgical treatment or the function of the reconstructed anorectal canal. In the latter case, a variety of factors are involved in bowel movement, such as the development of muscle complexes, rectal sensation, and reflexes. Even an improper diet may cause constipation or soiling.

Image studies such as ultrasound, MRI, contrast enemas, and manometry are the objective assessment methods commonly used to evaluate the function of the newly constructed anorectal canal. Ultrasound and MRI are studies concerning the anatomical structure (e.g. the position of the constructed anorectal canal) and the development of the muscle complex, whereas the enema and manometry provide valuable information about bowel movement. Recently, three-dimensional (3D) high-definition anorectal manometry has been believed to be a precise tool for assessing defecation function because it provides quantitative objective measurements in real-time and dynamically [5, 6]. It offers imaging and helps understand the functional and potential pathophysiology of functional anorectal disorders. In this chapter, we present our study of the use of 3D high-definition manometry in the evaluation of anal canal function in ARMs patients and their non-operative controls.

2. Materials and methods

2.1 Patients

2.1.1 Non-operative control

Non-operative control (CON) patients enrolled were those who underwent 3D manometry at Beijing Children's Hospital from November 2014 to January 2019. Inclusion criteria are as follows: patients without organic anorectal diseases (as determined by imaging studies and rectal mucosal biopsy) are included; and patients have normal bowel habits during clinical follow-up though they had manometry exams because of irregular bowel movements. Exclusion criteria included patients with Hirchsprung's disease (HD) and those with a history of anorectal-related surgery, with spinal cord or vertebral deformity. Of these controls, 71 children were selected as the age-matched CON when compared to patients with post-operative ARMs.

2.1.2 Congenital anorectal malformations patient

We conducted a retrospective review of all patients with ARMs admitted to Beijing Children's Hospital between January 2015 and December 2019. A total of 171 measurements were performed on 142 post-operative patients who received follow-up at our outpatient clinic. Among them, 10 patients who had previously undergone surgical repair at their local hospitals came to our clinic because of poor post-operative outcomes. The remaining 132 patients who underwent surgery at our hospital were subjected to routine follow-up starting 3 months after surgery, regardless of the presence of complications. Repeated manometric examinations were conducted on patients with impaired bowel function, either after conservative management or simply as they advanced in age.

Post-operative outcomes were rated as good, fair, or poor based on a patient's bowel movements. "Good" refers to the condition in which patients have regular bowel movements without any complaint of defecation. "Fair" refers to mild and controllable constipation and soiling conditions. In the former, constipation is treatable with oral medication or laxatives, while in the latter, only occasional episodes of dirty pants may occur during sleep, coughing, or diarrhea. "Poor" indicates severe constipation and frequent incontinence to the extent that regular bowel management is often needed.

2.1.3 Classification of patients

General information on the types of ARMs and their surgical management was obtained through an electronic medical record system. At the outpatient follow-up clinic, manometry measurement was conducted following a physical examination. Both CON and ARMs patients were asked to complete a questionnaire about their dietary and bowel habits. In manometric examination, non-operative CON were divided into four groups based on age: ≤1 month, 1–12 months, 1–4 years, and > 4 years. The rules of age grouping were quoted from our previous study [7] and those of others. The age divisions of less than 1 month and 1 month to a year were selected in accordance with Kumar's study [8], while the next dividing age four was originated from the Rome IV questionnaire [9]. The studies were approved by the Medical Ethics Committee of Beijing Children's Hospital (2018-K-129), and the patient consent requirement was waived.

2.2 Anorectal manometry

A high-definition manometry catheter (ManoScan 360HD, Sierra Scientific Instruments, Los Angeles, California) was used to determine the mean pressure of the anal canal with the implemented Smartmouse™ and its software algorithm (ManoView analysis software, Sierra Scientific Instruments, Los Angeles, California). The patient lays either supine or in a lateral position. A lubricated catheter (10.75 mm in diameter, 6.4 cm in length equipped with 256 pressure sensors in 16 rows and 16 circumferentially oriented) was inserted into the anus and the pressure was calibrated to the baseline position. When the proximal and distal ends of the high-pressure zone were established with the aid of the Smartmouse™, the following parameters were collected: (1) the length of the anorectal high-pressure zone (HPZ-length); (2) the mean resting pressure (HPZ-rest); (3) the mean squeeze pressure (HPZ-sqze), via measuring passive contractions induced by applying perianal pricks in patients under 4 years of age and voluntary contraction in those older than 4; (4) recto-anal inhibitory reflex (RAIR), RAIR was considered positive when a decrease of 25% or more in the resting pressure was achieved; (5) the strength distribution of the anal canal, as shown in Video 1 (https://bit.ly/3IkMJxs), in which the anal pressure and strength distribution could be viewed and calculated in the 2D topographic color plot of all pressure transducers when the 3D column plot was cut along the anterior line. Detailed anorectal manometry procedures can be quoted from our previous study [7]. All procedures were performed by the same registered nurse, and the results were analyzed by two senior physicians.

2.3 Statistical methods

All analyses were performed using SPSS, version 23.0 (IBM Corp, Armonk, NY), in which statistical significance was considered when the p-value was less than 0.05. Mean $\pm$ SD of numerical variable data between groups were compared using the Student's t-test. Fisher or $\chi 2$ test was used in categorical variable data, such as rate or proportion between group comparisons. Pearson or Spearman correlation coefficients and logistic regression analysis were applied to analyze the correlation as well as the impact factors on the postoperative anal function.

3. Results

3.1 Congenital anorectal malformations patients (ARMs)

One hundred forty-two patients (61 boys and 81 girls) ranging in age from 3 months to 15 years (median 1.71 years) were included in the surgery group. Based on the level of the rectum in relation to the levator ani muscle, the ARMs were classified into high (10%), intermediate (28%), and low type (62%) by Wingspread classification [10, 11]. Types of fistulas were classified as follows: no fistula (1%); anocutaneous fistula (42%); rectovestibular fistula (25%); rectobulbar-urethral fistula (17%); rectoprostatic-urethral fistula and rectovesical fistula (5%); rectovaginal fistula (6%); and cloaca (4%). Post-operative fecal continence was socially acceptable in 80% of the patients, 50% of whom having good functional outcomes, and 30% having fair ones. The remaining 20% were patients with poor outcomes, in which fecal incontinence and severe constipation were seen, with the former cases more than the latter. The detailed patient information presented in **Table 1** is derived from our previous study [12].

3.2 Anorectal manometry of the anorectal canal

3.2.1 General information of manometry in ARMs patients vs. CON

Quoted from our previous studies, the results of the correlation analysis between age and manometric parameters in non-operative CON revealed a positive correlation between age and manometric parameters, specifically HPZ-length, HPZ-rest, and HPZ-sqze measurements, indicating that anal length and pressure were influenced by

		Good (n = 72)	Fair (n = 42)		Poor (n = 28)	
			Constipation (n = 20)	Soiling (n = 22)	Severe constipation (n = 8)	Incontinence (n = 20)
Male:female		32:44	7:13	10:12	3:5	9:11
Low	Without fistula	1	0	0	0	1
	Anocutaneous fistula	34	11	10	2	3
	Anovestibular fistula	17	3	3	2	1
Intermediate	Without fistula	0	0	0	0	0
	Rectobulbar-urethral fistula	12	1	5	1	5
	Rectovestibular fistula	2	1	1	3	3
	Rectovaginal fistula	3	2	0	0	1
High	Without fistula	0	0	0	0	0
	Rectoprostatic-urethral fistula/ rectovesical fistula	2	0	2	0	3
	Rectovaginal fistula	0	0	1	0	1
Cloaca		1	2	0	0	2
Associated spinal/vertebral deformity		10	6	4	5	6

"Good" refers to regular bowel movement. "Fair" refers to constipation but could be solved by oral medication or laxatives, as well as occasional dirty pants occurred during sleep, cough, and diarrhea. "Poor" refers to severe constipation that bowel management (e.g., enema) was needed, whereas incontinence refers to a recurrent involuntary loss of liquid and/or solid stool in older children and frequent dirty pants in toddlers.

Table 1.
Characteristics of 142 ARMs patients and post-operative functional outcomes.

advancing age (**Figure 1**). When the reconstructed anal canal were compared with their age-matched non-operative CON, significantly lower HPZ-rest was observed in all post-operative groups (**Table 2**) [12].

In the study of anal strength distribution, asymmetric pressure distribution could be observed in both resting and contracting periods in patients, and even in the CON. Meanwhile, asymmetric strength distribution was also frequently seen in ARMs group regardless of surgical approaches taken (Video 2, https://bit.ly/3IkMJxs). When compared to CON, a significantly higher percentage of the asymmetric strength

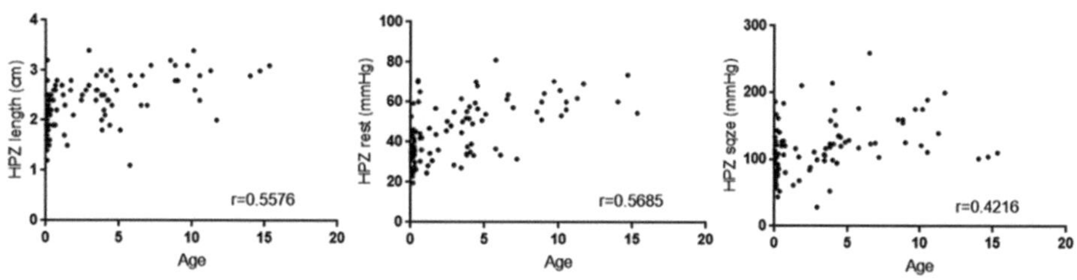

Figure 1.
Scatter plot with linear trend line for age and HPZ-length, HPZ-rest, and HPZ-sqze in CON.

Age group	Number	HPZ-length (cm)		P-value	HPZ-rest (mmHg)		P-value	HPZ-sqze (mmHg)		P-value
	ARMs:CON	ARMs	CON		ARMs	CON		ARMs	CON	
3–12 m	30:16	2.48 ± 0.46	2.32 ± 0.34	0.172	32.72 ± 12.30	43.94 ± 14.86	0.002*	108.11 ± 35.35	114.59 ± 34.60	0.525
1–4y	82:24	2.65 ± 0.52	2.45 ± 0.42	0.099	28.08 ± 10.54	43.05 ± 11.12	<0.001*	99.78 ± 35.13	107.90 ± 45.30	0.410
>4y	30:31	2.69 ± 0.60	2.64 ± 0.50	0.713	28.38 ± 11.90	55.97 ± 12.72	<0.001*	91.04 ± 29.74	141.46 ± 35.69	<0.001*
Total	142:71	2.57 ± 0.51	2.50 ± 0.45	0.307	30.43 ± 11.80	48.89 ± 14.03	<0.001*	102.61 ± 34.84	125.09 ± 41.21	<0.001*

The difference was statistically significant.
HPZ-length: the functional length of anorectal high-pressure zone; HPZ-rest: resting pressure of high-pressure zone; HPZ-sqze: squeeze pressure of high-pressure zone. Data was reported as mean ± standard deviation.

Table 2.
Comparison of basic manometric parameters between ARMs patients and non-operative CON.

distribution was seen in ARMs patients during both resting and squeezed phases (Video 3, https://bit.ly/3IkMJxs).

3.2.2 Comparison between good and poor functional outcomes in ARMs patients

Figure 2 shows our previous statistic results indicating that the incontinence ARMs individuals had significantly higher proportions of lower HPZ-rest, negative RAIR, and asymmetric distribution in the squeeze phase [12]. As there were no significant differences observed in the manometric parameters among adjacent age groups in ARMs patients, the mean values of each measurement were calculated and compared between the "Good + Fair" and "Poor" function groups, as well as CON. As shown in **Table 3**, all parameters of the functional "Good + Fair" group were comparable with CON, while significantly lower HPZ-rest and HPZ-sqze were observed in the functional "Poor" group.

3.2.3 Repeated manometry in ARMs patients with defection disorders

A total of 28 patients with ARMs had more than one measurement study, and 27 of them underwent their initial measurement study between 8 and 24 months of age during routine clinical follow-up. A female patient, who underwent primary surgery at birth at a local hospital, underwent her first manometry at the age of 6 due to chronic constipation. Subsequent examinations were performed as needed, either for

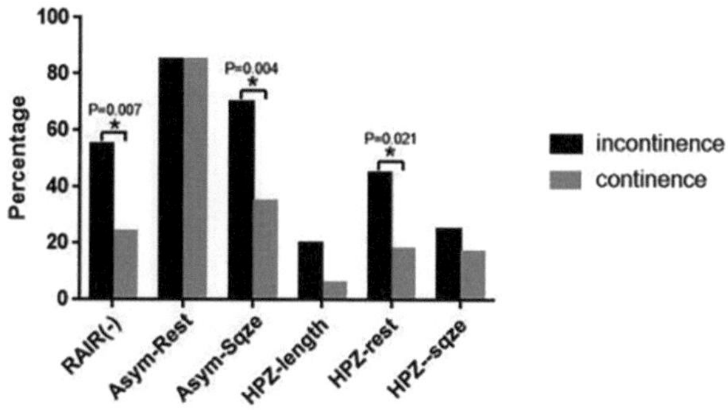

Figure 2.
Statistic results of comparing the patient number of the poor manometric parameter in ARMs between incontinence and continence group.

	HPZ-length (cm)	HPZ-rest (mmHg)	HPZ-sqze (mmHg)
Poor	2.775 ± 0.5961	26 ± 11.553*	90.57 ± 32.434*
Good + Fair	2.535 ± 0.4632	31.22 ± 11.569	104.87 ± 33.089
CON	2.50 ± 0.45	48.89 ± 14.03	125.09 ± 41.21

**The difference was statistically significant vs. Good + Fair.*
"Good" refers to regular bowel movement. "Fair" refers to constipation but could be solved by oral medication or laxatives, as well as occasional dirty pants occurred during sleep, cough, and diarrhea. "Poor" refers to severe constipation that bowel management (e.g., enema) was needed, whereas incontinence refers to a recurrent involuntary loss of liquid and/or solid stool in older children and frequent dirty pants in toddlers.

Table 3.
Comparison of basic manometric parameters between good and poor functional outcomes in ARMs patients.

Group	Manometry	Functional outcome					Abnormal Manometric parameters				Classification of ARMS			Associated spinal/ vertebral deformity		Contrast enema		Treatment	
		Good	Fair		Poor		HPZ-Length	HPZ-Rest	HPZ-Sqze	RAIR (−)	Low	Inter-mediate	High/ cloaca	Yes	No	Normal	Dilated Colon	Diet/Drug/ Biofeed-back	Surgical
			Consti-pation	Soil-ing	SC	IC													
Group 1 (N = 10)	Initial	10	0	0	0	0	—	<(N = 2)	—	1	10	0	0	N/A	N/A	N/A	N/A	Diet (N = 4)	0
	Repeated	10	0	0	0	0	—	<(N = 2)	—	1									
Group 2 (N = 9)	Initial	9	0	0	0	0	—	—	—	4	7	2	0	1	6	4	2	Diet (N = 7) Drug (N = 1) Biofeed-back (N = 1)	Biopsy (N = 3)
	Repeated	0	3	5	0	1	>(N = 1)	<(N = 6)	<(N = 3)	3									
Group 3 (N = 9)	Initial	0	5	3	0	1	>(N = 1)	<(N = 2)	—	6	3	4	1/1	3	6	5	4	Diet (N = 4) Biofeed-back (N = 2)	Curra-rino (N = 2) HD (N = 1)
	Repeated	3	4	1	0	1	—	<(N = 2)	<(N = 2)	4									

"—" indicates the values were comparable with mean; < represents the value was lower than mean-SD; > represents the value was higher than mean + SD
SC represents severe constipation; IC represents incontinence.

Table 4.
Clinical information of ARMs patients who had repeated manometric measurement.

the purpose of re-evaluation of impaired anal function or in response to parental requests as the child grew older. The details of these patients, categorized into three groups according to their functional and initial manometric assessments, are summarized in **Table 4**. Patients in Group 2 were those who had good bowel behavior at the time of initial follow-up. They came back to the clinic because of episodes of bowel movement problems. This could happen at any age. In this situation, repeated measurements were conducted. Comparing with their initial measurements, some of the measurements showed values lower than the mean-SD of their age-matched controls. Further subsequent investigations (such as X-ray, contrast enema, MRI, ultrasound, and biopsy) were conducted to rule out any associated pathology. The abnormal defecation in seven patients (four with dirty pants and three with constipation) was alleviated or improved through dietary adjustments, despite some of them having lower HPZ-rest or HPZ-sqze. Patients in Group 3 who had poor or fair function at the time of initial examination were those who required further investigation and treatment. Currarino syndrome was found in two cases of low-type ARMs with constipation who underwent a simple anoplasty procedure at birth at a local hospital. During physical examination, an incorrect position of the constructed anus was identified. Additionally, strange anal canal pressure distribution with an extra length of HPZ-length was seen in one of the patients (**Figure 3**). After surgical removal of the tumor, soiling rather than constipation occurred, and repeated manometry was performed at the age of 2 years. Results showed that the HPZ-sqze was considerably improved compared with the initial measurement, and anal canal strength distribution was also improved although there was still significant weakness seen in the posterior quadrant during squeezing. In another case, a 6-year-old girl, who came to our clinic for an

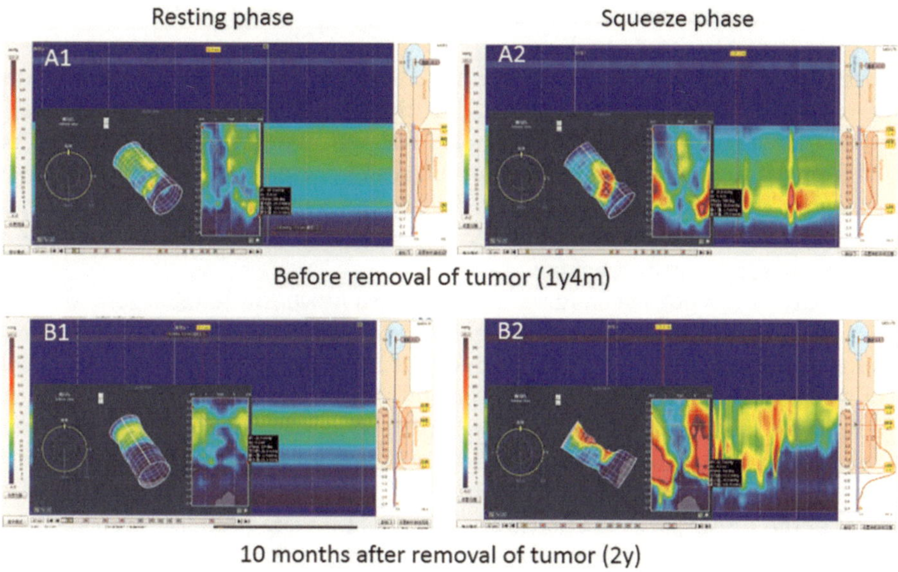

Figure 3.
3D and plane pressure maps of anal canal strength distribution in a post-operative AMRs patient associated with Currarino syndrome. A boy aged 1y4m presented with constipation and underwent primary simple ano-plasty at birth. A 6 × 5 × 3 cm anterior sacral mass (teratoma) and sacrococcygeal deformity were confirmed. Before tumor removal, an extra length of HPZ was observed in both resting (A1) and squeeze phases (A2). A manometric examination was repeated at the age of 2y (10 months after surgery) due to incontinence. The HPZ-length was comparable to the age-matched mean ± SD. Significant posterior weakness in strength distribution was observed in both resting (B1) and squeeze phases (B2).

initial examination, had been suffering from chronic constipation since her primary surgery for an intermediate type of rectalvestibular fistula in early infancy. The initial manometric measurements were comparable to the mean ± SD of her age-matched group, except for a negative RAIR. In subsequent investigations, sacrococcygeal malformations were observed on X-rays, and a dilated colon was identified during contrast studies. The diagnosis of HD was confirmed through rectal biopsy, followed by treatment with a pull-through procedure. Repeated post-treatment measurements showed a slightly lower HPZ-sqze, while other measurements remain comparable to the initial ones.

4. Discussion

Congenital anorectal malformations are developmental defects located at the end of the digestive tract that require surgical reconstruction of the anal canal to achieve defecation. The common long-term post-operative complications include constipation and fecal incontinence [13]. The clinical scoring systems commonly used for post-operative assessment of ARMs are inadequate in accurately assessing the function of the reconstructed anal canal and its role in defecation and continence. The reason is that defecation patterns can be influenced by multiple factors involved in the mechanism.

The anorectal manometric study is essential for evaluating restorative surgical procedures of the anorectal area for both adults and children, bearing the advantages of being non-invasive, safe, and intuitive [14, 15]. The development of solid catheters with sensors has enabled precise measurement (high definition), while 3D pressure modeling provides more accurate and detailed data that can be used to assess functional disorders of the anal canal.

Several studies have utilized manometry to evaluate the post-operative anal function among patients with different types of ARMs or different surgical procedures, but none of them was done with a non-operative control group [16, 17]. During the period from infancy to childhood, both physical and anatomical development proceeds rapidly before reaching a state of maturity and stability. Therefore, it is important to learn the functional capacity of the anal canal of a normal child at the same age before assessing a reconstructed one.

Our study of 104 normal children, ranging from newborns to teenagers, showed age-dependent increases in functional anal length, resting pressure, and squeezing pressure. A gradual increase in major manometric measurements was seen until the age of 4 years, suggesting that age is a crucial factor to consider when evaluating anal canal function in early childhood. Comparing mean manometric measurements without considering the age of the ARMs patient will not yield accurate statistical results, as post-operative complications can occur at any age.

Most of the ARMs patients in our recent study [12] were routinely followed up at the scheduled time after surgery, regardless of whether they had any complications or not. The manometric parameters collected could reflect the general situation of the "neo-anus" after reconstruction surgery. The results showed a comparable HPZ-length of with the non-operative CON ones in all age-matched groups, but a significantly lower HPZ-rest.

The high-pressure zone at the distal anus is believed to be the key mechanism of fecal continence. The high pressure required for anal continence is maintained by sphincter complexes, with the internal anal sphincter (IAS) contributing approximately 50–85% of resting phase pressure, while the external sphincter (EAS) and puborectalis working coordinately during the squeeze phase. This high-pressure zone is rather a functional structure than an anatomic one, which can be measured by the algorithm of analysis software and presented as the length of the area where the resting anal pressures exceed the resting intrarectal pressure by at least 5 mmHg in manometry. With this understanding, it is not difficult to explain our results in ARMs patients. However, significantly lower HPZ-rest values were observed in the majority of patients with incontinence ARMs compared to those with continence ARMs, indicating weak or degenerated IAS, regardless of whether this was due to poor primary development or damage from surgical dissection.

The external sphincter is a voluntary striated muscle that completely surrounds the anal canal and rectum and is divided into subcutaneous, superficial, and deep parts through the longitudinal and anal levator ani fibers. The HPZ-sqze is an indicator of voluntary contractions resulting from coordinate contractions in the unique triple-looped anatomy of the EAS complex and puborectalis. Any type of anal reconstructive surgery has the potential to affect local muscles and nerves. The selection of a surgical procedure should be based on the surgeon's experience in dealing with patients with different classifications of ARMs. One of the key steps is to place in the end of the rectum at the correct anatomical position so that it would be surrounded by the muscle complex. Statistical analysis of our study shows that functional outcomes were only correlated with the classification of the ARMs, not with surgical approaches. This indicates that the optimal functional outcome can be achieved with meticulous manipulation. If the effects of surgical manipulation are excluded, the underdeveloped anorectal structures, including sphincter muscle complexes and neural networks, seen more frequently in patients with high-type ARMs and cloacae, may be a major cause of inadequate functional outcomes. Conversely, factors other than abnormal embryonic development of the sphincter and nervous system should be considered in patients with ARMs who are not classified as high type but who claim incontinence. Extensive dissection or rough manipulation during surgery might result in damage to local muscles and nerves, while the incorrect placement of the anal canal would result in the risk of a newly reconstructed anus not properly surrounded by EAS.

With 3D models, asymmetry strength distribution of the anal canal was also seen in the non-operative CON as what has been observed in adults [18]. The reason for this may be attributed to the uneven development of different muscles leading to unbalanced sphincter complex response for maintaining the high pressure zone. In patients with ARMs, hypo-development of the anal sphincter complex in different degrees is common and may alter the pressure distribution. Image studies, such as MRI [19] and ultrasound [20], are recommended to identify the development of muscle complex and the location of the neo-anus in order to determine whether weakness is due to poor development or incorrect placement of the anal canal.

The mechanisms of RAIR and the neural pathways of reflex have remained unknown, though its prominent role in normal defecation and sensation is believed to depend upon the intrinsic intramural nerve network regulated by the sacral medullary [21]. A recent systematic review [22] concluded that the absence of RAIR indicated low quality or damage of the IAS, which might be due to poorly developed anorectal structures in ARMs patients with poor continence. In our series of ARMs studies, a higher incidence of negative RAIR and significantly lower HPZ-rest in the incontinence ARMs patients suggested poor sensation and weakness of their IASs. Negative RAIR is usually associated with an HD diagnosis. Although the coexistence of ARMs and HD is rare, accounting for only about 2% in ARMs patients according to a previous study [23], it is still necessary to rule out HD via biopsy, as reminded in our study in which one case of such combined symptoms was identified.

In a previous study [24] that compared four different scoring systems (Holschneider's, Rintala's, Krickenbeck's, and Peña's Questionnaires) based on anorectal manometry measurements, it was recommended that Holschneider's and Rintala's questionnaires be used in patients' follow-up, while Peña's and Krickenbeck's questionnaires in determining a proper bowel management program for patients rather than patients' follow up. Up to now, there is no widely accepted method for assessing the follow-up of patients with ARMs. Although it is difficult to identify the reasons for bowel functional outcomes using independent scoring systems, evaluations using questionnaires and scoring systems are certainly the first step. General information about bowel movement patterns should be collected ahead of any anorectal manometry. Very likely, patients or their parents may overstate the severity of "poor bowel functions" when completing a questionnaire. Therefore, it is important to ask detailed questions, such as daily diets (including any special food that may induce either constipation or soiling), medications taken, and other situations that may affect bowel movements. After a physical examination and clinical assessment, manometry and necessary radiographic studies should be performed to rule out other associated birth defects (spinal malformation or Currarino syndrome), and sometimes even a biopsy should be run to exclude HD. One fecal incontinence patient had comparable anorectal manometric parameters with her age-matched ARMs patients who having "Good and Fair" functional outcomes. Using this diagnostic algorithm, an infectious rectovestibular fistula was eventually diagnosed through careful physical examination, ultrasound, and contrast enema studies.

Conservative treatment is initially recommended for individuals with poor manometric measurements, which may include dietary fiber supplementation, stool modification drugs, biofeedback physiotherapy, trans-anal irrigation, or a combination of these interventions. After a certain period of treatment (at least 3 months), a subsequent manometric examination is conducted to assess the potential improvements in comparison with the previously measured parameters.

Fecal continence may be affected by extrinsic factors beyond the anorectum. The regulation and control of defecation (continence) depend upon the interaction between local anatomical structures, such as anorectum and pelvic floor musculature, and physiological systems, primarily involving nerves and cognitive. However, our current study is limited by the fact that most of our ARMs patients were relatively young, and only a few patients were able to complete such tests as defecation perception and simulated defecation.

Although anorectal manometry is now the most widely used investigational tool for detecting abnormalities in anorectal coordination and/or anal sphincter complex dysfunction, as stated in a recent systematic review on anorectal manometry in children who have undergone ARMs repair, it remains clinically challenging to determine the definitive thresholds for sphincter dysfunction that may lead to fecal incontinence [25].

According to their systematic review [25], manometric studies have been performed for the purpose of comparing different types of ARMs, evaluating operative techniques, assessing post-operative modalities, predicting bowel function, and investigating the pathophysiology and management of post-operative bowel dysfunction. Different manometric equipment, assessment protocols, and parameter definitions used in various studies have led to significant deviation in results. For example, in the efforts to identify abnormalities in anorectal function, what is considered "normal" was rarely provided or described in a clear definition. This makes it difficult to interpret the findings and compare data between different studies. Our current studies were based upon the understanding of the "normal" pediatric physiology, and such a criterion was held persistently from the design stage until post-operative determination of abnormalities. We recommend using the same measurement equipment or the same model and standardization procedure and having the same team collect and analyze the data to minimize confounding factors. In addition, the collection of manometry parameters of non-operative CON to establish a "normal"

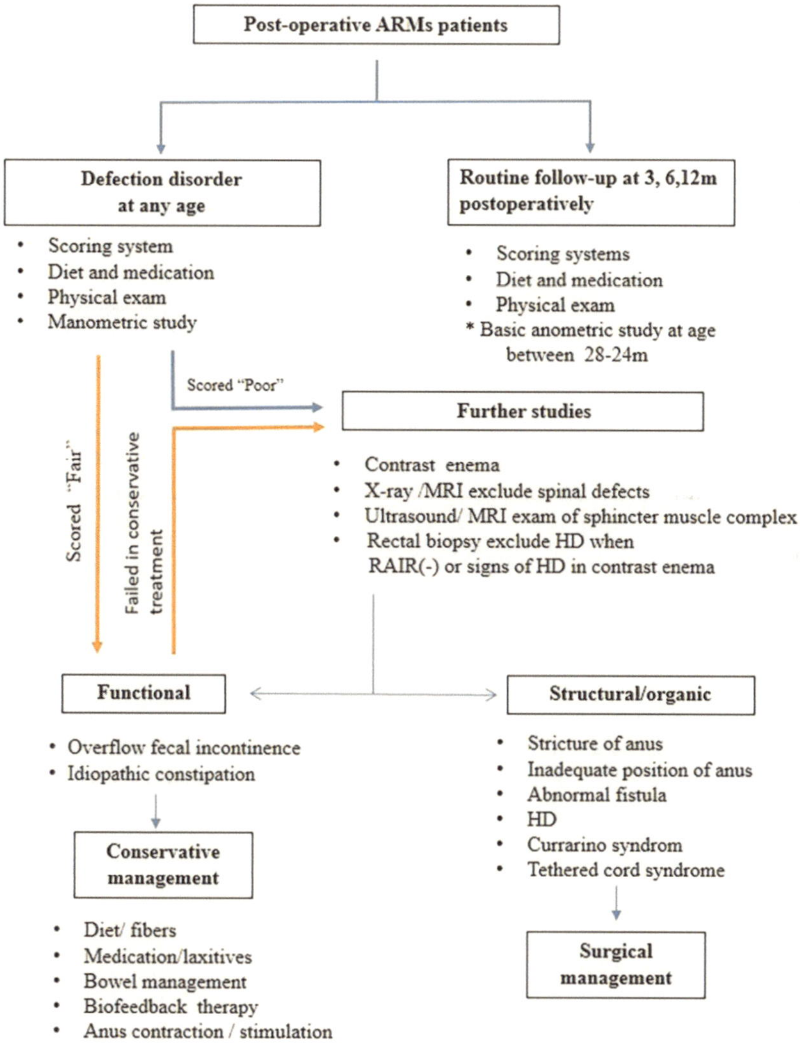

Figure 4.
*An algorithm presenting the proposed pathway for assessment of post-operative anal function. Routine follow-up at the outpatient clinic is recommended at 3, 6, 12 months after the operation. * One single manometric exam between 18 and 24 months of age is recommended to collect basic parameters of the anal canal even in the absence of any complications. Once defecation disorder occurs, patients classified as "Fair" with normal manometric results may be considered as having a functional disorder and initially managed with conservative treatment. Patients classified as "Poor", as well as those who failed with conservative treatment should undergo further investigations to exclude other associated disease or surgery-related structural problems.*

reference for future assessment of patients who may undergo any kind of anorectal surgeries and further prognostic training and evaluation. There is no need for frequent manometric studies in patients who underwent an anorectal surgery during early infancy, but even in the absence of any complications, one single manometric exam between the ages of 18–24 months is recommended. Within the first year of toddlerhood, the rapid physical development of the anal rectum is complete and the transition from formula to a solid food diet has been completed, making them ready for toilet training. Such a manometric record will provide basic information on the individuals with reconstructed anal canal in case of later occurrence of defecation disorder, since it may happen at any age (**Figure 4**). For those who have poor anal function, a long-term follow-up is necessary as the defecation problems may persist into adolescent or even adulthood. Therapeutic strategies should be carefully considered together with manometric findings. Manometric records provide valuable information regarding the actual origin of continence problems that may not always be clinically distinguished.

5. Conclusions

To conclude our study, age should be considered as an essential factor when evaluating post-operative anorectal function in ARMs patients. Classification of high-type and cloaca in ARMs and low HPZ-rest are two factors that affect post-operative functional outcomes. Different operative procedures or approaches do not affect the functional outcomes. 3D high-definition manometry is a valuable modality to provide accurate details of anal function based on age-matched non-operative CON in early childhood. The proper assessment will provide physicians with information on potential causes of complications, meanwhile, it will also provide the guidelines for the selection of adequate treatment modalities.

Acknowledgements

No funding was received to support this study. Weihong Guo designed the research study; Jiawei Zhao, Yanan Zhang, Yu Xiong, and Weihong Guo performed the research; Yanan Zhang, Weihong Guo interpreted data; Jiawei Zhao, Weihong Guo analyzed the data and wrote the paper.

Conflict of interest

The authors declare no conflict of interest.

Abbreviations

ARMs	anorectal malformations
HPZ	anorectal high-pressure zone
HPZ-length	the length of HPZ
HPZ-rest	the mean resting pressure of HPZ
HPZ-sqze	the mean squeeze pressure of HPZ

RAIR	recto-anal inhibitory reflex
HD	Hirschsprung's disease
IAS	internal anal sphincter
EAS	external anal sphincter

Author details

Weihong Guo*, Jiawei Zhao, Yanan Zhang, Yu Xiong and Jinshi Huang
Department of Neonatal Surgery, Beijing Children's Hospital, Capital Medical University, National Center for Children's Health, Beijing, China

*Address all correspondence to: guo_weihong@163.com

IntechOpen

© 2024 The Author(s). Licensee IntechOpen. This chapter is distributed under the terms of the Creative Commons Attribution License (http://creativecommons.org/licenses/by/3.0), which permits unrestricted use, distribution, and reproduction in any medium, provided the original work is properly cited.

References

[1] Yuan P, Qiao L, Dai L, et al. Spatial distribution patterns of anorectal atresia/stenosis in China: Use of two-dimensional graph-theoretical clustering. World Journal of Gastroenterology. 2009;**15**:2787-2793. DOI: 10.3748/wjg.15.2787

[2] Nah SA, Ong CCP, Safari SE, et al. Anorectal malformation & Hirschsprung's disease: A cross-sectional comparison of quality of life and bowel function to healthy controls. Journal of Pediatric Surgery. 2018;**53**:1550-1554. DOI: 10.1016/j.jpedsurg.2017.08.018

[3] Rintala R, Mildh L, Lindahl H. Fecal continence and quality of life for adult patients with an operated high or intermediate anorectal malformation. Journal of Pediatric Surgery. 1994;**29**: 777-780. DOI: 10.1016/0022-3468(94) 90368-9

[4] Holschneider A, Hutson J, Peña A, et al. Preliminary report on the international conference for the development of standards for the treatment of anorectal malformations. Journal of Pediatric Surgery. 2005;**40**: 1521-1526. DOI: 10.1016/j. jpedsurg.2005.08.002

[5] Carrington E, Knowles C, Grossi U, Scott S. High-resolution anorectal manometry measures are more accurate than conventional measures in detecting anal hypocontractility in women with fecal incontinence. Clinical Gastroenterology and Hepatology. 2019; **17**:477-485.e479. DOI: 10.1016/j. cgh.2018.06.037

[6] Ambartsumyan L, Shaffer M, Carlin K, Nurko S. Comparison of longitudinal and radial characteristics of intra-anal pressures using 3D high-definition anorectal manometry between children with anoretal malformations and functional constipation. Neurogastroenterology and Motility. 2021;**33**:e13971. DOI: 10.1111/nmo.13971

[7] Zhao J, Zhang Y, Xiong Y, et al. Three dimension high-definition manometry in evaluation of anorectal function in 104 normal infants and children: A clinical study from China. Neurogastro-enterology and Motility. 2022;**34**:e14395. DOI: 10.1111/nmo.14395

[8] Kumar S, Ramadan S, Gupta V, et al. Manometric tests of anorectal function in 90 healthy children: A clinical study from Kuwait. Journal of Pediatric Surgery. 2009;**44**:1786-1790. DOI: 10.1016/j.jpedsurg.2009.01.008

[9] Baaleman D, Velasco-Benítez C, Méndez-Guzmán L, Benninga M, Saps M. Functional gastrointestinal disorders in children: Agreement between Rome III and Rome IV diagnoses. European Journal of Pediatrics. 2021;**180**:2297-2303. DOI: 10.1007/s00431-021-04013-2

[10] Stephens F. Wingspread anomalies, rarities, and super rarities of the anorectum and cloaca. Birth Defects Original Article Series. 1988;**24**:581-585

[11] Wood R, Levitt M. Anorectal malformations. Clinics in Colon and Rectal Surgery. 2018;**31**: 61-70. DOI: 10.1055/s-0037-1609020

[12] Divarci E, Ergun O. General complications after surgery for anorectal malformations. Pediatric Surgery International. 2020;**36**:431-445. DOI: 10.1007/s00383-020-04629-9

[13] Carrington E, Brokjaer A, Craven H, et al. Traditional measures of normal anal

sphincter function using high-resolution anorectal manometry (HRAM) in 115 healthy volunteers. Neurogastroenterology and Motility. 2014;**26**:625-635. DOI: 10.1111/nmo.12307

[14] Banasiuk M, Banaszkiewicz A, Piotrowski D, et al. 3D high-definition manometry in evaluation of children after surgery for Hirschsprung's disease: A pilot study. Advances in Medical Sciences. 2016;**61**:18-22. DOI: 10.1016/j.advms.2015.07.008

[15] Brisighelli G, Macchini F, Consonni D, et al. Continence after posterior sagittal anorectoplasty for anorectal malformations: Comparison of different scores. Journal of Pediatric Surgery. 2018;**53**:1727-1733. DOI: 10.1016/j.jpedsurg.2017.12.020

[16] Bjørsum-Meyer T, Christensen P, Jakobsen M, Baatrup G, Qvist N. Correlation of anorectal manometry measures to severity of fecal incontinence in patients with anorectal malformations - A cross-sectional study. Scientific Reports. 2020;**10**:6016. DOI: 10.1038/s41598-020-62908-w

[17] Azpiroz F, Enck P, Whitehead WE. Anorectal functional testing: Review of collective experience. The American Journal of Gastroenterology. 2002;**97**: 232-240. DOI: 10.1111/j.1572-0241.2002.05450.x

[18] Li Y, Yang X, Xu C, Zhang Y, Zhang X. Normal values and pressure morphology for three-dimensional high-resolution anorectal manometry of asymptomatic adults: A study in 110 subjects. International Journal of Colorectal Disease. 2013;**28**:1161-1168. DOI: 10.1007/s00384-013-1706-9

[19] Gangopadhyay A, Pandey V, Gupta D, et al. Assessment and comparison of fecal continence in children following primary posterior sagittal anorectoplasty and abdominoperineal pull through for anorectal anomaly using clinical scoring and MRI. Journal of Pediatric Surgery. 2016;**51**:430-434. DOI: 10.1016/j.jpedsurg.2015.09.003

[20] Wang Z, Hu L, Jin X, Li X, Xu L. Evaluation of postoperative anal functions using endoanal ultrasonography and anorectal manometry in children with congenital anorectal malformations. Journal of Pediatric Surgery. 2016;**51**:416-420. DOI: 10.1016/j.jpedsurg.2015.09.024

[21] Espinosa-Medina I, Saha O, Boismoreau F, et al. The sacral autonomic outflow is sympathetic. Science. 2016;**354**:893-897. DOI: 10.1126/science.aah5454

[22] Rajasegaran S, Tan W, Ezrien D, et al. Utility of postoperative anorectal manometry in children with anorectal malformation: A systematic review. Pediatric Surgery International. 2022;**38**: 1089-1097. DOI: 10.1007/s00383-022-05152-9

[23] Nakamura H, Puri P. Concurrent Hirschsprung's disease and anorectal malformation: A systematic review. Pediatric Surgery International. 2020;**36**: 21-24. DOI: 10.1007/s00383-019-04580-4

[24] Mert M, Sayan A, Köylüoğlu G. Comparing the fecal continence scores of patients with anorectal malformation with anorectal manometric findings. Pediatric Surgery International. 2021;**37**:1013-1019. DOI: 10.1007/s00383-021-04884-4

[25] Evans-Barns HME, Tien MY, Trajanovska M, et al. Post-operative anorectal manometry in children following anorectal malformation repair: A systematic review. Journal of Clinical Medicine. 2023;**12**(7):2543. DOI: 10.3390/jcm12072543

Chapter 12

Surgical Treatment of Hemorrhoidal Disease

Goran Stanojević, Branko Branković, Milica Nestorović and Nikola Milutinović

Abstract

Hemorrhoidal disease (HD) is a condition characterized by enlarged normally present anal cushions or nodules accompanied by clinical symptoms. HD of grade I and II, is primarily treated conservatively with medication (creams and phlebotonics) as well as by office-based procedures, such as rubber band ligation, injection sclerotherapy, infrared coagulation, cryotherapy, and radiofrequency ablation. Indications for a surgical treatment of hemorrhoidal disease are: persistent and recurrent bleeding that does not respond to conservative treatment and office-based interventions, prolapse of hemorrhoids causing significant difficulties and discomfort (Grade III and IV), failure of conservative treatment methods, presence of complications (anemia, infection, or fistula). There are two types of surgical interventions, non-excisional and excisional. The group of non-excisional surgical procedures includes: stapled hemorrhoidopexy, Doppler-guided ligation of hemorrhoidal arteries and laser treatment of hemorrhoids. The group of excisional surgical procedures includes: open (Milligan-Morgan) hemorrhoidectomy, closed (Ferguson's) hemorrhoidectomy Ligasure and Harmonic hemorrhoidectomy and Park's hemorrhoidectomy. Non-excisional surgical methods represent potential options in the treatment of stage III hemorrhoids and patients with early stage IV disease. Non-excisional methods are characterized by lower postoperative pain intensity, faster recovery, and fewer postoperative complications, but they are also associated with a significantly higher rate of recurrence.Excisional methods in surgical treatment represent the method of choice for stage IV hemorrhoidal disease. They are characterized by intense postoperative pain and a higher frequency of complications such as bleeding, urinary retention, anal canal stenosis or stricture, and anal incontinence. There is no single best and most effective method for treating hemorrhoids.

Keywords: hemorrhoidal disease, surgical treatment, non excisional surgical procedure, excisional surgical procedures, complications

1. Introduction

Hemorrhoidal disease (HD) is a condition characterized by enlarged normally present anal cushions or nodules accompanied by clinical symptoms [1]. The prevalence of the disease varies depending on the data from the literature, but it is considered that 5% of the total world population over the age of 18, or 50% of individuals over the age of 50, experience various symptoms of HD. It is estimated that 90% of general population suffers from haemorrhoidal symptoms at least once in their life. The rectal bleeding incidence in human population related to haemorrhoidal bleeding is around 20% per year, compared to all kinds of rectal bleeding, while the prevalence of haemorrhoidal disease, according to different studies, varies between 4.4% and 86% It is more common in men than in women. In the United States, over 2.2 million outpatient visits for patients with hemorrhoidal disease are conducted annually [2].

The primary function of the hemorrhoidal plexus is to protect the anorectal muscles and ensure a complete closure of the anal canal during rest. Filled with blood, they assist in maintaining continence, especially during the retention of gas and liquid stool. During defecation, when straining occurs, they fill with blood and descend, acting like cushions in the upper part of the anal canal, thus protecting it from a mechanical injury. Regarding the pathophysiology of hemorrhoidal disease, there are several theories, but the most accepted one is the Thomson theory, which explains the development of the prolapse or "sliding" of anal cushions caused by weakening or laxity of the Treitz muscle due to the loss of elastic fibers, while hypertrophy and congestion of the vascular tissue occur secondarily [3, 4].

In everyday clinical practice, the most commonly used classification for staging hemorrhoidal disease is Goligher's classification (**Table 1**) [1].

In 2009, Nystrom and colleagues improved this classification by using a five-point questionnaire to assess the frequency of pain, discomfort, itching, staining of underwear (soiling), and the need for manual reduction of hemorrhoids. The frequency of symptoms was divided into four degrees: "never," "less than once a week," "1–6 times a week," and "daily" [5]. This classification system for hemorrhoidal disease has a limitation in that it does not capture the quality of life experienced by patients with hemorrhoidal symptoms. To address this limitation, Giordano and colleagues developed a questionnaire that measures bleeding, prolapse, need for manual reduction, pain, and discomfort during defecation (as a measure of quality of life) using scores ranging from 0 to 4. A score of 0 indicates no symptoms, while a score of 20 represents the most severe symptoms [6]. In 2019, Havard modified Nystrom's classification by replacing manual reduction with the frequency of hemorrhoidal prolapse occurrence. This modification makes it more adaptable to Goligher's classification [7].

The treatment includes:

1. Conservative treatment measures (diet, lifestyle changes, application of anti-hemorrhoidal creams or suppositories, phlebotonics, etc.).

Grade	Physical findings
I	Prominent hemorrhoidal vessels, no prolaps
II	Prolaps with Valsalva and spontaneous reduction
III	Prolaps with Valsalva requires manuel reduction
IV	Chronically prolapsed manuel reduction ineffective

Table 1.
Goligher's classification.

2. Office-based procedures (sclerotherapy of hemorrhoids, rubber band ligation, cryotherapy).

3. Surgical interventions, including non-excisional procedures (stapled hemorrhoidopexy, Doppler-guided arterial ligation, laser treatment) and excisional procedures (conventional hemorrhoidectomy, open Milligan-Morgan, closed Ferguson, submucosal hemorrhoidectomy according to Parks), are reserved for high-grade hemorrhoids when the conservative treatment has failed or complications have arisen [4].

Hemorrhoidal disease of grade I and II, according to the European Society of Coloproctology, is primarily treated conservatively with medication (creams and phlebotonics) as well as by office-based procedures, such as rubber band ligation (RBL), injection sclerotherapy, infrared coagulation, cryotherapy, and radiofrequency ablation [2]. The most commonly performed office-based procedure is rubber band ligation, as it has the lowest incidence of recurrent symptoms and the lowest need for retreatment. It is a relatively safe and painless procedure with minimal complications [8]. Additionally, in everyday proctology practice for patients with grade I and II hemorrhoidal disease, sclerotherapy is used, which involves injecting various sclerosing agents (such as 5% phenol, polidocanol foam, sodium tetradecyl sulfate, etc.) [9]. Only 10% of patients out of the total number of affected individuals with hemorrhoidal disease undergo surgical interventions.

Indications for a surgical treatment of hemorrhoidal disease:

1. Persistent and recurrent bleeding that does not respond to conservative treatment and office-based interventions.

2. Prolapse of hemorrhoids causing significant difficulties and discomfort (Grade III and IV).

3. Failure of conservative treatment methods (dietary modifications, topical creams or suppositories, and office-based procedures).

4. Presence of complications (anemia, infection, or fistula) [1].

2. Types of surgical interventions

2.1 Non-excisional procedures

2.1.1 Stapled hemorrhoidopexy (SH)

Stapled hemorrhoidopexy (SH) is a non-excisional procedure used in the treatment of hemorrhoids, initially introduced by Allegre in 1990 and later further developed by Maria Pecatoria [10]. However, it was Antonio Longo who achieved a widespread recognition of this method in 1998. It is also known as the procedure for prolapse and hemorrhoids (PPH) [11]. The treatment involves using a specialized stapler to excise the rectal tissue, specifically the mucosa and submucosa above the hemorrhoidal nodes, while preserving them and simultaneously lifting them upwards, creating a pexy of the hemorrhoids to prevent prolapse without disrupting the continence mechanism. Additionally, it reduces the arterial blood flow to the hemorrhoids and improves venous drainage [12].

The stapled hemorrhoidopexy (SH) procedure was developed as a response to the commonly used excisional techniques, such as the Milligan-Morgan and Ferguson procedures, in the treatment of hemorrhoids. The advantage of stapled hemorrhoidopexy is that it is associated with lower postoperative pain intensity and faster recovery. However, a drawback is that it has a higher recurrence rate compared to traditional hemorrhoidectomy. Numerous meta-analyses have compared the outcomes of stapled hemorrhoidopexy and conventional hemorrhoidectomy. One such study is the research by Burch et al. [13], which analyzed 27 randomized controlled trials involving 2279 patients. This study showed that SH was associated with lower postoperative pain intensity but had a higher rate of recurrence and the need for reintervention due to recurrent prolapse of hemorrhoids [13]. The results from the Cochrane Database published in 2010 confirmed the findings of the previous study and demonstrated a significantly higher recurrence rate after SH compared to conventional hemorrhoidectomy, as well as a higher need for additional surgical intervention during a longer-term follow-up [14].

In comparison to Doppler-guided hemorrhoidal artery ligation (DGHAL) or transanal hemorrhoidal dearterialization (THD), stapled hemorrhoidopexy (SH) shows similar results regarding overall postoperative complications and patient satisfaction. However, the percentage of recurrence in the short-term follow-up is higher in Doppler-guided ligation of hemorrhoidal arteries, while there are no differences in the long-term follow-up, as shown by the results of a meta-analysis comprising eight randomized controlled trials involving 977 patients (**Figures 1–3**) [15].

There are data in the literature describing varying frequencies of complications, ranging from 12.7% to 36.5%, following stapled hemorrhoidopexy. These complications may include: rectal bleeding, acute and chronic pain, thrombosed external piles, fecal impaction, proctitis, anal fissure, stricture, local abscess and fistula, perirectal hematoma, infections, complete rectal obliteration, rectovaginal fistulas, perforations, fecal incontinence, etc. Therefore, caution should be exercised when performing this procedure due to the potential risks and management of postoperative complications [16–19].

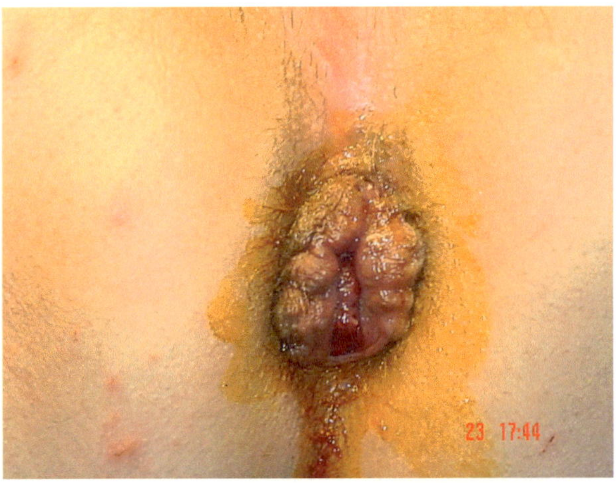

Figure 1.
Pre op hemorrhoids grade III.

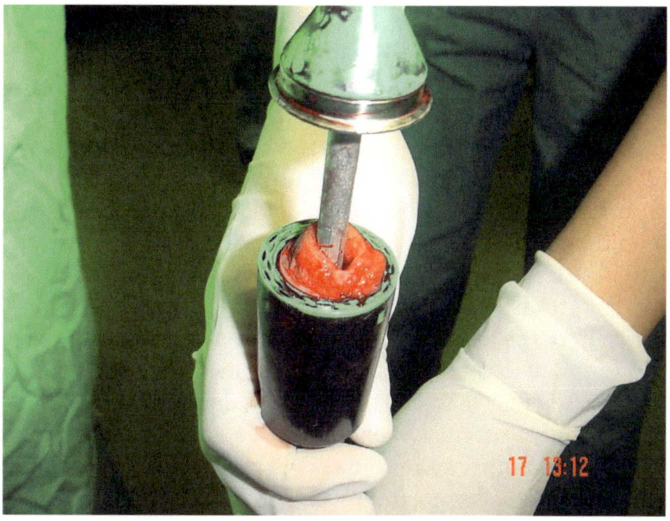

Figure 2.
PPH stapler with excised a ring as "donut" of redundant rectal mucosa and submucosa.

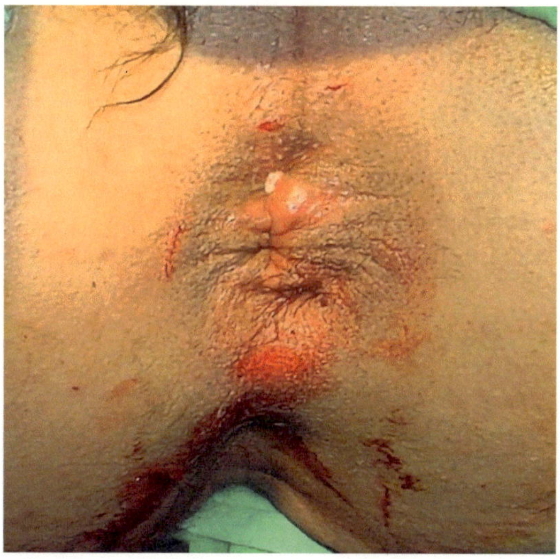

Figure 3.
After SH.

2.1.2 Doppler-guided ligation of hemorrhoidal arteries

Doppler-guided ligation of the terminal branches of hemorrhoidal arteries is a non-excisional surgical method used in the treatment of hemorrhoids. It is based on reducing the arterial blood flow to the hemorrhoids by identifying the terminal branches of the superior hemorrhoidal artery using Doppler ultrasound and consecutively selectively ligated. This is based on the theory that hemorrhoids occur when there is an imbalance in blood flow of the hemorrhoidal plexus. By arterial ligation the inflow is reduced, causing the plexus to diminish and the hemorrhoids to shrink. The Doppler identification of hemorrhoidal blood vessels was first used in 1993 by Jaspersen and colleagues during the sclerotherapy of hemorrhoids [20]. However, the first application of ligation of the branches of the hemorrhoidal artery for the treatment of hemorrhoids was performed by Kasumasa Morinaga in Japan in 1995. Excellent outcomes were reported in 50 out of 52 treated patients (96%). The surgeries were performed using the Moricorn device [21]. Subsequently, other devices have appeared on the market such as the KM 25 device, HAL-Doppler instrument, and more recently the transanal hemorrhoidal dearterialization (THD) instrument, promoted by Carlo Ratto from Italy [22].

Recent research in the field of surgical anatomy has shown that there are typically 6–10 (average 8) terminal branches of the superior hemorrhoidal artery. Ligating these branches leads to reduced arterial blood flow, decreased pressure within the hemorrhoidal node, and regeneration of connective tissue, resulting in a reduction in prolapse, bleeding, and other symptoms. The smaller branches of these arteries form a plexus in the corpus cavernosum recti. The procedure is performed using a set consisting of a proctoscope with a Doppler probe and absorbable suture (2–0) with a curved surgical needle (5/8). The Doppler probe is used to identify the terminal branches of the superior hemorrhoidal artery at two specific locations:

- Above the dentate line in the muscular layer of the rectum, at a distance of 4–6 cm from the anorectal junction.

- As well as at the site where it is most superficially positioned, at a distance of 1–2 cm above the dentate line.

Placement of the proctoscope in the patient in the lithotomy position, carefully advancing it up to 7 cm proximal to the rectum (**Figures 4** and **5**).

The course of the branches of the hemorrhoidal artery starts from the muscular layer of the upper part of the lower third of the rectum and descends to the dentate

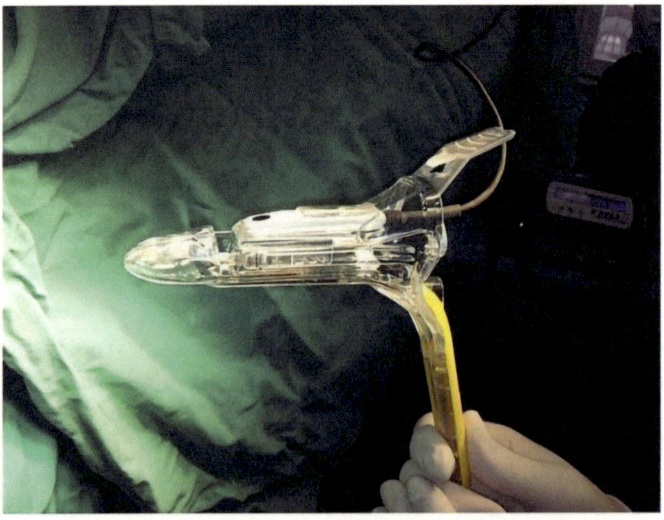

Figure 4.
THD slide® proctoscope.

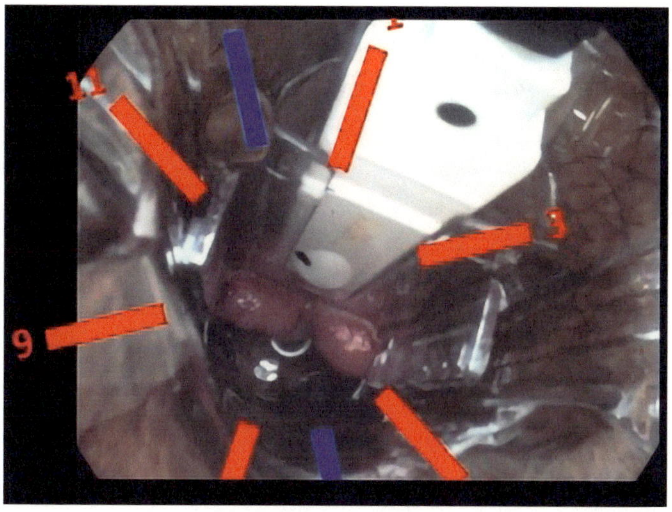

Figure 5.
Proctoscope inserted in the anal canal and the most frequent position of terminal branches of a hemorrhoidal is superior-marked in red.

line, where it becomes the most superficial and suitable for ligation. The identification of these points of ligation is performed using Doppler ultrasound, and they serve as the access points for ligating the blood vessel and, if necessary, for performing mucopexy in cases of hemorrhoid prolapse [23]. There can be variations in the pathway of the branches of the superior hemorrhoidal artery, making the use of a probe necessary for precision and speed during ligation.

There have been a number of studies on THD which show its early efficacy and safety for all grades of hemorrhoids, and recently THD has been acknowledged by the National Institute for Health and Care Excellence (NICE) as a safe and efficient alternative to conventional hemorrhoidectomies in Great Britain [24].

There are numerous publications on the application of Doppler-guided hemorrhoidal dearterialization, some of which are presented in **Table 2**.

In relation to patient satisfaction with THD, a retrospective study was conducted at our Department which included 70 patients with grade III et IV hemorrhoids, as well as grade II hemorrhoids, in whom the conservative treatment failed. The patients were contacted by phone 6 months after the surgery. In the course of this study we recorded the following parameters: gender, age, grade of hemorrhoids, duration of hospitalization, type of anesthesia, duration of the surgery, patient satisfaction, the combination of THD with other procedures and surgical complications. The results showed that 62.9% of the participants were satisfied, 27.1% moderately satisfied and 10% unsatisfied with this procedure [29].

Doppler-guided ligation of the terminal branches of hemorrhoidal arteries is not a completely painless procedure, especially when combined with mucopexy. Despite its popularity and the lower intensity of postoperative pain, THD is a procedure burdened with complications, primarily recurrence. Carlo Ratto, who pioneered this method, analyzed the results of 1000 operated patients in a study conducted in 2017 with a follow-up period of up to 5 years. About 10% of patients in the present series experienced recurrence of hemorrhoidal disease following the primary THD. The most significant risk factors for recurrence were identified as stage IV disease, patients under the age of 40, and high ligation of blood vessels (**Figure 6**) [30].

Authors	Type of procedure	Type of study	Number of patients	Grade of HB	Follow up	Results
Song et al. [15]	DGHAL[1] vs. SH[2]	Meta analysis	977	II–IV	3–36 months	Lower frequency of postoperative bleeding with DGHAL, but higher recurrence rates vs. SH
Denoya et al. [25]	THD[3] vs. CH[4]	Double blind RCT	40	III–IV	14 days	Decreased postoperative pain after THD
Sajid et al. [26]	THD vs. SH	Systematic review	150	—	—	Similar results, with less intensity of postoperative pain after THD
Brown et al. [27]	HAL[5] vs. RBL[6]	RCT	370	II–III	12 meseci	HAL higher intensity of post-op pain, lower percentage of recurrence, compared to RBL
Simillis et al. [28]	THD vs. SH THD vs. CH	Systematic review	291 203	III–IV	—	THD and SH were associated with decreased postoperative pain and faster recovery, but higher recurrence rate. CH resulted in fewer hemorrhoid recurrence

[1]*Doppler-guided hemorrhoidal artery ligation.*
[2]*Stapled hemorrhoidopexy.*
[3]*Transanal hemorrhoidal dearterialization.*
[4]*Conventional hemorrhoidectomy.*
[5]*Hemorrhoidal artery ligation.*
[6]*Rubber band ligation.*

Table 2.
Publications of comparative analysis of Doppler hemorrhoidal dearterialization.

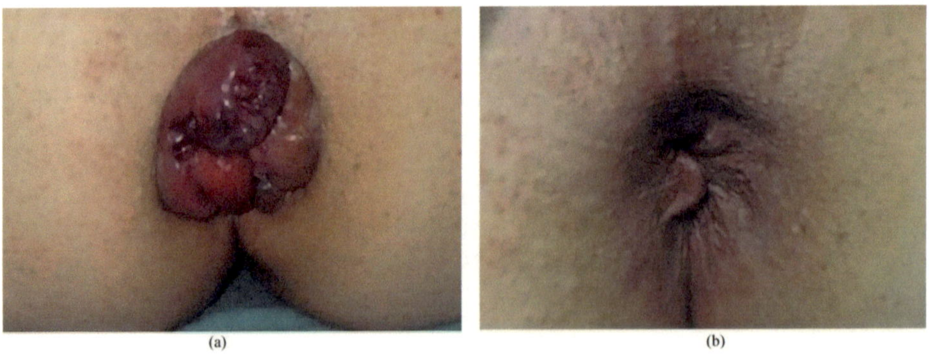

Figure 6.
(a) Before THD and (b) after THD.

Apart from recurrence, other complications are also described in the literature: postoperative bleeding, moderate pain, rarely constipation urinary retention and perianal fissure. Berkel and coauthors described brain abscess after THD as a case report 2013, as the most severe complication [31].

2.1.3 Laser treatment of hemorrhoids

The use of lasers in proctology began in the 1960s. Initially, CO_2, pulsed, and scanned lasers were used as an adjunct to open hemorrhoidectomy to address increased postoperative pain. It was observed that a laser treatment resulted in reduced postoperative pain and esthetically more pleasing scar tissue. In 2000, Plapler et al. [32] conducted studies on submucosal diode laser treatment in rats, which showed minimal changes in the interstitial tissue of the anal region. They also demonstrated that lasers could be used as a new surgical method for treating hemorrhoidal disease in primate tissue [32].

Laser Hemorrhoidoplasty, also known as Hemorrhoidal Laser Procedure (LHP and HeLP), was described by Plapler et al. [33]. It is based on the endovascular application of laser energy to the hemorrhoidal tissue, which leads to the destruction of submucosal blood vessels and their replacement with fibrous tissue, without damaging the mucosa. It is indicated for hemorrhoids of stages II and III, while for prolapsed hemorrhoids, it is recommended to be combined with mucopexy. The results of the laser energy application begin to be visible after 4 weeks from the surgery [33].

The HeLP procedure has shown, based on prospective studies that mostly included patients up to stage III of the disease, that intraoperative bleeding occurred in 8.7% of cases, which was resolved with sutures without the need for postoperative blood transfusion or blood product replacement. Postoperative bleeding was observed in 2.12% of patients, resulting in extended hospitalization, but none of them required blood transfusion or blood product replacement. Pain and analgesic use were minimal compared to open hemorrhoidectomy [34].

Based on prospective studies predominantly including patients with stage II and III disease, the LHP procedure has also demonstrated significantly less postoperative pain, minimal use of analgesics, negligible intraoperative bleeding, and no postoperative bleeding compared to open hemorrhoidectomy. However, described complications include postoperative edema (1.47%), abscess formation (0.36%), burns (0.73%), and the occurrence of skin tags (0.92%).

Laser procedures for the treatment of hemorrhoidal disease have been shown to be an effective therapeutic option for stage II and III cases, while in stage IV cases, they have demonstrated similar recurrence rates to open hemorrhoidectomy. They have been found to reduce hospital stay duration, have fewer postoperative complications, as well as lower incidence of urinary retention and anal stenosis [35].

2.2 Excisional procedures

2.2.1 Milligan-Morgan hemorrhoidectomy

Milligan-Morgan hemorrhoidectomy continues to be the gold standard in the treatment of stage III and IV hemorrhoids. The technique was pioneered in 1937 by two surgeons, Edward Campbell Milligan and Clifford Naughton Morgan, at St. Mark's Hospital in London [36].

The method involves the excision of hemorrhoidal nodules through a careful dissection technique between the mucosa and submucosa on one side, and the muscular layer on the other side. Dissection is performed to reach the root of the hemorrhoids, where the terminal branch of the superior hemorrhoidal artery is ligated. It is essential to leave "bridges" between the excised parts of the hemorrhoids to prevent stenosis or subtotal stenosis of the anal canal. This technique is primarily used for the

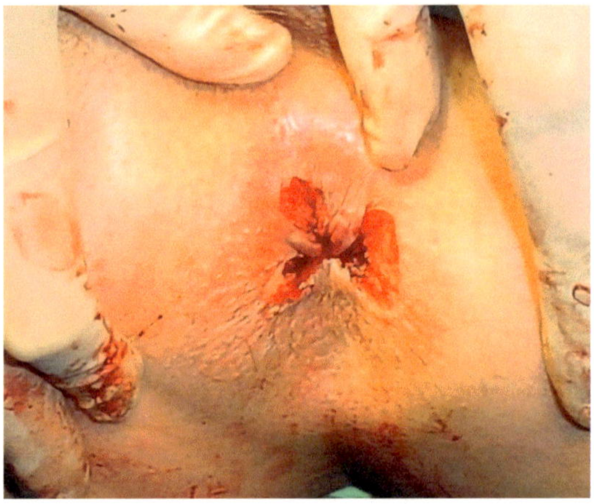

Figure 7.
Milligan-Morgan hemorrhoidectomy, appearance of the "three-leaf" clover.

removal of stage III and IV hemorrhoids at the 3, 7, and 11 o'clock positions, resulting in a "three-leaf" clover appearance after excision (**Figure 7**) [37].

However, Milligan-Morgan hemorrhoidectomy is associated with significant postoperative complications, including more intense pain, bleeding, longer hospital stay, anal canal stenosis, and the risk of anal incontinence. Numerous publications have examined the advantages and disadvantages of excisional procedures in the treatment of hemorrhoids. Simillis et al. [28] published a systematic review and meta-analysis in 2015, which included 98 randomized controlled trials involving 7827 patients. The results showed that classic hemorrhoidectomies (open and closed) were associated with higher intensity of postoperative pain, complications, and slower recovery, but significantly lower recurrence rates compared to other methods [28]. Regarding patient satisfaction, a French study demonstrated that out of 482 patients who underwent classical hemorrhoidectomy or Milligan-Morgan procedure, 90% were satisfied or very satisfied, and 93% responded that they would choose the same procedure again (**Table 3**) [41].

The surgeon's choice of specific procedures in the treatment of hemorrhoids depends on personal experience and patient preferences. An interesting study from

Guidelines	Grade	Level of evidence; grade of recommendation
Belgian consensus guideline on the management of hemorrhoidal disease [38]	III–IV	Agreement 100%. Grade A.
Consensus statement of the Italian society of colorectal surgery (SICCR): management and treatment of hemorrhoidal disease [39]	III–IV	Level of evidence: 1; Grade of recommendation: A
ASCRS Practical Guidelines for Management of Hemorrhoids [2]	III–IV	Grade of recommendation: strong recommendation based on high-quality evidence, 1A
Japanese Practice Guidelines for Anal Disorders I. Hemorrhoids [40]	III–IV	Grade of recommendation, A

Table 3.
Guidelines for good clinical practice with the level of recommendation for Milligan-Morgan hemorrhoidectomy.

the Netherlands published in 2018 analyzed a survey among 133 colorectal surgeons and specialists regarding their preferred methods for treating stage IV disease: 2% would perform laser therapy, only 21% would choose hemorrhoidopexy, 10% would opt for Doppler-guided ligation of hemorrhoidal vessels and mucopexy, 21% would prefer stapled hemorrhoidopexy, and 37% would still choose traditional hemorrhoidectomy [42]. It is clear that the choice of method varies for stage IV disease and, according to many, also for stage III disease, as demonstrated in a study by Altomare et al. published in 2018, which analyzed 34,000 patients operated on between 2000 and 2016 by 18 colorectal surgeons [43].

Therefore, it is necessary to thoroughly explain to the patient the advantages and disadvantages of excisional procedures through the process of obtaining informed consent prior to the surgical intervention.

2.2.2 Ferguson's hemorrhoidectomy

Ferguson's excisional hemorrhoidectomy is a similar method to the previous one, first published in 1955 in the United States by James Ferguson. The operation is performed in a very similar manner to the Milligan Morgan procedure, with the difference being greater preservation of the mucosa and closure of the edges of the previous excision with absorbable sutures, along with simultaneous ligation of the terminal branch of the superior hemorrhoidal artery (**Figure 8**) [36, 44].

Numerous published studies have focused on potential differences and similarities between these two methods. One of the well-known studies is a systematic review and meta-analysis of 11 randomized controlled trials (RCTs) involving 13,526 patients conducted by Bhatti et al. and published in 2016. The results are presented in **Table 4** [45].

Regardless of the existing minimal differences, Ferguson's hemorrhoidectomy also represents the gold standard for the treatment of stage III and IV hemorrhoids.

2.2.3 Ligasure and Harmonic hemorrhoidectomy

Excision of hemorrhoidal nodes can be performed using scissors, a knife, monopolar or bipolar cautery, radiofrequency knife, and more recently, Ligasure and Harmonic devices. The Ligasure system for vessel sealing has proven to be a very

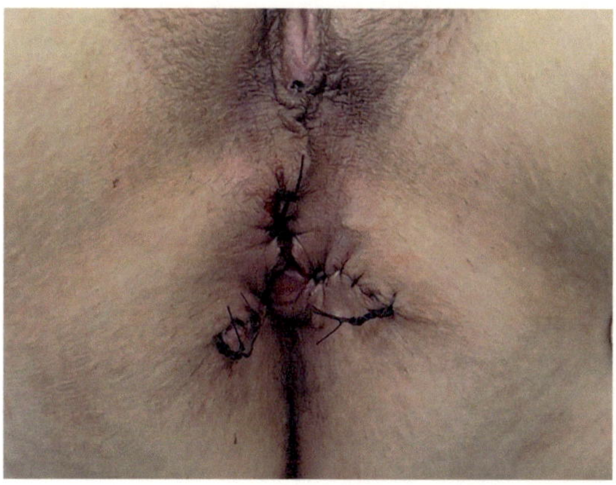

Figure 8.
Ferguson hemorrhoidectomy.

Clinical characteristics	Milligan-Morgan (open)	Ferguson (closed)
Postop pain	More intense	Less intense
Wound healing	Worse	Better
Bleeding	More	Less
Recurrence	ns*	ns
Postop complications	ns	ns
SSI	ns	ns
Lengths of stay	ns	ns

**Non-significant.*

Table 4.
Differences between Milligan Morgan and Ferguson hemorrhoidectomy.

effective method in reducing pain compared to traditional hemorrhoidectomy. The technique allows for complete coagulation of vessels up to 7 mm in diameter, with a minimal thermal spread. The thermal spread is limited to 2 mm of the adjacent tissue, which prevents anal spasm and reduces pain (**Figures 9** and **10**) [46, 47].

This treatment method is relatively new and has shown a low recurrence rate, as well as a reduction in postoperative pain, without a clear difference in the occurrence of complications such as bleeding, urinary retention, stenosis, or abscesses [48]. A randomized controlled study on 44 patients conducted by Tan et al. [49], comparing the results of Ligasure hemorrhoidectomy with open diathermy hemorrhoidectomy, demonstrated significant advantages of Ligasure hemorrhoidectomy. A publication in the Cochrane Database of Systematic Reviews with 12 randomized controlled trials and 1142 patients demonstrated lower intensity of postoperative pain immediately after the operation and up to 14 days postoperatively, shorter duration of the operation, less intraoperative bleeding, and statistically significantly lower frequency of urinary retentions [50].

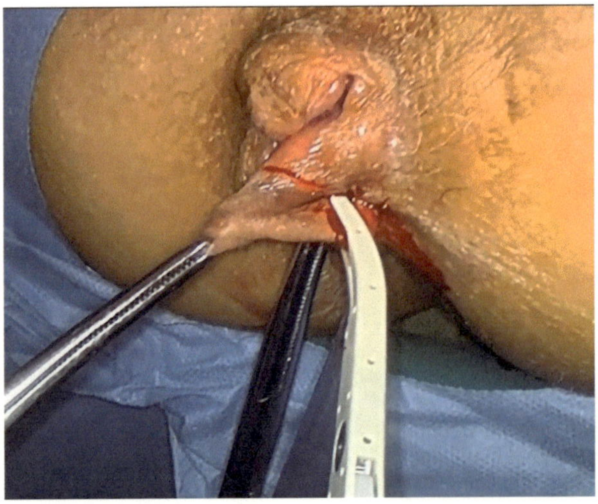

Figure 9.
Ligasure hemorrhoidectomy.

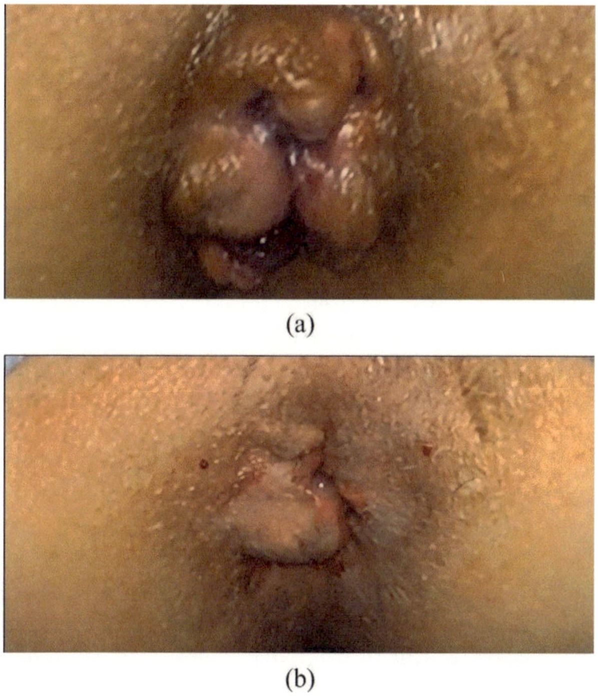

Figure 10.
(a) Before and (b) after Ligasure hemorrhoidectomy.

A randomized controlled trial conducted by Tsunoda et al. [51] compared Ligasure and Harmonic devices in the treatment of 60 patients with stage III and IV hemorrhoidal disease. In the Ligasure group, the surgical procedure was statistically significantly shorter in duration, there was less blood loss, and a smaller amount of postoperative analgesics was required. The length of hospital stay, patient satisfaction, and intensity of postoperative pain were similar between the two groups [50]. In any case, the use of Ligasure or Harmonic scalpel in the excision technique yields better results compared to standard methods of hemorrhoid coagulation and cutting [51].

2.2.4 Park's hemorrhoidectomy

Parks' hemorrhoidectomy is a method that was first described by Sir Alan Guyatt Parks from St. Mark's Hospital in London in 1956. It was developed as an alternative to the traditional Milligan Morgan procedure, which was associated with significant postoperative complications such as pain, bleeding, and large resection of the rectal mucosa. Parks' approach aimed to spare the mucosa of the distal colon by performing a high ligation of the terminal branches of the superior hemorrhoidal artery. The original method involves a Y-shaped incision, measuring 3–5 cm in length, starting from the mucocutaneous junction between the mucosa of the upper anal canal and the anorectal junction. The hemorrhoidal node is dissected and separated from the muscular layer of the anal canal and rectum. The terminal branch of the superior hemorrhoidal artery is ligated. The ligated area is then covered with a mucosal flap, while the skin incision is left open for potential drainage. Parks' hemorrhoidectomy is a relatively lengthy surgical procedure compared to other excision techniques, with a slightly higher risk of anal incontinence due to the long lasting application of the Parks self-retractor placed in the anal canal. However, the competing Milligan Morgan technique remains the method of choice to this day, and Parks' hemorrhoidectomy could not overshadow the popularity of the open excision procedure [36].

3. Conclusion

Non-excisional surgical methods (such as stapled hemorrhoidopexy, Doppler ligations, and mucopexy of the terminal branches of the superior hemorrhoidal artery) represent potential options in the treatment of stage III hemorrhoids and patients with early stage IV disease. Non-excisional methods are characterized by lower postoperative pain intensity, faster recovery, and fewer postoperative complications, but they are also associated with a significantly higher rate of recurrence. Excisional methods in surgical treatment (Milligan-Morgan—open, Ferguson—closed, Parks' submucosal hemorrhoidectomy) represent the method of choice for stage IV hemorrhoidal disease. They are characterized by intense postoperative pain and a higher frequency of complications such as bleeding, urinary retention, anal canal stenosis or stricture, and anal incontinence. Hemorrhoidectomy performed using Ligasure or Harmonic devices represents an alternative excisional method that reduces the intensity of postoperative pain. It is necessary to thoroughly explain to the patient the advantages and disadvantages of all potential procedures as part of the informed consent process, as the treatment of hemorrhoids should be personalized. There is no single best and most effective method for treating hemorrhoids.

Acknowledgements

We would like to express our gratitude to Mrs. Gorjana Djordjevic, for meticulous proofreading and assistance with the English text.

Author details

Goran Stanojević[1,2*], Branko Branković[1,2], Milica Nestorović[1,2] and Nikola Milutinović[2]

1 Department of Surgery, Medical Faculty, University of Niš, Serbia

2 Clinic for Digestive Surgery, University Clinical Center Niš, Serbia

*Address all correspondence to: stgoran1964@gmail.com

IntechOpen

© 2023 The Author(s). Licensee IntechOpen. This chapter is distributed under the terms of the Creative Commons Attribution License (http://creativecommons.org/licenses/by/3.0), which permits unrestricted use, distribution, and reproduction in any medium, provided the original work is properly cited.

References

[1] Lohsiriwat V. Treatment of hemorrhoids: A coloproctologist's view. World Journal of Gastroenterology. 2015;**21**:9245-9252. DOI: 10.3748/wjg.v21.i31.9245

[2] Bradley RD, Lee-Kong SA, Migaly J, Feingold DL, Steele SR. The American Society of Colon and Rectal Surgeon clinical practice guidelines for the management of hemorrhoids. Diseases of the Colon and Rectum. 2018;**61**:284-229. DOI: 10.1097/DCR.0000000000001030

[3] Aigner F, Gruber H, Conrad F, Eder J, Wedel T, Zelger B, et al. Revised morphology and hemodynamics of the anorectal vascular plexus: Impact on the course of hemorrhoidal disease. International Journal of Colorectal Disease. 2009;**24**:105-113. DOI: 10.1007/s00384-008-0572-3

[4] Lohsiriwat V. Hemorrhoids: From basic pathophysiology to clinical management. World Journal of Gastroenterology. 2012;**18**:2009-2017. DOI: 10.3748/wjg.v18.i17.2009

[5] Nyström PO, Qvist N, Raahave D, Lindsey I, Mortensen N. Randomized clinical trial of symptom control after stapled anopexy or diathermy excision for haemorrhoid prolapse. British Journal of Surgery. 2009;**97**(2):167-176. DOI: 10.1002/bjs.6804

[6] Giordano P, Nastro P, Davies A, Gravante G. Prospective evaluation of stapled haemorrhoidopexy versus transanal haemorrhoidal dearterialization for stage II and III haemorrhoids: Three-year outcomes. Techniques in Coloproctology. 2011;**15**:67-73. DOI: 10.1007/s10151-010-0667

[7] Rørvik HD, Styr K, Ilum L, McKinstry GL, Dragesund T, et al. Hemorrhoidal disease symptom score and short health scale HD: New tools to evaluate symptoms and health-related quality of life in hemorrhoidal disease. Diseases of the Colon and Rectum. 2019;**62**:333-342. DOI: 10.1097/DCR.0000000000001234

[8] Ramzisham AR, Sagap I, Nadeson S, Ali IM, Hasni MJ. Prospective randomized clinical trial on suction elastic band ligator versus forceps ligatorin the treatment of haemorrhoids. Asian Journal of Surgery. 2005;**28**:241-245. DOI: 10.1016/S1015-9584(09)60353-5

[9] Cocorullo G, Tutino R, Falco N, Licari L, Orlando G, et al. The non-surgical management for hemorrhoidal disease. A systematic review. Il Giornale di Chirurgia. 2017;**38**:5-14. DOI: 10.11138/gchir/2017.38.1.005

[10] Pescatori M, Favetta U, Dedola S, Orsini S. Transanal stapled excision of rectal mucosal prolapse. Techniques in Coloproctology. 1997;**1**:96-98

[11] Longo A. Treatment of haemorrhoidal disease by reduction of mucosa and haemorrhoidalprolase with a circular stapling device: A new procedure—6th World Congress of Endoscopic Surgery. MundozziEditore. 1998:777-784

[12] Tjandra JJ, Chan MK. Systematic review on the procedure for prolapse and hemorrhoids (stapled haemorrhoidopexy). Diseases of the Colon and Rectum. 2007;**50**:878-892. DOI: 10.1007/s10350-006-0852-3

[13] Burch J, Epstein D, Baba-Akbari AS, Weatherly H, Jayne J, Fox D, et al. Stapled

haemorrhoidopexy for the treatment of haemorrhoids: A systematic review. Colorectal Disease. 2009;**11**:233, 244. DOI: 10.1111/j.1463-1318.2008.01638.x

[14] Lumb KJ, Colquhoun PH, Malthaner R, Jayaraman S. Stapled versus conventional surgery for hemorrhoids (review). Cochrane Database of Systematic Reviews. 2010;**4**:CD005393. DOI: 10.1002/14651858.CD005393.pub2

[15] Song Y, Da M, Chen H, Yang F, Zeng Y, He Y, et al. Transanal hemorrhoidal dearterialization versus stapled hemorrhoidectomy in the treatment of haemorrhoids. A PRISMA-compliant updated meta-analysis of randomized control trials. Medicine. 2018;**97**(29):e11502. DOI: 10.1097/MD.0000000000011502

[16] Popivanov G, Fedeli P, Cirocchi R, Lancia M, Mascagni D, Giustozzi M, et al. Perirectal hematoma and intra-abdominal bleeding after stapled hemorrhoidopexy and STARR—A proposal for a decision-making algorithm. Medicine. 2020;**56**:269-281. DOI: 10.3390/medicina56060269

[17] Park JI. Pneumoretroperitoneum after procedure for prolapsed hemorrhoid. Annals of Coloproctology. 2013;**29**:256-258. DOI: 10.3393/ac.2013.29.6.256

[18] McCloud JM, Jameson JS, Scott AN. Life-threatening sepsis following treatment for haemorrhoids: A systematic review. Colorectal Disease. 2006;**8**:748-755. DOI: 10.1111/j.1463-1318.2006.01028.x

[19] Pescatori M, Gagliardi G. Postoperative complications after procedure for prolapsed hemorrhoids (PPH) and stapled transanal rectal resection (STARR) procedures. Techniques in Coloproctology. 2008;**12**:7-19. DOI: 10.1007/s10151-008-0391-0

[20] Jaspersen D, Koerner T, Schorr W, Hammar CH. Proctoscopic ultrasound in diagnostics and treatment bleeding haemorrhoids. Diseases of the Colon and Rectum. 1993;**36**(10):942-945

[21] Morinaga K, Hasuda K, Ikeda T. A novel therapy for internal hemorrhoids: Ligation of the hemorrhoidal artery with a newly devised instrument (Moricorn) in conjunction with a doppler flowmeter. The American Journal of Gastroenterology. 1995;**90**:610-613

[22] Ratto C, Donisi L, Parello A, Litta F, Zaccone G, De Simone V. Distal doppler-guided dearterialization' is highly effective intreating hemorrhoids by transanal hemorrhoidal dearterialization. Colorectal Disease. 2012;**14**:e786-e789. DOI: 10.1111/j.1463-1318.2012.03146.x

[23] Ratto C. THD doppler procedure for hemorrhoids: The surgical technique. Techniques in Coloproctology. 2014;**18**:291-298. DOI: 10.1007/s10151-013-1062-3

[24] Pucher PH, Sodergren MH, Lord AC, Darzi A, Ziprin P. Clinical outcome following doppler-guided hemorrhoidal artery ligation: A systematic review. Colorectal Disease. 2013;**15**:e284-e294. DOI: 10.1111/codi.12205

[25] Denoya PI, Fakhoury M, Chang K, Fakhoury J, Bergamaschi R. Dearterialization with mucopexy versus haemorrhoidectomy for grade III or IV haemorrhoids: Short-term results of a double-blind randomized controlled trial. Colorectal Disease. 2013;**15**:1281-1288. DOI: 10.1111/codi.12303

[26] Sajid MS, Parampalli U, Whitehouse P, Sains P, McFall BMK. A systematic review comparing transanal

haemorrhoidal dearterialisation to stapled haemorrhoidopexy in the management of haemorrhoidal disease. Techniques in Coloproctology. 2012;**16**:1-168. DOI: 10.1007/s10151-011-0796-z

[27] Brown S, Tiernan J, Biggs K, Hind D, Shephard N, et al. The HubBLe trial: Haemorrhoidal artery ligation (HAL) versus rubber band ligation (RBL) for symptomatic second—An third-degree haemorrhoids: A multicentre randomized controlled trial and health-economic evaluation. Health Technology Assessment. 2016;**20**:1-150. DOI: 10.3310/hta20880

[28] Simillis C, Thoukididou SN, Slesser AAP, Rasheed S, Tan E, Tekkis P. Systematic review and network meta-analysis comparing clinical outcomes and effectiveness of surgical treatments for haemorrhoids. BJS. 2015;**102**:1603-1618. DOI: 10.1002/bjs.9913

[29] Branković B, Nestorović M, Stanojević G, Petrović D, Mihajlović D, Golubović I. Patients 'contentment with transanal hemorrhoidal dearterialization. Facta Universitatis Series: Medicine and Biology. 2019;**21**:25-28. DOI: 10.22190/FUMB190507007B

[30] Ratto C, Campennì P, Papeo F, Donisi L, Litta F, Parello A. Transanal hemorrhoidal dearterialization (THD) for hemorrhoidal disease: A single-center study on 1000 consecutive cases and a review of the literature. Techniques in Coloproctology. 2017;**21**:953-962. DOI: 10.1007/s10151-017-1726-5

[31] Berkel AEM, Witteb ME, Koopa R, Hendrixc MGR, Klaasea JM. Brain abscess after transanal hemorrhoidal dearterialization: A case report. Case Reports in Gastroenterology. 2013;7:208-213. DOI: 10.1159/000351817

[32] Plapler H. A new method for hemorrhoid surgery: Experimental model of diode laser application in monkeys. Photomedicine and Laser Surgery. 2008;**26**:143-146. DOI: 10.1089/pho.2007.2121

[33] Plapler H, Hage R, Duarte J, Lopes N, Masson I, Cazarini C, et al. A new method for hemorrhoid surgery: Intrahemorrhoidal diode laser, does it work? Photomedicine and Laser Surgery. 2009;**27**:819-823. DOI: 10.1089/pho.2008.2368

[34] Trigui A, Rejab H, Akrout A, Trabelsi J, Zouari A, Majdoub Y, et al. Laser utility in the treatment of hemorrhoidal pathology: A review of literature. Lasers in Medical Science. 2022;**37**:693-699. DOI: 10.1007/s10103-021-03333-x

[35] Lie H, Caesarini EF, Purnama AA, Irawan A, Sudirman T, Jeo WS, et al. Laser hemorrhoidoplasty for hemorrhoidal disease: A systematic review and meta-analysis. Lasers in Medical Science. 2022;**37**:3621-3630. DOI: 10.1007/s10103-022-03643-8

[36] Pata F, Gallo G, Pellino G, Vigorita V, Podda M, et al. Evolution of surgical management oh hemorrhoidal disease: An historical overview. Frontiers in Surgery. 2021;**8**:2-11. DOI: 10.3389/fsurg.2021.727059

[37] Miligan S, Morgan C. Surgical anatomy of the anal canal with special reference to anorectal fistulae. The Lancet. 1937;**230**:1150-1156

[38] De Schepper H, Coremans G, Denis MA, Dewint P, Duinslaeger M, et al. Belgian consensus guideline on the management of hemorrhoidal disease. Acta Gastro-Enterologica Belgica. 2021;**84**:101-120. DOI: 10.51821/84.1.497

[39] Gallo G, Martellucci J, Sturiale A, Clerico G, Milito G, et al. Consensus

statement of the Italian society of colorectal surgery (SICCR): Management and treatment of hemorrhoidal disease. Techniques in Coloproctology. 2020;**24**:145-164. DOI: 10.1007/s10151-020-02149-1

[40] Yamana T. Japanese practice guidelines for anal disorders I. Hemorrhoids. Journal of the Anus, Rectum and Colon. 2017;**1**:89-99. DOI: 10.23922/jarc.2017-018

[41] Bouchard D, Abramovitz L, Castinel J, Suduca M, Staumont G, et al. One-year outcome of haemorrhoidectomy: A prospective multicentre French study. Colorectal Disease. 2013;**15**:719-726. DOI: 10.1111/codi.12090

[42] Van Tol R, Bruijnen MPA, Melenhorst J, van Kuijk SMJ, Laurents PS, Stassen LPS, et al. A national evaluation of the management practices of hemorrhoidal disease in the Netherlands. International Journal of Colorectal Disease. 2018;**33**:577-588. DOI: 10.1007/s00384-018-3019-5

[43] Altomare DF, Picciariello A, Pecorella G, Milito G, Naldini G, Amato A, et al. Surgical management of haemorrhoids: An Italian survey of over 32000 patients over 17 years. Colorectal Disease. 2018;**20**:1117-1124. DOI: 10.1111/codi.14339

[44] Rakinic J, Poola VP. Hemorrhoids and fistulas: New solutions to old problems. Current Problems in Surgery. 2014;**51**:98-137. DOI: 10.1067/j.cpsurg.2013.11.002

[45] Bhatti MI, Sajid SM, Baig MK. Milligan-Morgan (open) versus Ferguson Haemorrhoidectomy (closed): A systematic review and meta-analysis of published randomized, controlled trials. World Journal of Surgery. 2016;**40**:1509-1519. DOI: 10.1007/s00268-016-3419-z

[46] Thorbeck CV, Montes MF. Haemorrhoidectomy: Randomised controlled clinical trial of Ligasure compared with Milligan-Morgan operation. The European Journal of Surgery. 2002;**168**:482-484. DOI: 10.1080/110241502321116497

[47] Palazzo FF, Francis DL, Clifton MA. Randomized clinical trial of Ligasure versus open haemorrhoidectomy. The British Journal of Surgery. 2002;**89**:154-157. DOI: 10.1046/j.0007-1323.2001.01993.x

[48] Bulus H, Tas A, Coskin A, Kucukazman M. Evolution of two Haemorrhoidectomy techniques: Harmonic scalpel and Ferguson with electrocautery. Asian Journal of Surgery. 2014;**37**:20-23. DOI: 10.1016/j.asjsur.2013.04.002

[49] Tan KY, Zin T, Sim HL, Poon PL. Randomized clinical trial comparing LigaSure haemorrhoidectomy with open diathermy haemorrhoidectomy. Techniques in Coloproctology. 2008;**12**:93-97. DOI: 10.1007/s10151-008-0405-y

[50] Nienhuijs SW, de Hingh IHJ. Conventional versus LigaSure hemorrhoidectomy for patients with symptomatic hemorrhoids (review). Cochrane Database of Systematic Reviews. 2009;**21**:CD006761. DOI: 10.1002/14651858.CD006761.pub2

[51] Tsunoda A, Sada H, Sugimoto T, Kano N, Kawana M, Sasaki T, et al. Randomized controlled trial of bipolar diathermy vs ultrasonic scalp el for closed hemorrhoidectomy. World Journal of Gastrointestinal Surgery. 2011;**3**:147-152. DOI: 10.4240/wjgs.v3.i10.147

Chapter 13

Anal Fistula: From Diagnosis and Classification to Surgical Management

Jerry Xiao, Erin Santos, Nana-Yaw Bonsu, Woihwan Kim, Michael Eisenberg, Marianne Cusick and Jeffrey Van Eps

Abstract

In this chapter, we discuss the classification and diagnosis of anal fistulas and the surgical approaches for fistula repair. According to the Parks classification, there are four main fistula types based on the location of the fistula tract in relation to the external sphincter: intersphincteric, transsphincteric, suprasphincteric, and extrasphincteric. One of the conventional repair techniques for low transsphincteric fistulas involves cutting open the tract by lay open fistulotomy. Control of a complex fistula tract with a draining seton is used as the first of a two-stage repair or as definitive therapy in patients with contraindications to repair such as concomitant fecal incontinence or active Crohn's disease. Sphincter-preserving techniques for high transsphincteric fistulas include ligation of the intersphincteric fistula tract (LIFT) and endorectal or anodermal advancement flap with largely equivalent expected results. Biologic adjuncts such as platelet-rich plasma (PRP), acellular matrix (AM) material, and mesenchymal stem cells (MSC) represent a promising area for possibly augmenting healing of complex fistulas. Additional novel treatment techniques being developed for complex fistulas including Video-Assisted Anal Fistula Treatment (VAAFT), Fistula Tract Laser Closure (FiLaC), and Over the Scope Clip (OTSC) are also described.

Keywords: anal fistula, transsphincteric, fistula repair, LIFT, advancement flap, biologic adjuncts, platelet-rich plasma (PRP), acellular matrix (AM), mesenchymal stem cells (MSC), video-assisted anal fistula treatment (VAAFT), fistula tract laser closure (FiLaC), over the scope clip (OTSC)

1. Introduction

Anal fistula is defined as a pathological, epithelial-lined tract connecting the perianal skin with the anal canal [1, 2]. The cryptoglandular theory dominates notions of anal fistula etiology, suggesting that obstruction of the glands within anal crypts by stool or debris and subsequent infection is the root cause. These crypts/glands exist within the base of the columns of Morgagni at the dentate line with an average of six glands per person (range 3–12) and are concentrated at the posterior anus [3]. Gland ducts penetrate the submucosa for a variable distance, with two thirds penetrating the internal sphincter muscle and the remaining glands terminating within the intersphincteric plane [3, 4]. This anorectal gland anatomy explains the predilection for anal fistulas to have posterior anal internal openings and the prevalence of intersphincteric fistulas as the most common subtype overall, since obstructed glands can form unmitigated abscesses within this space. Chronic infection and epithelialization of the abscess tract can result in fistula formation [1, 5–7]. The reported incidence varies in literature but up to 76% of patients with anorectal abscess are found to harbor or later develop anal fistula [8, 9]. Although the vast majority (90%) of fistulas are cryptoglandular in origin, they also are a hallmark of the fistulizing phenotypic subtype of Crohn disease (3%) or may develop as a result of postoperative/traumatic events (3%), tuberculosis (1%) or other rare causes such as radiation or malignancy [5].

The incidence of anal fistula ranges from 1.04 to 2.32 per 10,000 people per year while the prevalence ranges from 2.8 to 23.2 patients per 100,000 people [2, 10]. Significant variation in epidemiology worldwide exists, possibly influenced by the different health systems. Reported rates may also be underestimated from patient aversion to seeking care related to the sensitive nature of the symptoms and involved body area [7]. Patients presenting for evaluation and treatment of anal fistula have a mean age of 40 for both biological sexes and are uncommon in children. Men are affected more than women at a 2:1 male to female ratio [6, 7].

Anal fistulas have afflicted patients and physicians since antiquity, with little innovation in treatment for centuries until the last several decades. Hippocrates (460–375 BC) is credited as the first to treat anal fistula. He recognized the importance of timely drainage of anal abscesses to minimize the risk of fistula formation. He described the original seton, lint wrapped in horsehair, placed through the fistula tract and periodically tightened to act as a cutting seton and unroof the tract, as well as use of alum as a fistula plug [11–13]. In 1835, Frederick Salmon, a British surgeon who treated Charles Dickens for anal fistula, established the seven bed "Benevolent Dispensary for the Relief of the Poor Afflicted with Fistula and Other Diseases of the Rectum and Lower Intestines." With increasing recognition in the field, the institution later moved to larger facilities in 1851 and renamed "St Mark's Hospital for Fistula and other Diseases of the Rectum" [14–16]. Salmon discussed his recommendation for fistulotomy on the Lancet in 1844 and opined its low risk for hemorrhage from his nearly two decades of experience in proctology at the time [17]. Sir Lockhart-Mummery (1929) summarized the difficulties that surgeons encountered in treating anal fistula when he said, "Probably more reputations have been damaged by the unsuccessful treatment of cases of fistula than by excision of the rectum or gastro-enterostomy. Perhaps that is why the largest surgical fee in history was paid for the performance of an operation for fistula!" [18].

Perhaps the most famous case of anal fistula is that of the 17th century King Louis XIV, known as the Sun King, who developed a fistula after recurrent anal abscesses. The king's physicians tried numerous treatments, including enemas, poultices, and bloodletting. Repeated barbaric treatments with a red-hot iron made the anal cavity larger. Plagued by pain and chronic drainage, Louis turned into an ill-tempered hermit, no longer participating in court and changing clothes three times a day. At that time, surgeons were viewed purely as technicians and inferior to physicians. However, given the failure of multiple treatments, the king obtained the opinion of the surgeon-barber and Surgeon of the Court, Charles-Francois Felix, for surgical repair. Felix worked hard to develop a long, silver probe known as a bistoury and practiced the operation on patients from Versailles hospitals, some reportedly dying and buried in secret in the early morning. His operation, a fistulotomy over the bistoury, took 3 hours but reportedly provided significant relief. The king ultimately required two additional debridements for "uneven healing" and another operation to achieve final success. Fame spread of his operation and reportedly courtiers lined up to have the same operation whether they had a fistula or not. This event changed how surgeons were viewed and sparked significant subsequent surgical advancement, including establishment of the first academy of surgery [19–21].

Like the distress experienced by King Louis XIV, patients with anal fistula have reported overall reduction in quality of life (QoL) compared to controls using the well-known short form 36 (SF-36) questionnaire on health status [22, 23]. Increased fistula complexity corresponded to worsened QoL. In a 2018 study of nearly 100 fistula patients to validate a new fistula-specific QoL tool, Anal Fistula Questionnaire (QoLAF-Q), moderately graded decreases in QoL were found, with significantly worse values in patients with recurrent disease vs. primary disease [24]. Such functional decrement has been mirrored anecdotally in our own practice but remains poorly defined. Despite advancement since the time of King Louis, these elements highlight the desperate need for further innovation for anal fistula repair. In this chapter, we will discuss current and novel treatments for anal fistula with a focus on cryptoglandular fistula.

2. Classification, diagnosis and the role of preoperative testing

2.1 Anal fistula classification

The easiest and most frequently discussed categorization of anal fistula is simple versus complex, with simple referring to a fistula treatable by fistulotomy without incurring incontinence and complex meaning the fistula requires an alternative technique for repair. Complex fistulas include: fistulas traversing >30% of anal sphincter mechanism, recurrent fistula after prior attempted repair, the presence of multiple branching tracts or a blind sinus tract, any anterior fistula in a female, horseshoe fistula, and any fistula in the presence of trauma, malignancy, inflammatory bowel disease, or history of pelvic radiation or immunosuppression. The formal classification of fistula-in-ano has evolved since it was first attempted in 1934 by Milligan and Morgan. This original classification system distinguished several types based on anatomic relation to the anorectal ring [25]. Parks et al. later amended this in 1976 in a published study of over 400 anal fistula cases [26]. This has become the most widely used classification system and characterizes fistulas based on the tract(s) course in Ref. to the external sphincter complex, given its crucial importance in choosing a treatment technique. The Parks system not only established a common nomenclature, but it dictated treatment based on the type of fistula encountered. The five types established by this system include superficial (subcutaneous), intersphincteric, transsphincteric, suprasphincteric, and extrasphincteric (**Figure 1**).

Intersphincteric fistulas travel within the intersphincteric space and penetrate the anorectum without traversing the external sphincter. This has been reported as the most common fistula subtype, making up 20–45% of all anorectal fistula [27]. Parks further defined seven subsets of intersphincteric fistula based on the presence of a high tract and location of openings (simple intersphincteric, high blind tract, high tract with opening in the lower rectum, high tract with no rectal opening, high tract

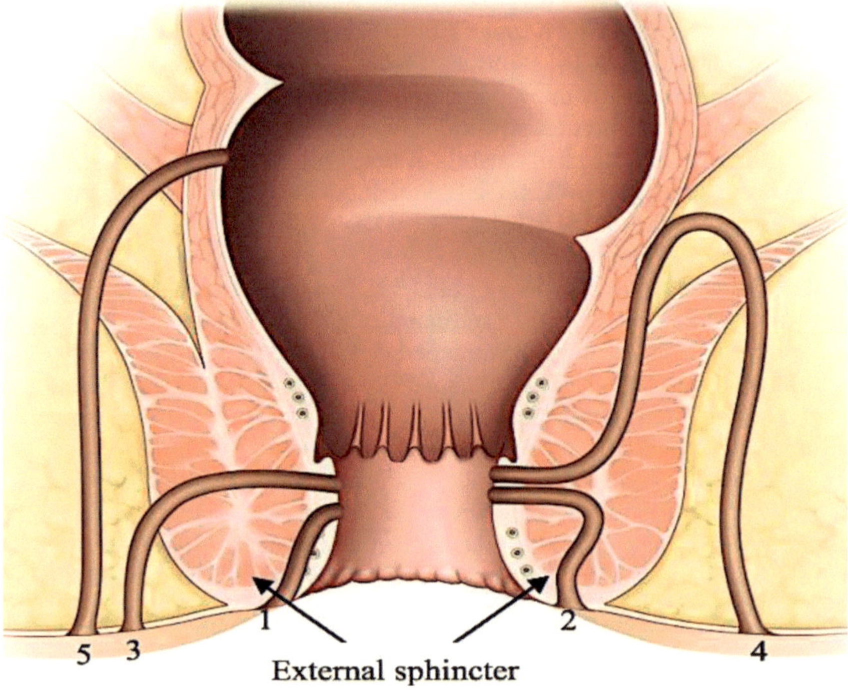

Figure 1.
Parks classification of anal fistula. Superficial (1), Intersphincteric (2), Transsphincteric (3), Suprasphincteric (4), Extrasphincteric (5). Illustration used with permission from park, M. Y., et al. (2021).

with no perineal opening, extra-rectal extension and secondary to pelvic disease). Treatment of intersphincteric fistulas ranges from fistulotomy to advancement flap depending on risk of incontinence.

Transsphincteric fistulas traverse the external anal sphincter (EAS) at some point below the level of the puborectalis muscle and through the ischiorectal fossa to exit the perianal skin. These are further classified based on where the tract crosses the EAS in Ref. to the puborectalis muscle and the presence or absence of a blind sinus tract. With the latter, care must be taken when exploring as the blind tract may take a high trajectory into the ischiorectal fossa or through the levator plate. Low transsphincteric fistula involve 30% or less of the sphincter complex and are generally considered likely safe for treatment by lay-open fistulotomy, especially in males with longer anal canals, but treatment must be personalized based on individuals' risk for postoperative incontinence. High transsphincteric fistula are complex and require a more nuanced sphincter-sparing repair like ligation of intersphincteric fistula tract (LIFT) or advancement flap, discussed later in the text. Many clinicians have adopted verbiage referencing a third anatomic category of mid-height transsphincteric fistula, involving more than 30% of the sphincter complex but not abutting the puborectalis/levator plate at the internal opening. These similarly require a sphincter-sparing complex repair.

Suprasphincteric fistulas course over the top of the puborectalis muscle in the intersphincteric space and then down through the levator plate and ischiorectal fossa before exiting the perianal skin. Fistulas of this nature cannot simply be divided as this would cause incontinence. Given the location in the supralevator space, abscesses that form here might only be palpated on rectal exam. Progression of an infection here can result in a horseshoe abscess to form in the deep space around the rectum. The high curvilinear tract in these cases can be difficult to successfully cannulate for draining seton placement.

Extrasphincteric fistulas progress from the perineal skin through the ischiorectal fat and levator muscle into the rectum above the dentate line and anorectal ring, completely avoiding the external sphincteric complex. It is the least common type of fistula, with an incidence of 5% in the Parks study. These are further classified based on their etiology. They can form spontaneously, or secondary to trauma, retained foreign bodies, inflammatory bowel disease, malignancy or inflammation from the pelvis that tracks down through the levators to the perineum (such as in diverticulitis, ruptured appendicitis), or iatrogenically from aggressive probing of a blind tract in a transsphincteric fistula. Division of this fistula would lead to incontinence and their anatomy make repair by LIFT or flap often very difficult if not impossible, leaving alternative repair options of fistula plug or more recently, over-the-scope clip for an internal opening far enough above the anorectal ring. This is discussed in more detail later in this chapter.

With the advent of MRI, Morris et al. developed a system of classification that provides a more precise definition referred to as St. James Hospital University classification [28]. There are five grades increasing in complexity given the presence of multiple fistulous tracts or associated abscesses. Grades I and II are considered simple fistulas while Grade III–V are complex (III–IV are transsphincteric, and V is supralevator/extrasphincteric). More recently, Garg et al. proposed a new five-grade classification system based on a retrospective cohort study of 440 patients and their preoperative MRI and operative findings, comparing established classification systems [29]. This Garg classification was found to be more accurate than prior schemes in terms of appropriate treatment for the various grades but has not been widely adopted.

2.2 Diagnosis and imaging

It is estimated that up to 76% of patients who present with peri-rectal abscess either have an underlying fistula or will develop one [8, 9]. On rare occasions, an underlying anal fistula may be diagnosed on computed tomography (CT) imaging done to evaluate an acute abscess and a fraction of anal fistula are diagnosed at the time of surgical abscess drainage. A high-quality examination under anesthesia (EUA) is sufficient in most fistula cases and remains the surgical standard and it is the authors' routine practice to always assess for fistula at the time of incision and drainage. With an anal retractor in place, the area of abscess is palpated, and purulent drainage within the anorectal lumen is the first clue to the presence of a fistula. To confirm, a diagnostic substance is instilled under pressure into the abscess cavity such as hydrogen peroxide, methylene blue dye, or even milk whilst directly viewing the distal anorectum by anoscopy. The presence of diagnostic fluid within the anorectal lumen signifies the presence of an underlying fistula tract. Gentle probing of the wound base can also be performed with a fistula probe, being careful not to create any false tracts. If a fistula is diagnosed by the methods above, the fistula probe is placed typically from external to internal opening, allowing assessment of the amount of sphincter muscle involved and either primary fistulotomy over the probe or placement of a draining seton as part of a 2-stage repair (discussed later). However, sometimes the acute soft tissue inflammation present with an acute abscess prevents an underlying fistula from being recognized. The fistula may heal or scar with adequate drainage alone, but more frequently reveals itself weeks to years later with the presence of recurrent peri-rectal abscess or a draining sinus with or without chronic granulation tissue at the external skin opening.

Fistula-specific factors that are higher risk for surgical failure and recurrence in a complex primary fistula include fistula height/length and the presence of multiple branching tracts or unrecognized blind-ending sinus. Thin-slice magnetic resonance imaging (MRI) is regarded as the most sensitive entity for soft tissue evaluation including characterization of anal fistula. However, the cost of MRI can be prohibitive and most clinicians including the authors will reserve cross-sectional evaluation with MRI judiciously for preoperative characterization only in diagnostic conundrums, very high-risk or otherwise difficult cases. Some examples include patients with blind sinus suggested by probing at the time of first-stage draining seton placement, those who suffer an early fistula recurrence, or those who demonstrate ongoing/recurrent signs of infection after seton placement like abscess, indurated soft tissues or heavy drainage. Preoperative evaluation by MRI prior to second stage fistula repair should be strongly considered in such cases. Endorectal ultrasound (ERUS) is also an effective diagnostic modality for the diagnosis and characterization of anal fistula but is especially operator-dependent and not commonly done for this purpose. Fistulography can be effective to diagnose and define fistula anatomy but may not be available at all locations and may require clinician assistance for performance, making it a rarely used diagnostic entity overall.

3. Surgical management

3.1 Fistulotomy and Seton

3.1.1 Overall treatment goals

The overarching goals of treatment of perianal fistulas are preventing systemic infection, closure of the fistula tract, maintain fecal continence by preserving sphincter function, and minimize recurrence [5]. To accomplish this goal, proper drainage of acute infection is crucial, followed by tailored surgical treatment that considers both fistula anatomy and patient-specific factors that risk postoperative functional decrement or recurrence, as no two fistulas are created equal.

3.1.2 Fistulotomy

As previously stated, simple fistulas are those amenable to treatment by primary lay-open fistulotomy, whereby the external and internal openings are connected by transecting the overlying soft tissues between them. These include subcutaneous fistulas, most low transsphincteric fistulas, and some intersphincteric fistulas. This class of fistula makes up a significant proportion of those encountered clinically, often estimated at 50% or more [5]. The primary concern when performing primary fistulotomy is iatrogenic functional complications of sphincter incompetence and fecal incontinence. The commonly reported absolute maximum amount of sphincter muscle that can be transected with a fistulotomy is 30%. This must be individualized to the patient and their baseline continence and sphincter function, as a history of prior traumatic vaginal birth can severely compromise sphincter tone and preclude safe treatment with fistulotomy. An informed digital rectal exam provides a quality initial assessment but when in doubt, anatomic sphincter defects can be defined using endorectal ultrasound and function characterized with anorectal manometry. At least one novel classification system uses MRI to predict amenability to fistulotomy. Patients with sizable deficits should be counseled extensively on the risk of proceeding or a sphincter-sparing approach should be employed like those described later in this text.

After cannulating the tract with a probe, the overlying tissues are transected sharply (**Figure 2**). Underlying granulation tissue and debris is removed with a bone curette and hemostasis obtained with electrocautery. Some clinicians prefer to marsupialize the exposed fistulotomy wound edges with absorbable suture to assure healing by secondary intention. Multiple randomized trials have demonstrated benefits of marsupialization, including decreased wound healing time, and decreased postoperative bleeding and [30–33]. Patients should be counseled that fistulotomy wounds may take 8–12 weeks to fully heal. Fistulotomy is regarded as the preferred treatment option for fistula because of its low failure rate, commonly reported as 10% or less [34, 35]. In our practice, we commonly quote patients an expected success rate of 95% or more for fistulotomy treatment. Incontinence is the most feared complication of fistulotomy, but true incidence rates are difficult to reliably predict. Incidence of incontinence varies according to several factors including fistula complexity/height and surgeon experience and covers a wide range of severity from minor (e.g., temporary gas incontinence) to major incontinence as defined by a validated scoring system. A systematic review by Litta et al. of 66 studies and 4883 patients undergoing fistulotomy by some means found an overall weighted average healing rate of 93 and 12.7% incidence of any

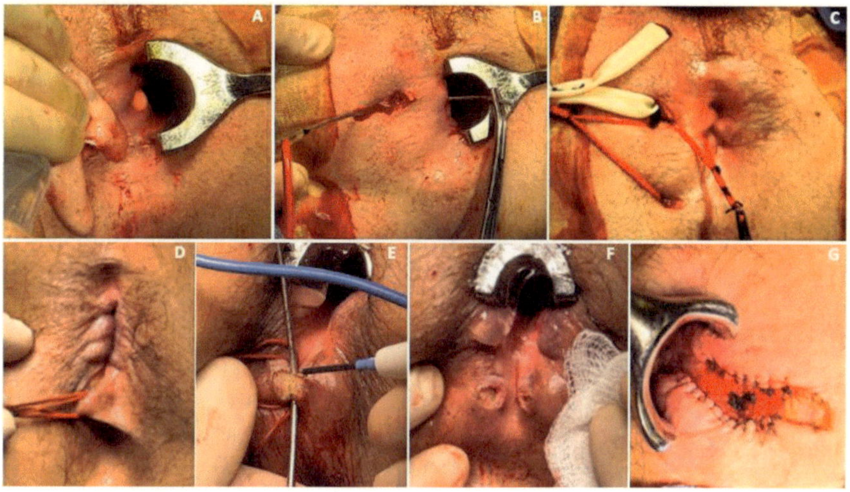

Figure 2.
Seton and fistulotomy technique. (A) the candidate external opening or site of abscess drainage is injected with a diagnostic substance like hydrogen peroxide. Presence of the substance within the anorectum signifies presence of a fistula. (B) a probe is used to cannulate the tract and assess the degree of sphincter muscle involvement. (C) a loose, draining seton is brought through the tract and secured to itself. Large underlying abscess cavities may require counter-drainage as shown with a penrose style drain or another silastic seton. (D) Longstanding setons can act as a modified cutting seton over time to transpose the fistula to a lower position, which may convert a patient into a candidate for (E-F) second-stage fistulotomy and (G) marsupialization. Pictures care of Jeff Van Eps, MD, and Mark Pidala, MD, UT physicians colon & rectal clinic.

postoperative continence impairment, which directly correlated to self-reported decrement in quality of life [36]. Female sex, multiple prior abscess drainage procedures or other anorectal surgeries, high fistulas, and surgical fistulotomy versus cutting seton have been associated with incontinence [5].

3.1.3 Seton

Fistulas that are too complex for single-stage treatment by fistulotomy because of fistula-specific factors like involvement of over 30% of the sphincter or patient-specific factors like active Crohn-related proctitis require control of the tract with a drain to prevent recurrent abscess and potential further complex evolution of the fistula with branching. This involves placement of some material through the tract and secured to itself as a draining seton. Materials used range from a simple silk suture tie, penrose-style rubber drain, pediatric feeding tube or most commonly, a silastic vessel loop. With the patient in either prone jackknife or lithotomy position depending on surgeon preference and anatomic location, a diagnostic substance is instilled under pressure into the suspected external opening to identify the internal fistula opening with a retractor in the anus (**Figure 2**). Various substances have been utilized, including hydrogen peroxide (H_2O_2), methylene blue, or even milk. Chronic tracts often have granulation tissue externally and the corresponding internal anal pit may be identified as a depression with or without active drainage with abscess compression. Cannulation with a fistula probe and a guiding finger in the anus may be used as an alternative or in addition to solution, but care must be taken not to create an iatrogenic false passage. Patience is paramount and probing should never be forced. Once the tract is defined, a seton is pulled through the tract and its ends secured together with silk ties. Seton placement is frequently combined with a partial fistulotomy, whereby the tract is opened over a probe from the external opening up to the edge of the external sphincter muscle. This effectively shortens the tract for second-stage repair, which has been shown to improve outcomes [37, 38].

Setons may be either the loose, non-cutting or cutting type. A cutting seton is purposely applied snugly and is often tightened sequentially over time, with a purpose of using pressure and tension necrosis to slowly work its way through the overlying tissues to unroof a fistula essentially as a slow fistulotomy. Cutting setons have been shown to have essentially equivalent outcomes to surgical fistulotomy regarding healing and incontinence rates [39, 40]. Non-cutting setons maintain drainage of the fistula to prevent recurrent abscess as fibrosis occurs. For Crohn-associated fistulas, seton placement may be the definitive, permanent treatment or used as a bridge until medical control of underlying proctitis can be achieved to make the patient a candidate for fistula repair, albeit with counseling on the increased risk of surgical failure. Seton drains can also be useful for complex fistulas in the presence of other perianal pathology and/or complex perineal soft tissue disease, such as necrotizing soft tissue infection (NSTI), hidradenitis, or pilonidal disease (**Figure 3**).

3.2 Ligation of intersphincteric fistula tract (LIFT)

3.2.1 Background and indications

The ligation of intersphincteric fistula tract (LIFT) procedure is designed to treat complex perianal fistula while simultaneously sparing as much of the anal sphincter

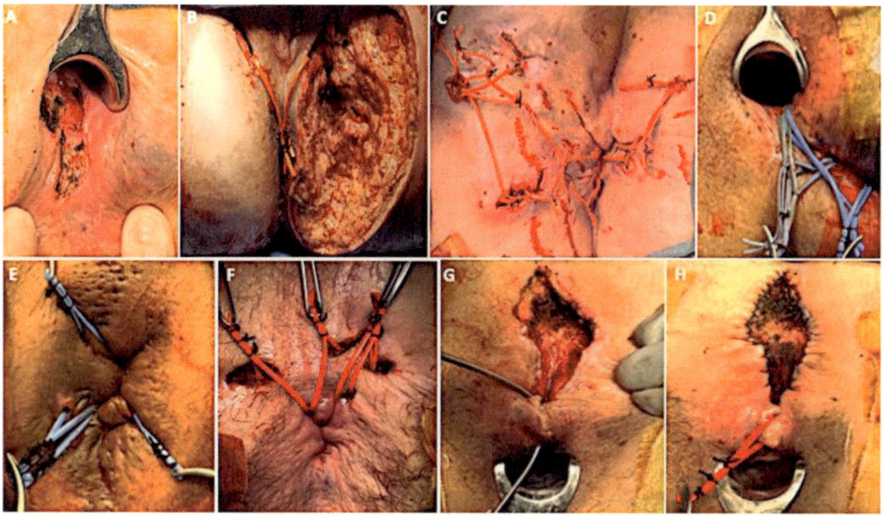

Figure 3.
Fistulotomy and seton special conditions and circumstances. A fistula in conjunction with (A) anal fissure may mandate treatment by fistulotomy, treating both conditions well. Complex perineal infections from (B) necrotizing soft tissue infection (NSTI) and (C) hidradenitis suppurativa can present with complex fistulizing networks involving the soft tissues and the anorectum. (D) Multiple setons may be placed within the same tract when encountering one particularly long or difficult to successfully cannulate, but more than two setons is unnecessary. Multiple drains were removed in this case to simplify. Non-Crohn cryptoglandular fistulas may present as (E) multifocal, complex locations requiring multiple draining setons, or as (F) branching tracts with multiple external or, more rarely, multiple internal openings like this patient with both types. Pilonidal cysts may rarely present as part of a complex anal fistula and should be treated by (G) excision/unroofing with or without (H) marsupialization and possibly negative pressure wound therapy prior to second-stage treatment. Pictures care of Jeff Van Eps, MD, UT physicians colon & rectal clinic.

complex as possible to decrease the likelihood of postoperative incontinence. The procedure was first pioneered in Thailand in 2007 by Rojanasakul and colleagues [41]. This section will discuss indications for the LIFT procedure, operative details of the procedure, and outcomes compared to flap repair.

The LIFT procedure is considered an appropriate surgical treatment of complex fistulas of mid- and high height (see "Classification" Section 2) for which traditional fistulotomy would result in an unacceptable risk of post-operative incontinence. While no absolute contraindications to the procedure have been identified in the literature, certain factors have been found to increase the risk of surgical failure. These include patient factors such as obesity, smoking, and diabetes mellitus which may impair wound healing and characteristics that increase the complexity of the fistula and the resulting operation (i.e. previous operations, active infection/perianal collections, increased length of the fistula tract) [42, 43]. Fistula with a particularly deep course within the intersphincteric plane such as suprasphincteric fistulas should be approached with caution for LIFT repair as a much larger incision may be required and a high-quality ligation can be particularly difficult. While prior attempted repair of a fistula by LIFT is not an absolute contraindication, scarred tissues within the intersphincteric space may increase the difficulty or risk of injury with the operation and an alternative approach like advancement flap should be considered. The senior author specifically finds a LIFT approach ideal to repair radial fistulas that have the external and internal openings both lateral to the anatomic midline.

3.2.2 LIFT operative technique

As with any complex fistula repair, the LIFT procedure should be approached in a staged fashion. The first stage addresses the acute infectious/inflammatory process with drainage of any local fluid collections and seton placement [44]. This allows for the initial infection and local inflammation to abate and meanwhile facilitates tract maturation to make it not only more easily identifiable during dissection, but also robust enough to tolerate suture ligation.

To begin the operation, the patient is positioned in accordance with fistula location. Anterior fistulas are treated in the prone, jack-knife position whereas posterior fistulas are treated with the patient in lithotomy position. A lacrimal probe is then inserted through the fistula to use as a visual/tactile aid and confirm that the tract depth is amenable to repair by LIFT. The intersphincteric groove is palpated and a 3-4 cm curvilinear incision is made following this landmark with the incision centered on the fistula tract (**Figure 4**). Using a combination of blunt dissection and electrocautery, the tract is isolated within the intersphincteric space where it is suture ligated.

It is crucial to remain within the intersphincteric plane during this phase of the operation. Deviation can cause injury to the internal or external sphincters, increasing the risk of post-operative incontinence. Using the lacrimal probe as a guide, overlying soft tissue is transected and the fistula tract is isolated as it traverses the intersphincteric plane with a window created immediately underneath. A right-angle clamp is helpful during this portion of the dissection and to pull suture ties into place for ligation. After excising anorectal mucosa immediately around the internal fistula opening, it is closed at the level of the internal sphincter muscle using absorbable suture. The adequacy of closure is confirmed by injecting hydrogen peroxide under pressure into the external opening(s) without bubbling at the anorectum and

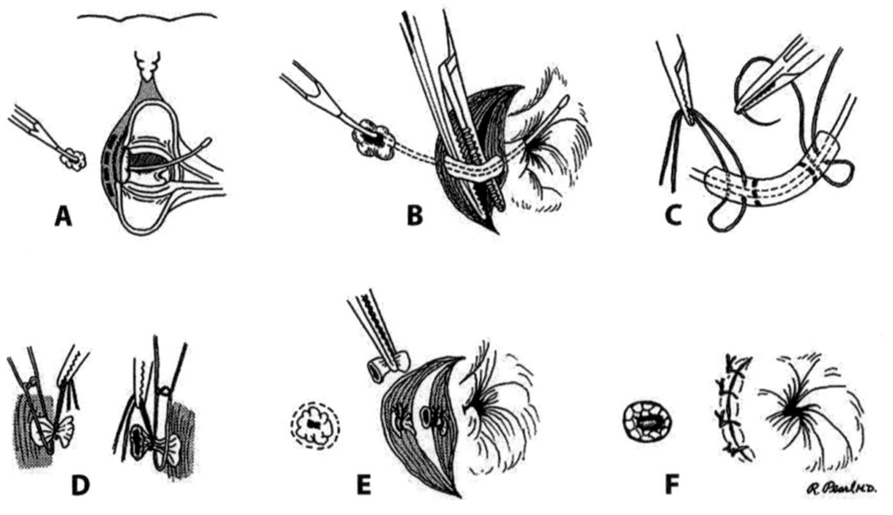

Figure 4.
LIFT operative technique schematic. Illustration used with permission from Abcarian, AM, et al. (2012). (A) the intersphincteric groove is identified and dissected with a probe through the tract to assist with (B) circumferential dissection of the tract in that space. (C-D) the medial and lateral exposed intersphincteric margins of the tract are suture ligated, and (E) the intervening portion can be excised along with fistulectomy of the external opening before (F) closing the incision with suture.

additional sutures can be placed as needed. The adjacent anorectal mucosa/submucosa can be closed over the closure site for reinforcement. The previously placed suture ties are used to ligate the fistula medially and laterally, close to the respective sphincters. It is not uncommon for one of the ties to be inadvertently cut when transecting the ligated tract with a scalpel, so it is the senior author's practice to err well medially toward the internal sphincter with the initial ligation. Any remaining opening defect in the external sphincter can be easily identified by placing the fistula probe from the external skin opening and ligating around the probe. Some authors have reported reinforcing this ligation with a biologic matrix (discussed later in the text, **Figure 5**). Finally, the intersphincteric site is closed in layers with interrupted absorbable suture and the previous external opening can be excised by fistulectomy to promote drainage if so desired.

3.2.3 LIFT outcomes

A recent updated meta-analysis of 26 studies by Emile et al. found pooled LIFT success rates of 76% and identified specific factors associated with surgical failure including horseshoe fistulas, Crohn-associated fistulas, and recurrent fistulas after prior repair attempt [45]. As previously stated, both the LIFT procedure and endorectal or anodermal advancement flap are acceptable procedures for the treatment of complex perianal fistula. There have been conflicting results in the literature regarding outcomes of the two procedures. In a randomized control trial by Kumar et al., LIFT was compared to endorectal advancement flap in the treatment of high anal fistula. LIFT was found to have significantly higher healing rate (76.2 vs. 54.7%) and lower operative time (46 vs. 90 minutes), but the authors' reported healing rate for endorectal advancement flap was lower than the average reported elsewhere [46, 47].

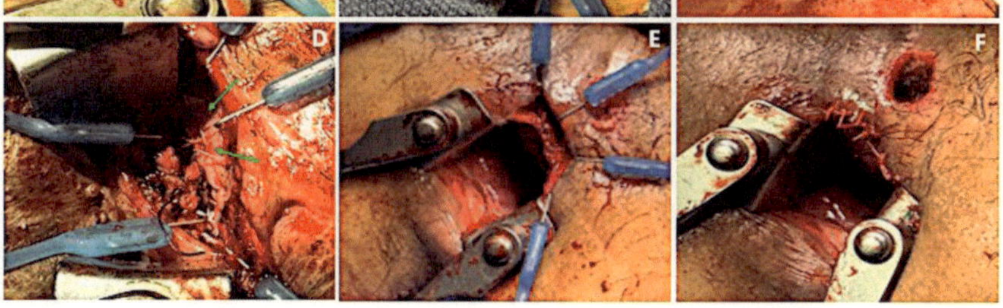

Figure 5.
LIFT repair operative technique. After seton removal and tract debridement the intersphincteric groove is identified and dissected sharply (A). The primary internal opening is closed with suture (not pictured). The mature fistula tract is encircled circumferentially within the intersphincteric space (B) and isolated with suture for ligation(C). In special cases or within a clinical trial, tract ligation can be reinforced by placement of an acellular scaffold as a bio-LIFT procedure, (D, matrix denoted by green arrows). The intersphincteric space is closed in layers (E), followed by the anoderm with possible fistulectomy of the external fistula opening to promote external drainage (F). Pictures care of Jeff Van Eps, MD, UT physicians colon & rectal clinic.

In comparison, Tan et al. found in a retrospective review that endorectal advancement flap had a significantly higher success rate compared to LIFT (93.5 vs. 62.5%) [48]. Others have not been able to consistently demonstrate a significant difference in success rate between the two procedures [49, 50]. A 2019 meta-analysis of 30 studies found no statistically reliable difference between the two procedures for surgical success or recurrence, but LIFT was found to have slightly higher postoperative incontinence rates (7.8 vs. 1.6%) [51]. No direct comparison has been specifically made of anodermal advancement flap to LIFT. Various modifications to the classic LIFT procedure have been developed including but not limited to: LIFT with fistula plug, LIFT with advancement flap, LIFT with bioprosthetic mesh, etc. There is a general paucity of literature directly comparing any of these procedural variations and more data is needed but this is discussed in more detail in subsequent sections regarding biologic augmentation [52].

3.3 Advancement flap

3.3.1 Background and theory

It is thought that failure to control the internal fistula opening at the anorectal lumen is the primary cause of surgical failure and fistula recurrence. This dynamic area with at times questionable tissue viability experiences mechanical and pressure forces that risk reopening after simple suture closure. Repair of complex fistula by local tissue advancement flap prevents ongoing contamination by reinforcing this deep suture closure of the internal fistula opening with a well-vascularized adjacent tissue transfer. There are two general types of advancement flap—endorectal flaps (also termed anorectal, transanal, etc.) whereby the proximal anorectal tissue is moved downward/caudally or "up to down," and anodermal flaps whereby adjacent anodermal soft tissue is moved upward/cranially or "out to in" to cover the internal opening. Specific techniques described in literature vary widely regarding the depth of tissue layers incorporated, flap size and configuration, and preparation of the recipient site prior to securing the flap. This section will describe the indications/contraindications for advancement flaps, provide some expansion on technical details of the procedure, and compare flap repair to the ligation of intersphincteric fistula tract (LIFT) procedure.

3.3.2 Indications and contraindications

Advancement flaps are generally considered a 'sphincter-sparing' approach and are indicated to treat fistulas in which traditional fistulotomy would be associated with an unacceptably high risk of post-operative incontinence. As previously defined in the section on fistula classification, a 'high' anal fistula is defined as involving greater than one-third of the internal anal sphincter. Simple fistulotomy in such patients is associated with unacceptably high rates of incontinence (2–63%) and require a more nuanced approach [53]. Other fistula subtypes or special situations that might call for flap repair include a high or mid-height intersphincteric fistula in a patient with tenuous continence or sphincter function (e.g., women with history of traumatic vaginal birth). These are not candidates for LIFT repair and are ideal candidates for anodermal flap repair. In reality, however, calling advancement flaps sphincter-sparing is a misnomer. No modality of complex fistula repair can avoid all muscular injury, even if it includes just a portion of the subcutaneous portion of external sphincter.

Bleeding diatheses and active infection at the site of the fistula (heavy purulent drainage, indurated local tissues) are contraindications to any fistula repair. Contraindications specific to advancement flap repair follow similar constraints as tissue transfer at other anatomic sites. Active smoking status, history of pelvic/perineal radiation, and severe, poorly controlled diabetes can all cause microvascular disease that threatens flap viability through mechanisms such as local ischemia and would be considered by some to be contraindications to flap repair—particularly by anodermal advancement, which is a true pedicled flap. For modifiable risks such as smoking and glucose control, it is important to optimize patients during prolonged seton drainage prior to any attempt at fistula repair.

It can often be difficult to determine the best approach for fistula repair using in-office examination alone in a conscious patient with a flexible seton drain in place, as full muscular relaxation under anesthesia is often required to determine tract depth and the level of the internal opening in Ref. to the dentate line, as it can transpose distally after prolonged seton drainage. It is the practice of the senior author to prepare these patients for repair by LIFT versus flap to be determined when under anesthesia. In our practice broadly speaking, advancement flaps are preferred for fistula with tracts coursing deeply within the intersphincteric plane or those with midline internal openings, particularly anterior midline fistulas in females, as the anterior sphincter mechanism is known to be anatomically variable and may be incompletely developed even if nulliparous [54, 55]. When deciding between an endorectal or anodermal approach, surgeon preference usually dominates, but the height of the internal opening is also very important. Anodermal flaps can work well to cover internal openings at or below the lower border of the dentate line, particularly in females who tend to have shorter anal canals by rule compared to males. However, in patients with a long anal canal or a primary opening just above the dentate, this can place an anodermal flap at risk for failure from flap retraction or necrosis secondary to undue tension and is better suited for endorectal flap coverage from above. Conversely, low to mid-height fistula repaired by endorectal flap from above risk complications of mucosal ectropion and increased urgency or incontinence secondary to muscular injury with flap harvest.

3.3.3 Staged repair of perianal fistula and preparation of flap site

Patients with perianal fistula undergoing advancement flap repair are typically treated via a two-stage approach. The first stage typically addresses the acute septic foci with incisional drainage of any perianal abscess and placement of a non-cutting seton through the fistula tract to prevent abscess reaccumulation and promote tract maturation. Having ensured adequate drainage, the fistula tract is allowed to 'cool-down' for a minimum period of 6–8 weeks. It is our practice to allow first-stage seton drainage for a minimum of 12 weeks prior to final repair or until physical exam confirms a mature tract and uninfected perineum with softened, pliable tissues and drainage that is more fibrinous than purulent. Rare patients with refractory inflamed tissues and/or heavy purulence despite appropriate seton drainage may require cross-sectional imaging to rule out occult blind-ending sinus and possible preoperative oral antibiotic treatment. In a retrospective review specifically evaluating endorectal advancement flap repair of high transsphincteric fistula, Van Onkelen et al. found that pre-operative seton drainage did not significantly affect outcomes [56]. However, most clinicians would have significant concerns for flap failure if performing a local advancement flap in the setting of an acute infectious process and this should be approached with caution.

3.3.4 Flap technique: positioning and preparation of flap site

Once the acute infectious process has resolved and the tract has matured, the patient may undergo second stage repair. The patient is positioned in accordance with the location of the fistula. Posterior fistulas are best approached with the patient in lithotomy positioning. Anterior fistulas are best approached with the patient in a prone jack-knife position. A fistula probe is passed through the fistula tract following the course of the pre-existing seton and the seton is removed. The tract is de-epithelialized and cleared of granulation and debris using a curette or umbilical tape and flushed with hydrogen peroxide or saline. Electrocautery is used to circumferentially core out denuded mucosa immediately surrounding the tract internal opening down to the internal sphincter muscle to ensure that healthy mucosa will be incorporated into the final repair. The internal opening is then closed primarily with interrupted absorbable suture, confirmed by instilling hydrogen peroxide under pressure at the external opening with adequate closure signaled by a lack of bubbling at the closure site.

3.3.5 Flap technique: endorectal advancement flap

Having prepared the fistula site for flap coverage, the next step involves selecting an appropriate flap technique. Literature surrounding advancement flaps in the treatment of perianal fistula focuses primarily on endorectal advancement flaps. With this technique, a 'U' shaped flap is raised from the rectal wall with the tip distal to the internal opening of the fistula. Dissection is continued 4–6 cm proximally taking care to leave the base wider than the tip of the flap (**Figure 6**). Care should be taken to raise a flap with a base twice as wide as the tip as a rough measurement to prevent flap ischemia. Regarding flap thickness, multiple studies

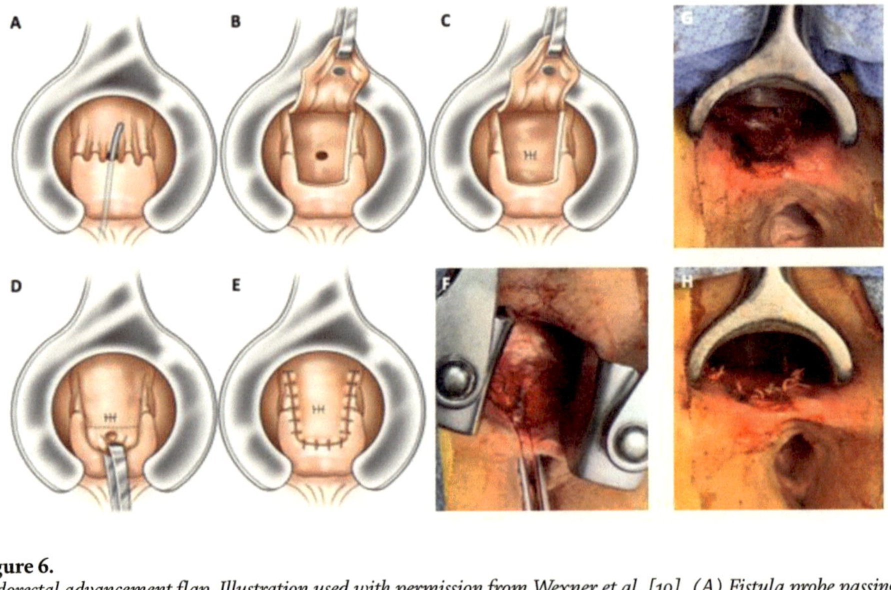

Figure 6.
Endorectal advancement flap. Illustration used with permission from Wexner et al. [10]. (A) Fistula probe passing through internal opening. (B) a partial-thickness rectal flap is raised. (C) Suture ligation of internal opening. (D) Excision of non-viable tissue from around internal opening. (E) Approximation of flap over tissue defect with interrupted sutures. An operative example of endorectal flap repair for low rectovaginal fistula is shown with (F) early flap mobilization and suture closure of primary opening, (G) partial-thickness flap containing some muscle partially secured with suture before (H) fully secured, care of Jeff Van Eps, MD, UT physicians colon & rectal clinic.

have demonstrated superiority of both full-thickness flaps (the entire rectal wall) and partial-thickness flaps (mucosa, submucosa, and a portion of the internal sphincter) compared to mucosal flaps (mucosa and submucosa only) [57, 58]. The apical area of the flap with poor quality mucosal and submucosal tissues that previously surrounded the fistula is transected and excised back to healthy, bleeding tissue. After a sufficient flap is raised to allow for tension-free closure, the flap is then re-approximated to the distal edge of mucosa using intermittent absorbable sutures. Retrospective study has shown durable healing rates several years of about 72% after repair without significant impact on fecal continence and failed patients were able to undergo repeat reparative attempt(s) with variable success without serious quality of life decrement [59].

3.3.6 Flap technique: anodermal advancement flap

Anodermal advancement flap is better studied in the treatment of anal stenosis and anal fissure but may provide certain advantages in select patients with perianal fistula. Unlike endorectal advancement flap, this technique represents a true pedicled tissue flap. The internal fistula opening site is prepared and closed in identical fashion as previously described. With this technique, a tissue island is raised in diamond or house-shaped configuration from the cranial tip immediately adjacent to the internal fistula opening down to the base, which extends caudally distal to the anal verge onto and including the perianal skin (**Figure 7**). The flap is dissected through all layers of superficial tissue down to the underlying sphincter muscle and into deep perianal subcutaneous fat. It is vitally important not to bevel this dissection underneath the harvested flap and to take care when dissecting the caudal flap base not to compromise the feeding vasculature at this site. Failure to follow these principles can lead to a thin, ischemic flap and treatment failure. Zimmerman et al. found that anodermal advancement flaps were successful in 78% of patients who had no or only one previous attempt at repair [60]. Results deteriorated significantly in patients who had 2 or more previous attempts at repair. This technique may facilitate repair for patients in whom an endorectal advancement flap is challenging such as those with large body habitus or anatomically narrow anal canal, or as a fresh alternative in patients who have failed prior repair at the same site.

3.4 Biologic augmentation

3.4.1 Background and need

Given the propensity for failure of complex fistula repair as previously stated, any adjuncts that provide improved surgical success could theoretically translate to profound impacts on patients' health-related quality of life (HRQoL) and healthcare spending. Biologic additives that have been investigated for augmented fistula repair with promising potential include injection of platelet-rich plasma (PRP), stem cells, or implanted acellular matrix (AM) material.

3.4.2 Platelet-rich plasma (PRP)

The biologic milieu within alpha granules and the provisional matrix provided by PRP provide an optimal environment for soft tissue wound regeneration and have demonstrated anti-bacterial and anti-inflammatory effects to decrease infection and

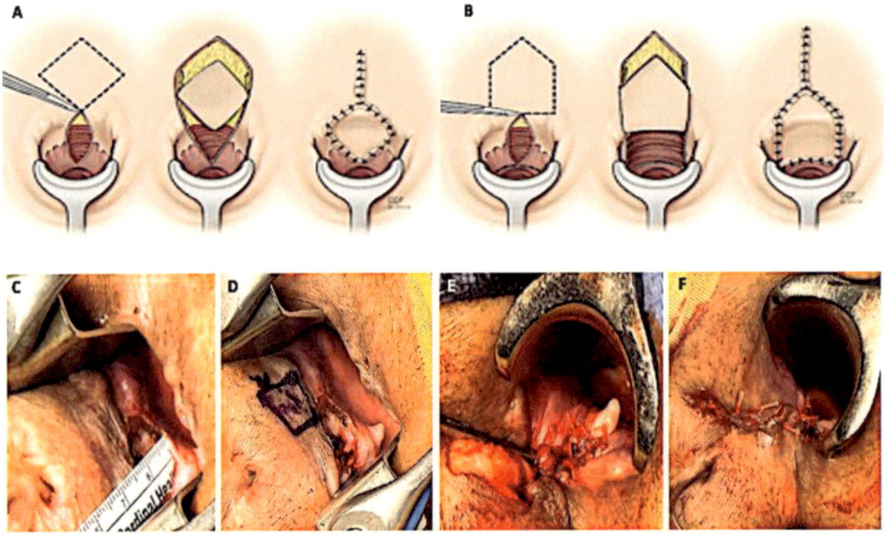

Figure 7.
Anodermal advancement flap. (A) Diamond and (B) house shaped anodermal advancement flap. Illustration demonstrates technique for purposes of anal fissure repair, used with permission from Shawki and Costedio [8]. An example is shown of anodermal advancement flap repair for anterior anal fistula and adjacent anal fissure. After anal seton removal and tract cleaning and closure of the internal opening, (C) the remaining internal defect is measured and (D) a diamond-shaped piece of adjacent anodermal skin is marked and mobilized by sharp dissection before (E) securing it with suture over the internal defect and (F) closure of the flap harvest site and possible external opening fistulectomy. Pictures care of Jeff Van Eps, MD, UT physicians colon & rectal clinic.

postoperative pain [51, 61, 62]. Platelets assist in the healing of complex fistula tracts by initiating the immune cascade through interaction with neutrophils and leukocytes via surface toll-like receptors and P-selectins [61, 63, 64]. This activation causes alpha granules to release their contents, flooding the nearby area with bioactive factors and chemokines that culminate in neovascularization, type II macrophage phenotypic polarization, and stem cell and fibroblast recruitment/retention [61, 65, 66]. Some studies have demonstrated enhanced healing of chronic wounds and anti-bacterial effects both in vitro and in vivo including randomized trials of sternal and skin closure after major vascular operations [61, 67, 68].

There is a dearth of high-quality data for the use of PRP in anal fistula repair, with most studies performed as prospective cohort studies with insufficient power or controls and often employed in non-traditional techniques rather than an augmenting agent to standard repairs. Of the available evidence however, one prospective cohort study evaluated flap repair augmented by PRP in 25 patients noted an 83% success rate at a mean follow-up beyond 2 years [69]. A separate study evaluating augmented flap repair using adipose-derived stromal vascular fraction with PRP in 45 patients witnessed an 84% success rate (38/45 patients) [70]. At the time of this writing, only a single RCT exists with greater than 10 patients, which evaluated LIFT surgical repair augmented with PRP compared to LIFT alone. This demonstrated significant improvement in overall fistula healing at 1 year in the LIFT + PRP group (42/49 vs. 32/49 patients, $p = 0.03$) [71]. There is some evidence that the anti-inflammatory effects of PRP can diminish postoperative pain [71] but whether this can translate to improved postoperative QoL for augmented anal fistula repair remains undefined.

3.4.3 Mesenchymal stem cells (MSC)

Although the exact mechanism by which mesenchymal stem cells (MSC) exert therapeutic effects for anal fistula repair is unknown, it is likely mediated via a local immunomodulatory and regenerative response [72, 73]. The application of MSC is primarily reserved for patients with perianal fistulizing Crohn disease (PFCD) who fail to respond to other medical therapies. Most studies utilize adipose-derived MSC and include direct injection both at the muscular level during simple suture closure of the internal opening as well as into the soft tissues surrounding the tract walls. Alternative sources of MSC such as bone marrow-derived mesenchymal stem cells (bm-MSC) have also demonstrated efficacious results in smaller studies [72, 74, 75]. The largest trial evaluating MSC effects in Crohn disease was the ADMIRE-CD (Adipose-Derived Mesenchymal Stem Cells for Induction of Remission in Perianal Fistulizing Crohn's Disease) trial [72, 76]. This was a randomized, double-blind, placebo-controlled study comparing injection of Cx601 (a solution of 120 million adipose-derived MSC) into the fistula versus a placebo saline solution in a 1:1 fashion [72, 76]. Treatment success at 1 year, defined as closure of external opening(s) and absence of internal collections >2 cm on MRI imaging, occurred in 58/103 (56.3%) patients in the MSC treatment arm compared to 39/101 (38.6%) in the control arm ($p = 0.010$) [77]. A similar trial, ADMIRE-CD-II, is ongoing in the U.S. and a European registry has been established to follow the safety and efficacy of an MSC product being used for fistula commercially [72].

A systematic review by Ciccocioppo et al. of 23 studies including 4 RCT found 64% fistula closure in MSC treated patients versus 37% in control (OR 1.54) without significant safety events [78]. Two other systematic reviews by Cheng and Huang et al. evaluated 7 and 13 trials respectively and found similarly consistent improvement in fistula healing for PFCD patients without increased adverse events. In the first review, patients receiving MSC were twice as likely to heal in pooled results (OR 2.05) overall compared to control while also noting that the source of MSC is important, with autologous stem cells outperforming allogeneic (79% healing vs. 57%) [79]. Their second review examined over 730 patients from 7 RCT and found a similar pooled overall increase in healing with MSC treatment (OR 2.03) that differed depending on individual study definitions of fistula healing, with a range of OR 1.77–5.92 [79]. Included in this review is one of the rare trials of MSC treatment for non-Crohn cryptoglandular fistula, which demonstrated improved healing as well with OR 2.98 compared to control. Also, an interesting subset of MSC application with fibrin glue displayed improved healing with an odds ratio of 3.27, suggesting there may be a role for combining MSC with different biologic matrices or carriers to enhance their regenerative effect. Additional studies are warranted to address optimal dosing and treatment protocols; however the use of MSC is likely to remain an important adjunct once widely available [72]. As the process and cost of MSC isolation is streamlined, there is exciting potential for well-designed trials of MSC application to augment repair of non-Crohn cryptoglandular fistula as well.

3.4.4 Acellular matrix scaffold

Another alternative therapeutic adjunct is biologic acellular matrix (AM), which act as scaffolding for recruited cells and regenerative tissue to build upon. Evidence suggests that AM also induce anti-inflammatory, pro-regenerative effects at the molecular level [80]. Use of AM has increased in popularity since their introduction in 1994, stemming from widespread use in breast surgery beginning in 2001, and their indications continue to expand. A variety of different brands, decellularization processes, and tissue sources (animal-derived vs. cadaveric, dermis vs. small intestine vs. urinary bladder) are now commercially available for use in a multitude of operations ranging from burn and breast surgery to abdominal wall reconstruction [81, 82]. These AM have traditionally only been available as a solid implantable sheet, but more recently micronized powder formulations have been introduced, capable of lining a wound bed or even direct tissue injection after reconstitution. The concept of utilizing biocompatible material to fill fistulous tracts was first investigated using fibrin glue in gynecologic literature in 1982 [83]. Within the realm of anorectal surgery, AM have been used as a biologic 'plug' to fill the fistula tract or as an additional barrier augmenting the LIFT procedure, with varying degrees of success. Most commonly, this matrix plug is secured with suture at the primary internal opening using an internal cuff and customizable tail(s) trimmed to fit the individual tract length at the secondary external opening thereby filling in the previous tract (**Figure 8**).

Success of this method occurs approximately 40–50% per utilization, with limitations including plug extrusion and fistula recurrence [84–86]. The primary advantage of using a plug repair is a low-risk potential high-reward opportunity for healing with minimal risk of incontinence or further morbidity given a lack of tissue disruption. Indications for the use of a matrix plug may include patients with impaired fecal continence at baseline, or the presence of a long, high extrasphincteric fistula tract. When assessing the available literature as a whole, fibrin glue and fistula plugs are generally regarded as relatively ineffective treatment modalities.

The first reported study detailing the use of AM for anal fistula completed by Champagne and colleagues applied a porcine small intestinal submucosa (Surgisis®) 'plug' to fill the fistula tract [87]. They reported an 83% healing rate after follow up of

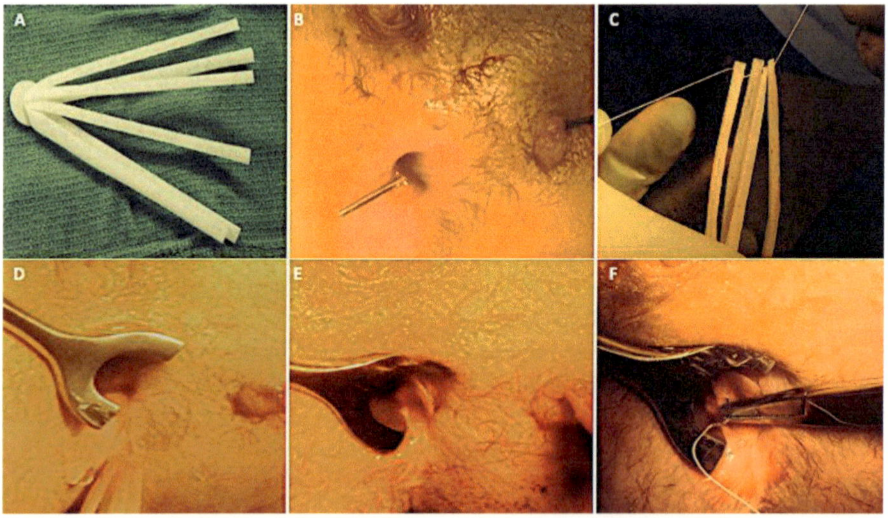

Figure 8.
Anal fistula plug repair. (A) Ex vivo picture of the Gore® bio-a® fistula plug prior to implantation. (B) after seton removal, the fistula tract is cannulated and cleaned of debris. (C) Control of plug using suture through tails. (D) Suture used to pull customized plug through fistula tract. (E) Plug pulled snugly within tract. (F) Plug cuff secured with suture at the internal opening at the anal sphincter. Pictures care of Michael Snyder, MD, UTHealth, UT physicians colon & rectal clinic (CRC).

6–24 months [87]. Subsequent efforts to replicate these results have been unsuccessful, and the combination of non-reproducible results coupled with unclear clinical indications for the optimal type of anal fistula to benefit from a biologic 'plug' have led the technique to largely fall out of favor among clinicians [88–91]. However, subsequent prospective cohort studies have reported promising outcomes when combining standard repairs with AM. Notably, Ellis et al. utilized a Bio-LIFT procedure whereby a biologic matrix was secured within the intersphincteric space after fistula tract ligation with a 94% success rate (29/31 patients) at one-year follow up [92]. This was corroborated by Han and colleagues who also witnessed excellent success rates, (95% success, 20/21 patients) by modified bio-LIFT procedure with a biologic fistula plug placed within the external sphincter portion of the fistula tract following proximal intersphincteric ligation [93].

3.4.5 Future considerations

The overall optimistic but inconclusive results from using biologic agents in the limited number of studies available provide a glimmer of hope for improving the historically unacceptable failure rates of complex anal fistula repair. With the added cost of applying biologic adjuncts, defining their cost utility with consideration for patient-centered impacts on HRQoL will be crucial. Looking to the future, well-designed and adequately powered randomized clinical trials comparing biologic augmentation to standard technique are required to define the indications, if any, for their routine use in complex fistula repair. Our research group is currently trying to address that need with a factorial, randomized controlled clinical trial [94].

4. New and alternative fistula treatments

4.1 Background and clinical need

High recurrence rates of 25–30% or more with advancement flap and LIFT repair and difficult cases like extrasphincteric fistula that preclude standard repair with these approaches have prompted ongoing efforts to develop novel sphincter-sparing approaches. These alternative techniques are in different stages of development and availability but are important tools to keep in mind as anal fistula surgery continues to evolve.

4.2 Video-assisted anal fistula treatment (VAAFT)

Accurate diagnosis and characterization of an anal fistula is crucial, as undetected additional tracts contribute to recurrence. However, complex cross-sectional imaging such as pelvic MRI is an expensive diagnostic modality that is not indicated for most anal fistula. Motivated by these principles, Meinero and Mori introduced the idea of direct fistula visualization through VAAFT [95]. First described in 2006, this sphincter sparing technique involves two phases—diagnostic and operative. In the diagnostic phase, a fistuloscope is inserted through the external opening with continuous glycine-mannitol irrigation and advanced slowly to the internal opening with the assistance of an obturator to straighten the tract (**Figure 9**). Stay sutures are placed in the internal opening illuminated by the fistuloscope but not tied. The goal is to reliably identify the internal opening as well as any secondary tracts or abscess cavities.

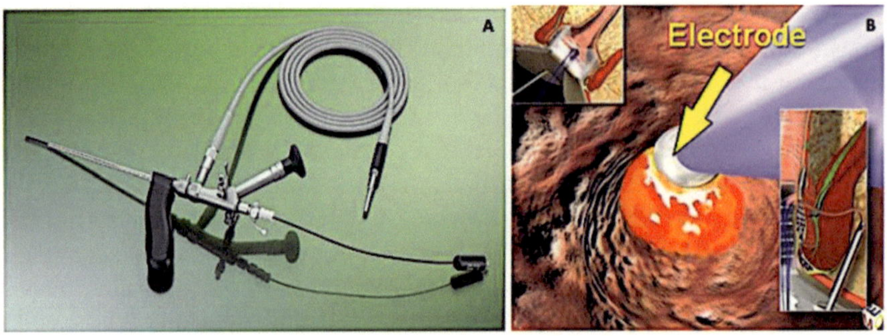

Figure 9.
Video-assisted anal fistula treatment (VAAFT). (A) Standard rigid fistuloscope. (B) Schematic of the VAAFT procedure with cauterization of the fistula tract by the VAAFT electrode. Reused with permissions from Meinero et al. [95].

In the operative phase, the tract is destroyed internally with an electrode under direct visualization working toward the internal opening, removing debris with a brush. The internal opening is then closed either with suture alone, circular stapler, or with a local advancement flap. Meinero and Mori report reinforcing this site of closure using 0.5 mL of cyanoacrylate in the soft tissue just deep to the internal opening applied using a small catheter, leaving the remainder of the treated tract to drain. Their initial series of 136 cases yielded a success rate of 74% at 3 months and 87% at 1 year, but less than half of patients followed up for this duration. Although not measured with a validated scoring tool no patients reported new or worsened fecal incontinence.

According to multiple systematic reviews, VAAFT demonstrates success rates between 76 and 86% [96, 97] with the most recent study reporting a weighted mean success rate of 83% on pooled analysis. Some important differences exist in the likelihood of treatment success according to the method of internal opening closure and fistula type. Zelic evaluated recurrence rates according to closure method and reports recurrence rates of 21% with staple closure, 19% with suture closure, and 24% with advancement flap [98]. Regarding fistula type, Stazi showed short term success rates at 77 and 64% for simple (n = 52) and complex fistulas (n = 172) respectively [99]. Romaniszyn reports long-term success rates (mean of 31 months) by fistula type with 80% (n = 30) of simple transsphincteric fistulas healing, while only 39% (n = 38) of complex fistulas healed [100].

VAAFT has several purported strengths. It is a sphincter sparing procedure with relatively rare and minor complications (creation of false tract, scrotal edema, bleeding, prolonged discharge, itching, allergic reaction, cellulitis, and problems related to spinal anesthesia) [95, 101]. Procedure time is relatively short at an average of 42 to 52 minutes [96, 101], patients report less postoperative pain compared to traditional fistulotomy [96, 102], and quick recovery to baseline function of three to 5 days [103, 104]. Its diagnostic capabilities are emphasized, both with the ability to identify and treat secondary tracts/cavities and identification of a primary internal opening in 79–98% of cases [95, 96, 101].

Reported drawbacks include variable success depending on fistula pathology, rigid construction, and wide diameter of the fistuloscope, and difficulty adequately ablating wide fistula tracts [95, 100]. The rigid nature of the fistuloscope makes traversal of angulated fistula tracts particularly difficult. Prior anal surgery or treatment of a recurrent fistula is associated with treatment failure after VAAFT [101, 105]. Lastly, VAAFT is not currently widely available in the U.S. as it has not been FDA approved at the time of this writing, making our evaluation of its potential utility reliant upon non-randomized international studies often insufficiently controlled or powered.

4.3 Fistula tract laser closure (FiLaC)

Persistent fistula epithelium or granulating tissue contributes to fistula persistence or recurrence [106]. In the pilot study of FiLaC [107], Wilhelm sought to improve success rates of the advancement flap technique by following internal closure of the internal opening by flap with subsequent ablation of the epithelial layer of the fistula using a radial emitting laser probe to shrink and seal the tract by denaturation (**Figure 10**). Since then the FiLaC procedure has been described both independently as the laser ablative portion and in conjunction with the closure of the internal opening (e.g., via advancement flap, staple, suture closure).

Primary healing rates of this technique are 63–67% based on pooled calculations from two systematic reviews performed to date [108, 109]. Elfeki et al. reported a 67% healing rate but 117 of the 454 patients were treated with additional closure of the internal opening (mainly by advancement flaps) compared to the rest that underwent FiLaC alone. The 117 patients were from Wilhelm's study which reported a 64% healing rate [110].

Interestingly, FiLaC has similar treatment success for Crohn's fistula. A systemic review of studies that employed FiLaC to fistulizing Crohn's disease reports a pooled primary healing rate of 68% [111]. Wilhelm found that intersphincteric fistulas showed superior success rates compared to transsphincteric, suprasphincteric, and extrasphincteric fistulas [106].

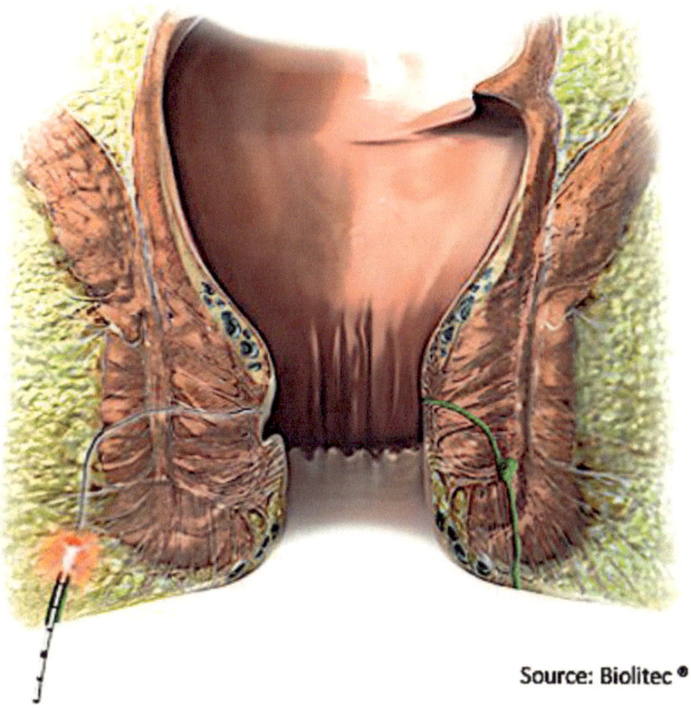

Figure 10.
FiLAC procedure schematic. Source: Biolitec®, used with permissions.

The nature of failure after FiLaC in most cases is one of persistence rather than recurrence [108]. Patients who fail treatment will have persistent drainage that does not resolve in the acute period [112]. Repeat FiLaC does not portend lower chances of success in subsequent attempts, meaning it can be repeated liberally without apparent significant morbidity [110–113].

Proponents of pre-procedural seton placement argue that it allows the fistula tract to mature, allowing homogenous formation of granulation tissue for consistent FiLaC treatment [111]. Giamundo et al. reported a trend toward greater success after seton drainage, however, it was not a significant difference [112]. It is not clear whether fistula length is a predictor of success as discrepant opinions exist. Giamundo claims anecdotally that longer fistulas (>4 cm) produce the best results and shorter tracts (<2 cm) should not be candidates for FiLaC [112]. Conversely, Lauretta et al. found in their small retrospective study (n = 30) that fistulas <3 cm actually had superior outcomes compared to longer fistulas with healing rates 58 vs. 16% [114]. These results should be taken with a modicum of skepticism given their low overall success rate of 33% compared to figures reported in the literature.

There are several strengths to FiLaC. It has comparable efficacy whether the fistula is of Crohn's or cryptoglandular etiology. FiLaC is repeatable without accumulation of negative effects or morbidities and complications are rare with a pooled rate of 4% [108] and usually minor in nature (e.g., minor soiling, temporary postoperative pain, abscess, bleeding) [106, 108]. The average reported procedure is 20 minutes [108, 110] with an average learning curve of only five procedures [115]. Patients report minimal postop pain and early return to work [116].

The disadvantage of FiLaC is that it is a blind procedure which could lead to missed identification of secondary tracts. The laser fiber is also not FDA approved in the United States at the time of writing.

4.4 Over the scope clip (OTSC)

OTSC is an endoscopic technique developed in 2008 to enhance efficient control of gastrointestinal bleeding and iatrogenic perforations, as it utilizes a clip much larger than is allowable by the endoscope working channel [117, 118]. Indications expanded to include usage for anastomotic leaks and fistulas, particularly anal fistulas with the OTSC Proctology device (Ovesco Endoscopy GmbH, Tübingen, Germany) (**Figure 11**). This technique involves curetting the fistulous tract with a wire brush followed by irrigation and dissection of a circumferential area of anoderm from around the internal opening to expose the internal sphincter muscle. Two U-stitches are placed through or adjacent to the internal opening for clip applier guidance over the sutures to allow positioning at the base of the internal opening. The clip—made of biocompatible nitinol—is deployed, and the external opening is widened to ensure easy drainage of the fistula tract. There is no evidence-based data regarding how long the clip should remain in place and it is frequently left in place indefinitely unless the patient experiences symptoms.

The largest current study is a series of 100 procedures by Prosst et al. with the vast majority indicated for cryptoglandular fistula and 11 associated with IBD [120]. The median length of procedure was 32 minutes with a length of stay between three and 4 days [120]. They report an overall success rate of 65% with differential outcomes based on indication. Treatment for an initial fistula showed a 79% healing rate compared to the dismal 26% in those treated for recurrence, and 45% for the 11 IBD patients. The same group reported the most comprehensive review to date

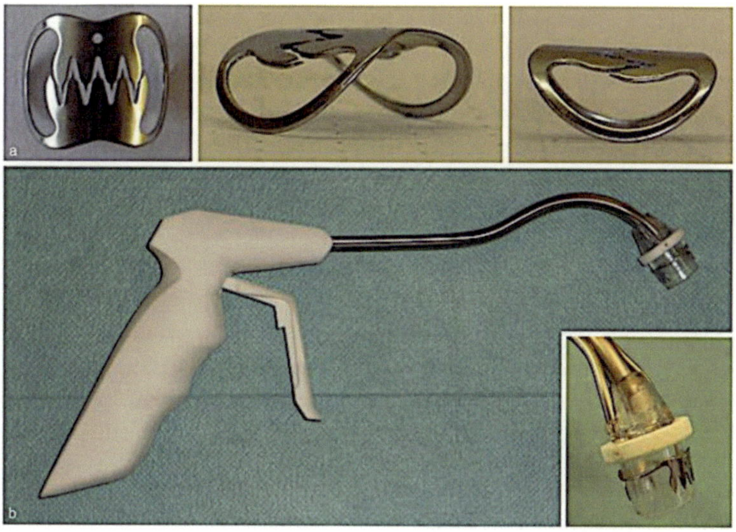

Figure 11.
Over the scope clip (OTSC) equipment. (a) Representation of the "bear claw" clip that is deployed and (b) the OTSC proctology device. Reused from Prosst et al. [119] with permissions from Taylor and Francis.

summarizing the ten available published studies [119] and a total of 236 procedures. Apart from Prosst's largest study (n = 100), the studies have very small sample sizes ranging from single case reports to case series of 35 procedures. Predictors of failure included application on a recurrent fistula, early clip detachment prior to 4 weeks, and IBD [119].

OTSC treatment of anal fistulas seems to be safe and painless. Multiple studies report the surprisingly high level of patient tolerance with application despite the full thickness force of the clip [119–121]. Proponents of this technique emphasize the clip's ability to apply constant pressure in between its jaws despite the dynamic changes in the tissue throughout the healing process. This is especially pronounced when compared to the static nature of a simple suture [117, 120, 121].

Many questions remain to be answered as robust data is currently lacking for OTSC. IBD fistulas seem to have inferior outcomes, but larger studies are needed [119, 120]. Management the clip postoperatively also needs to be clarified. Prosst was able to identify clips in 15 patients postoperatively at 6 months and they were not removed [120]. The risks should be considered as there is no long-term data on the effect of clips remaining *in situ*.

5. Conclusion

Anorectal fistulas represent a difficult and complex spectrum of disease that continues to plague surgical patients and clinicians alike with impacts on quality of life and high rates of surgical failure. Successful surgical treatment aims to control infection while maximizing healing and safeguarding anorectal function. This requires an intimate knowledge of anorectal anatomy and fistula classification, along with experience in management of simple and complex fistulas, and an ever-growing armamentarium of tools and techniques to promote successful outcomes through individualized treatment. Surgical dogma of fistulotomy for simple, low fistulas and two-stage sphincter-sparing approaches for complex, high fistulas remain the rule. A truly skilled fistula specialist is comfortable with a variety of treatments ranging from seton placement to LIFT, to advancement flap and more importantly, discerns when each is appropriate. However, the surgical landscape is ever-changing, and the future is bright for fistula surgery, with the promise of improved outcomes potentially coming with the advent of new biologic augmentations, fistula-specific instruments, and minimally-invasive techniques as outlined in this text.

Conflict of interest

Dr. Van Eps is the primary investigator on the BIO RAMP clinical trial currently underway to investigate biologic augmentation of complex fistula repair, which is supported by ACell (Integra) with donated biologic matrix material only.

Notes/thanks/other declarations

Thanks to our partners and colleagues within the UT Health Colon & Rectal Clinic (CRC) for supporting this effort and specifically to Mark Pidala, MD, Scott McKnight, MD, and Michael Snyder, MD for contributing operative images used in our figures.

Author details

Jerry Xiao[1], Erin Santos[2], Nana-Yaw Bonsu[1], Woihwan Kim[2], Michael Eisenberg[2], Marianne Cusick[2,3] and Jeffrey Van Eps[2,3*]

1 Department of Surgery, Houston Methodist Hospital, Houston, TX, USA

2 Department of Surgery, UT Health at Houston, McGovern Medical School, Houston, TX, USA

3 UT Physicians Colon & Rectal Clinic, Houston, TX, USA

*Address all correspondence to: jeffrey.l.vaneps@uth.tmc.edu

IntechOpen

© 2024 The Author(s). Licensee IntechOpen. This chapter is distributed under the terms of the Creative Commons Attribution License (http://creativecommons.org/licenses/by/3.0), which permits unrestricted use, distribution, and reproduction in any medium, provided the original work is properly cited. (cc) BY

References

[1] Gaertner WB, Burgess PL, Davids JS, et al. The American Society of Colon and Rectal Surgeons clinical practice guidelines for the management of anorectal abscess, fistula-in-ano, and rectovaginal fistula. Diseases of the Colon and Rectum. 2022;**65**(8):964-985. DOI: 10.1097/DCR.0000000000002473

[2] Sarveazad A, Bahardoust M, Shamseddin J, Yousefifard M. Prevalence of anal fistulas: A systematic review and meta-analysis. Gastroenterology and Hepatology From Bed to Bench. 2022;**15**(1):1-8

[3] Carmichael JC, Mills S. Anatomy and embryology of the colon, rectum, and anus. In: The ASCRS Textbook of Colon and Rectal Surgery. New York: Springer International Publishing; 2022. pp. 3-27

[4] Lilius HG. Fistula-in-ano, an investigation of human foetal anal ducts and intramuscular glands and a clinical study of 150 patients. Acta Chirurgica Scandinavica. Supplementum. 1968;**383**:7-88

[5] Davis BR, Kasten KR. Anorectal abscess and fistula. In: Steele SR, Hull TL, Read TE, Saclarides TJ, Senagore AJ, Whitlow CB, editors. The ASCRS Textbook of Colon and Rectal Surgery. New York: Springer International Publishing; 2016. pp. 215-244. DOI: 10.1007/978-3-319-25970-3_14

[6] Abcarian H. Anorectal infection: Abscess-fistula. Clinics in Colon and Rectal Surgery. 2011;**24**(1):14-21. DOI: 10.1055/s-0031-1272819

[7] Włodarczyk M, Włodarczyk J, Sobolewska-Włodarczyk A, Trzciński R, Dziki Ł, Fichna J. Current concepts in the pathogenesis of cryptoglandular perianal fistula. The Journal of International Medical Research. 2021;**49**(2):300060520986669. DOI: 10.1177/0300060520986669

[8] Chrabot CM, Prasad ML, Abcarian H. Recurrent anorectal abscesses. Diseases of the Colon and Rectum. 1983;**26**:105-108. DOI: 10.1007/BF02562586

[9] Ramanujam PS, Prasad ML, Abcarian H, Tan AB. Perianal abscesses and fistulas. Diseases of the Colon and Rectum. 1984;**27**(9):593-597. DOI: 10.1007/BF02553848

[10] Zanotti C, Martinez-Puente C, Pascual I, Pascual M, Herreros D, García-Olmo D. An assessment of the incidence of fistula-in-ano in four countries of the European Union. International Journal of Colorectal Disease. 2007;**22**(12):1459-1462. DOI: 10.1007/s00384-007-0334-7. Epub 2007 Jun 7

[11] Smith WDH. Biography, Works, & Facts. Britannica. Available from: https://www.britannica.com/biography/Hippocrates; [Accessed: October 12, 2023]

[12] Corman ML. Classic articles in colon and rectal surgery. Hippocrates: On fistulae. Diseases of the Colon and Rectum. 1980;**23**(1):56-59. DOI: 10.1007/BF02587204

[13] Tsamis D. The origin of cure for fistula in ano: Technique of hippocrates. Techniques in Coloproctology. 2015;**19**(8):489-490. DOI: 10.1007/s10151-015-1338-x

[14] Banov L. Frederick salmon-surgeon who founded St. Mark's Hospital. Diseases of the Colon & Rectum.

1968;**11**(6):447-451. DOI: 10.1007/BF02616775

[15] Tsoucalas G. British surgeon Frederick Salmon (1796-1868) and his "trans-fixing pins and excision" surgical procedure for the "rectum prolapsus". Surgical Innovation. 2018;**25**(1):88-89. DOI: 10.1177/1553350617731384

[16] St Marks Hospital Foundation. The History of St Mark's Hospital and Founder Frederick Salmon. St Marks Hospital Foundation. Available from: https://www.stmarkshospitalfoundation.org.uk/about/history/ [Accessed: October 12, 2023]

[17] Salmon F. On the treatment of fistula: To the editor of the lancet. The Lancet (British edition). 1845:**45**(1122):248-248

[18] Lockhart-Mummery JP. Discussion on fistula-in-ano. Proceedings of the Royal Society of Medicine. 1929;**22**(9):1331-1358. DOI: 10.1177/003591572902200960

[19] Fry RD. History of anal fistulas. Seminars in Colon and Rectal Surgery. 2014;**25**(4):173-175. DOI: 10.1053/j.scrs.2014.08.003

[20] Schouten WR. Anorectal abscess and fistula. In: Keighley, Williams, editors. Surgery of the Anus, Rectum and Colon. 4th ed. Boca Raton: CRC Press, Taylor & Francis; 2018

[21] Jørum E. The sun king's anal fistula. Tidsskrift for Den norske legeforening. 23 Aug 2016;**136**(14):1244-1247. Available from: https://tidsskriftet.no/2016/08/sun-kings-anal-fistula [Accessed: October 21, 2023]

[22] Owen HA, Buchanan GN, Schizas A, Cohen R, Williams AB. Quality of life with anal fistula. Annals of the Royal College of Surgeons of England. 2016;**98**(5):334-338. DOI: 10.1308/rcsann.2016.0136

[23] Ware JE, Sherbourne CD. The MOS 36-item short-form health survey (SF-36): I. Conceptual framework and item selection. Medical Care. 1992;**30**(6):473-483. Available from: https://www.jstor.org/stable/3765916 [Accessed: October 22, 2023]

[24] Ferrer-Márquez M, Espínola-Cortés N, Reina-Duarte Á, Granero-Molina J, Fernández-Sola C, Hernández-Padilla JM. Analysis and description of disease-specific quality of life in patients with anal fistula. Cirugía Española (English Edition). 2018;**96**(4):213-220. DOI: 10.1016/j.cireng.2017.12.006

[25] Morgan CN, Thompson HR. Surgical anatomy of the anal canal with special reference to the surgical importance of the internal sphincter and conjoint longitudinal muscle. Annals of the Royal College of Surgeons of England. 1956;**19**(2):88-114

[26] Parks AG, Gordon PH, Hardcastle JD. A classification of fistula-in-ano. British Journal of Surgery. 1976;**63**(1):1-12. DOI: 10.1002/BJS.1800630102

[27] Sileri P, Cadeddu F, D'Ugo S, Franceschilli L, Del Vecchio Blanco G, De Luca E, et al. Surgery for fistula-in-ano in a specialist colorectal unit: A critical appraisal. BMC Gastroenterology. 2011;**11**:120. DOI: 10.1186/1471-230X-11-120

[28] de Criado JM, del Salto LG, Rivas PF, del Hoyo LFA, Velasco LG, M Isabel Díez Pérez Vacas de las , et al. MR imaging evaluation of perianal fistulas: Spectrum of imaging features. Radiographics. 2012;**32**(1):175-194. DOI:10.1148/RG.321115040

[29] Garg P. Comparing existing classifications of fistula-in-ano in

440 operated patients: Is it time for a new classification? A retrospective cohort study. International Journal of Surgery. 2017;**42**:34-40. DOI: 10.1016/J.IJSU.2017.04.019

[30] Anan M et al. Fistulotomy with or without marsupialisation of wound edges in treatment of simple anal fistula: A randomised controlled trial. Annals of the Royal College of Surgeons of England. 2019;**101**(7):472-478

[31] Ho YH et al. Marsupialization of fistulotomy wounds improves healing: A randomized controlled trial. The British Journal of Surgery. 1998;**85**(1):105-107

[32] Jain BK et al. Comparison of a fistulectomy and a fistulotomy with marsupialization in the management of a simple anal fistula: A randomized, controlled pilot trial. Journal of the Korean Society of Coloproctology. 2012;**28**(2):78-82

[33] Pescatori M et al. Marsupialization of fistulotomy and fistulectomy wounds improves healing and decreases bleeding: A randomized controlled trial. Colorectal Disease. 2006;**8**(1):11-14

[34] Abbas MA, Jackson CH, Haigh PI. Predictors of outcome for anal fistula surgery. Archives of Surgery. 2011;**146**(9):1011-1016

[35] Hall JF et al. Outcomes after operations for anal fistula: Results of a prospective, multicenter, regional study. Diseases of the Colon and Rectum. 2014;**57**(11):1304-1308

[36] Litta F et al. Simple fistula-in-ano: Is it all simple? A systematic review. Techniques in Coloproctology. 2021;**25**(4):385-399

[37] Sugrue J et al. Sphincter-sparing anal fistula repair: Are we getting better? Diseases of the Colon & Rectum. 2017;**60**(10):1071-1077

[38] Liu WY et al. Long-term results of ligation of intersphincteric fistula tract (LIFT) for fistula-in-ano. Diseases of the Colon and Rectum. 2013;**56**(3):343-347

[39] Ritchie R, Sackier J, Hodde J. Incontinence rates after cutting seton treatment for anal fistula. Colorectal Disease. 2009;**11**(6):564-571

[40] Garcia-Aguilar J et al. Cutting seton versus two-stage seton fistulotomy in the surgical management of high anal fistula. Journal of British Surgery. 1998;**85**(2):243-245

[41] Rojanasakul A et al. Total anal sphincter saving technique for fistula-in-ano; the ligation of Intersphincteric fistula tract. Journal of the Medical Association of Thailand. 2007;**90**(3):581

[42] Alasari S, Kim NK. Overview of anal fistula and systematic review of ligation of the intersphincteric fistula tract (LIFT). Techniques in Coloproctology. 2014;**18**(1):13-22

[43] Vergara-Fernandez O, Espino-Urbina LA. Ligation of Intersphincteric fistula tract: What is the evidence in a review? World Journal of Gastroenterology: WJG. 2013;**19**(40):6805-6813

[44] Amato A et al. Evaluation and management of perianal abscess and anal fistula: SICCR position statement. Techniques in Coloproctology. 2020;**24**(2):127-143

[45] Emile SH, Khan SM, Adejumo A, Koroye O. Ligation of intersphincteric fistula tract (LIFT) in treatment of anal fistula: An updated systematic review, meta-analysis, and meta-regression

of the predictors of failure. Surgery. 2020;**167**(2):484-492

[46] Kumar P et al. Ligation of Intersphincteric fistulous tract vs endorectal advancement flap for high-type fistula in ano: A randomized controlled trial. Journal of the American College of Surgeons. 2023;**236**(1):27-35

[47] Soltani A, Kaiser AM. Endorectal advancement flap for cryptoglandular or Crohn's fistula-in-ano. Diseases of the Colon & Rectum. 2010;**53**(4):486-495

[48] Tan K-K et al. To lift or to flap? Which surgery to perform following seton insertion for high anal fistula? Diseases of the Colon & Rectum. 2012;**55**(12):1273-1277

[49] Madbouly KM et al. Ligation of intersphincteric fistula tract versus mucosal advancement flap in patients with high transsphincteric fistula-in-ano: A prospective randomized trial. Diseases of the Colon & Rectum. 2014;**57**(10):1202-1208

[50] van Praag EM et al. Ligation of the Intersphincteric fistula tract and endorectal advancement flap for high perianal fistulas in Crohn's disease: A retrospective cohort study. Journal of Crohn's and Colitis. 2020;**14**(6):757-763

[51] Stellingwerf ME, Van Praag EM, Tozer PJ, Bemelman WA, Buskens CJ. Systematic review and meta-analysis of endorectal advancement flap and ligation of the intersphincteric fistula tract for cryptoglandular and Crohn's high perianal fistulas. BJS Open. 2019;**3**(3):231-241

[52] Sirany A-ME, Nygaard RM, Morken JJ. The ligation of the Intersphincteric fistula tract procedure for anal fistula: A mixed bag of results. Diseases of the Colon & Rectum. 2015;**58**(6):604-612

[53] Ommer A et al. Continence disorders after anal surgery—A relevant problem? International Journal of Colorectal Disease. 2008;**23**(11):1023-1031

[54] Bollard RC, Gardiner A, Lindow S, Phillips K, Duthie GS. Normal female anal sphincter: Difficulties in interpretation explained. Diseases of the Colon & Rectum. 2002;**45**:171-175

[55] Starck M, Bohe M, Fortling B, Valentin L. Endosonography of the anal sphincter in women of different ages and parity. Ultrasound in Obstetrics & Gynecology. 2005;**25**(2):169-176

[56] van Onkelen Robbert S, Gosselink Martijn P, Sjoerd T, Schouten WRMD. Predictors of outcome after transanal advancement flap repair for high transsphincteric fistulas. Diseases of the Colon & Rectum. 2014;**57**(8):1007-1011. DOI: 10.1097/DCR.0000000000000154

[57] Khafagy W et al. Treatment of anal fistulas by partial rectal wall advancement flap or mucosal advancement flap: A prospective randomized study. International Journal of Surgery (London, England). 2010;**8**(4):321-325

[58] Dubsky PC et al. Endorectal advancement flaps in the treatment of high anal fistula of cryptoglandular origin: Full-thickness vs. mucosal-rectum flaps. Diseases of the Colon & Rectum. 2008;**51**(6):852-857

[59] Jarrar A, Church J. Advancement flap repair: A good option for complex anorectal fistulas. Diseases of the Colon & Rectum. 2011;**54**(12):1537-1541

[60] Zimmerman DDE, Briel JW, Gosselink MP, et al. Anocutaneous advancement flap repair of transsphincteric fistulas. Diseases of the

Colon and Rectum. 2001;**44**:1474-1477. DOI: 10.1007/BF02234601

[61] Fernandez-Moure JS, Van Eps JL, Cabrera FJ, et al. Platelet-rich plasma: A biomimetic approach to enhancement of surgical wound healing. The Journal of Surgical Research. 2017;**207**:33-44. DOI: 10.1016/j.jss.2016.08.063

[62] Le ADK, Enweze L, DeBaun MR, Dragoo JL. Current clinical recommendations for use of platelet-rich plasma. Current Reviews in Musculoskeletal Medicine. 2018;**11**(4):624-634. DOI: 10.1007/s12178-018-9527-7

[63] Clark SR, Ma AC, Tavener SA, et al. Platelet TLR4 activates neutrophil extracellular traps to ensnare bacteria in septic blood. Nature Medicine Apr 2007;13(4):463-469. DOI: 10.1038/nm1565

[64] Wang HB, Wang JT, Zhang L, et al. P-selectin primes leukocyte integrin activation during inflammation. Nature Immunology. 2007;**8**(8):882-892. DOI: 10.1038/ni1491

[65] Nasirzade J, Kargarpour Z, Hasannia S, Strauss FJ, Gruber R. Platelet-rich fibrin elicits an anti-inflammatory response in macrophages in vitro. Journal of Periodontology. 2020;**91**(2):244-252. DOI: 10.1002/jper.19-0216

[66] Heffron SP, Weinstock A, Scolaro B, et al. Platelet-conditioned media induces an anti-inflammatory macrophage phenotype through EP4. Journal of Thrombosis and Haemostasis. 2021;**19**(2):562-573. DOI: 10.1111/jth.15172

[67] Khalafi RS, Bradford DW, Wilson MG. Topical application of autologous blood products during surgical closure following a coronary artery bypass graft. European Journal of Cardio-Thoracic Surgery. 2008;**34**(2):360-364. DOI: 10.1016/j.ejcts.2008.04.026

[68] Saratzis N, Saratzis A, Melas N, Kiskinis D. Non-activated autologous platelet-rich plasma for the prevention of inguinal wound-related complications after endovascular repair of abdominal aortic aneurysms. The Journal of Extra-Corporeal Technology. 2008;**40**(1):52-56

[69] Göttgens KW, Vening W, van der Hagen SJ, et al. Long-term results of mucosal advancement flap combined with platelet-rich plasma for high cryptoglandular perianal fistulas. Diseases of the Colon and Rectum. 2014;**57**(2):223-227. DOI: 10.1097/dcr.0000000000000023

[70] Schouten WR, Arkenbosch JHC, van der Woude CJ, et al. Efficacy and safety of autologous adipose-derived stromal vascular fraction enriched with platelet-rich plasma in flap repair of transsphincteric cryptoglandular fistulas. Techniques in Coloproctology. 2021;**25**(12):1301-1309. DOI: 10.1007/s10151-021-02524-6

[71] Madbouly KM, Emile SH, Issa YA, Omar W. Ligation of intersphincteric fistula tract (LIFT) with or without injection of platelet-rich plasma (PRP) in management of high trans-sphincteric fistula-in-ano: Short-term outcomes of a prospective, randomized trial. Surgery. 2021;**170**(1):61-66. DOI: 10.1016/j.surg.2020.12.025

[72] Vasudevan A, Bruining DH, Loftus EV Jr, Faubion W, Ehman EC, Raffals L. Approach to medical therapy in perianal Crohn's disease. World Journal of Gastroenterology. 2021;**27**(25):3693-3704. DOI: 10.3748/wjg.v27.i25.3693

[73] Carvello M, Lightner A, Yamamoto T, Kotze PG, Spinelli A. Mesenchymal stem cells for perianal Crohn's disease. Cell. 2019;**8**(7):764. DOI: 10.3390/cells8070764

[74] Dietz AB, Dozois EJ, Fletcher JG, et al. Autologous mesenchymal stem cells, applied in a bioabsorbable matrix, for treatment of perianal fistulas in patients with Crohn's disease. Gastroenterology. 2017;**153**(1):59-62.e2. DOI: 10.1053/j.gastro.2017.04.001

[75] Barnhoorn MC, Wasser M, Roelofs H, et al. Long-term evaluation of allogeneic bone marrow-derived mesenchymal stromal cell therapy for Crohn's disease perianal fistulas. Journal of Crohn's & Colitis. 2020;**14**(1):64-70. DOI: 10.1093/ecco-jcc/jjz116

[76] Turner D, Ricciuto A, Lewis A, et al. STRIDE-II: An update on the selecting therapeutic targets in inflammatory bowel disease (STRIDE) initiative of the International Organization for the Study of IBD (IOIBD): Determining therapeutic goals for treat-to-target strategies in IBD. Gastroenterology. 2021;**160**(5):1570-1583

[77] Panés J, García-Olmo D, Van Assche G, et al. Long-term efficacy and safety of stem cell therapy (Cx601) for complex perianal fistulas in patients with Crohn's disease. Gastroenterology. 2018;**154**(5):1334-1342. e4

[78] Ciccocioppo R, Klersy C, Leffler DA, Rogers R, Bennett D, Corazza GR. Systematic review with meta-analysis: Safety and efficacy of local injections of mesenchymal stem cells in perianal fistulas. JGH Open. 2019;**3**(3):249-260. DOI: 10.1002/jgh3.12141

[79] Cheng F, Huang Z, Li Z. Mesenchymal stem-cell therapy for perianal fistulas in Crohn's disease: A systematic review and meta-analysis. Techniques in Coloproctology. 2019;**23**(7):613-623. DOI: 10.1007/s10151-019-02024-8

[80] Badylak SF, Freytes DO, Gilbert TW. Extracellular matrix as a biological scaffold material: Structure and function. Acta Biomaterialia. 2009;**5**(1):1-13

[81] Debels H, Hamdi M, Abberton K, Morrison W. Dermal matrices and bioengineered skin substitutes: A critical review of current options. Plastic and Reconstructive Surgery. Global Open. 2015;**3**(1):e284. DOI: 10.1097/gox.0000000000000219

[82] Petrie K, Cox CT, Becker BC, MacKay BJ. Clinical applications of acellular dermal matrices: A review. Scars, Burns & Healing. 2022;**8**:20595131211038313. DOI: 10.1177/20595131211038313

[83] Hjortrup A, Moesgaard F, Kjaergård J. Fibrin adhesive in the treatment of perineal fistulas. Diseases of the Colon and Rectum. 1991;**34**(9):752-754. DOI: 10.1007/bf02051064

[84] Hansen MS, Kjær ML, Andersen J. Efficacy of plug treatment for complex anorectal fistulae: Long-term Danish results. Annals of Coloproctology. 2019;**35**(3):123-128. DOI: 10.3393/ac.2018.07.14

[85] Almeida IS, Wickramasinghe D, Weerakkody P, Samarasekera DN. Treatment of fistula in-ano with fistula plug: Experience of a tertiary care Centre in South Asia and comparison of results with the west. BMC Research Notes. 2018;**11**(1):513. DOI: 10.1186/s13104-018-3641-x

[86] Tan KK, Kaur G, Byrne CM, Young CJ, Wright C, Solomon MJ. Long-term outcome of the anal fistula plug for

anal fistula of cryptoglandular origin. Colorectal Disease. 2013;**15**(12):1510-1514. DOI: 10.1111/codi.12391

[87] Champagne BJ, O'Connor LM, Ferguson M, Orangio GR, Schertzer ME, Armstrong DN. Efficacy of anal fistula plug in closure of cryptoglandular fistulas: Long-term follow-up. Diseases of the Colon and Rectum. 2006;**49**(12):1817-1821. DOI: 10.1007/s10350-006-0755-3

[88] Christoforidis D, Etzioni DA, Goldberg SM, Madoff RD, Mellgren A. Treatment of complex anal fistulas with the collagen fistula plug. Diseases of the Colon and Rectum. 2008;**51**(10):1482-1487. DOI: 10.1007/s10350-008-9374-5

[89] Ky AJ, Sylla P, Steinhagen R, Steinhagen E, Khaitov S, Ly EK. Collagen fistula plug for the treatment of anal fistulas. Diseases of the Colon and Rectum. 2008;**51**(6):838-843. DOI: 10.1007/s10350-007-9191-2

[90] Safar B, Jobanputra S, Sands D, Weiss EG, Nogueras JJ, Wexner SD. Anal fistula plug: Initial experience and outcomes. Diseases of the Colon and Rectum. 2009;**52**(2):248-252. DOI: 10.1007/DCR.0b013e31819c96ac

[91] Garg P, Song J, Bhatia A, Kalia H, Menon GR. The efficacy of anal fistula plug in fistula-in-ano: A systematic review. Colorectal Disease. 2010;**12**(10):965-970. DOI: 10.1111/j.1463-1318.2009.01933.x

[92] Ellis CN. Outcomes with the use of bioprosthetic grafts to reinforce the ligation of the intersphincteric fistula tract (BioLIFT procedure) for the management of complex anal fistulas. Diseases of the Colon and Rectum. 2010;**53**(10):1361-1364. DOI: 10.1007/DCR.0b013e3181ec4470

[93] Han JG, Yi BQ, Wang ZJ, et al. Ligation of the intersphincteric fistula tract plus a bioprosthetic anal fistula plug (LIFT-plug): A new technique for fistula-in-ano. Colorectal Disease. 2013;**15**(5):582-586. DOI: 10.1111/codi.12062

[94] Van Eps JL. BIOlogic Augmented Repair of Complex Anal Fistula Using Acellular Matrix and/or Autologous Platelet-Rich Plasma (BIO RAMP): National Library of Medicine; 2023. Available from: clinicaltrials.gov

[95] Meinero P, Mori L. Video-assisted anal fistula treatment (VAAFT): A novel sphincter-saving procedure for treating complex anal fistulas. Techniques in Coloproctology. 2011;**15**(4):417-422

[96] Garg P, Singh P. Video-assisted anal fistula treatment (VAAFT) in Cryptoglandular fistula-in-ano: A systematic review and proportional meta-analysis. International Journal of Surgery. Elsevier Ltd. 2017;**46**:85-91

[97] Tian Z, Li YL, Nan SJ, Xiu WC, Wang YQ. Video-assisted anal fistula treatment for complex anorectal fistulas in adults: A systematic review and meta-analysis. Techniques in Coloproctology. 2022;**26**(10):783-795

[98] Zelić M, Karlović D, Kršul D, Bačić Đ, Warusavitarne J. Video-assisted anal fistula treatment for treatment of complex cryptoglandular anal fistulas with 2 years follow-up period: Our experience. Journal of Laparoendoscopic & Advanced Surgical Techniques. Part A. 2020;**30**(12):1329-1333

[99] Stazi A, Izzo P, D'Angelo F, Radicchi M, Mazzi M, Tomassini F, et al. Video-assisted anal fistula treatment in the management of complex anal fistula: A single-center experience. Minerva Chirurgica. 2018;**73**(2):142-150

[100] Romaniszyn M, Walega P. Video-assisted anal fistula treatment: Pros and

cons of this minimally invasive method for treatment of perianal fistulas. Gastroenterology Research and Practice. 2017:1-7

[101] Emile SH, Elfeki H, Shalaby M, Sakr A. A systematic review and meta-analysis of the efficacy and safety of video-assisted anal fistula treatment (VAAFT). Surgical Endoscopy. 2018;**32**(4):2084-2093

[102] Liu H, Tang X, Chang Y, Li A, Li Z, Xiao Y, et al. Comparison of surgical outcomes between video-assisted anal fistula treatment and fistulotomy plus seton for complex anal fistula: A propensity score matching analysis—retrospective cohort study. International Journal of Surgery. 2020;**75**:99-104

[103] Meinero P, Mori L, Gasloli G. Video-assisted anal fistula treatment: A new concept of treating anal fistulas. Diseases of the Colon and Rectum. 2014;**57**(3):354-359

[104] Kochhar G, Saha S, Andley M, Kumar A, Saurabh G, Pusuluri R, et al. Video-assisted anal fistula treatment. Journal of the Society of Laparoendoscopic Surgeons. 2014;**18**(3):1-5

[105] Mei Z, Li Y, Wang Q, Shao Z, Du P, Zhu J, et al. Risk factors for postoperative recurrence of anal fistula identified by an international, evidence-based Delphi consultation survey of surgical specialists. International Journal of Surgery. 2021;**92**:106038

[106] Wilhelm A. A new technique for sphincter-preserving anal fistula repair using a novel radial emitting laser probe. Techniques in Coloproctology. 2011;**15**(4):445-449

[107] Lunniss PJ, Sheffield JP, Talbot IC, Thomson JP, Phillips RK. Persistence of idiopathic anal fistula may be related to epithelialization. The British Journal of Surgery. 1995;**82**(1):32-33. DOI: 10.1002/bjs.1800820112

[108] Elfeki H, Shalaby M, Emile SH, Sakr A, Mikael M, Lundby L. A systematic review and meta-analysis of the safety and efficacy of fistula laser closure. In: Techniques in Coloproctology. Vol. 24. New York: Springer; 2020. pp. 265-274

[109] Frountzas M, Stergios K, Nikolaou C, Bellos I, Schizas D, Linardoutsos D, et al. Could FiLaCTM be effective in the treatment of anal fistulas? A systematic review of observational studies and proportional meta-analysis. Colorectal Disease. 2020;**22**(12):1874-1884

[110] Wilhelm A, Fiebig A, Krawczak M. Five years of experience with the FiLaCTM laser for fistula-in-ano management: Long-term follow-up from a single institution. Techniques in Coloproctology. 2017;**21**(4):269-276

[111] Cao D, Li W, Ji Y, Wang X, Cui Z. Efficacy and safety of FiLaCTM for perianal fistulizing Crohn's disease: A systematic review and meta-analysis. In: Techniques in Coloproctology. Vol. 26. Berlin: Springer Science and Business Media Deutschland GmbH; 2022. pp. 775-781

[112] Giamundo P, Esercizio L, Geraci M, Tibaldi L, Valente M. Fistula-tract laser closure (FiLaCTM): Long-term results and new operative strategies. Techniques in Coloproctology. 2015;**19**(8):449-453

[113] Wolicki A, Jäger P, Deska T, Senkal M. Sphincter-saving therapy for fistula-in-ano: Long-term follow-up after FiLaC®. Techniques in Coloproctology. 2021;**25**(2):177-184

[114] Lauretta A, Falco N, Stocco E, Bellomo R, Infantino A. Anal fistula laser closure: The length of fistula is the Achilles' heel. Techniques in Coloproctology. 2018;**22**(12):933-939

[115] Giamundo P, Geraci M, Tibaldi L, Valente M. Closure of fistula-in-ano with laser - FiLaCTM: An effective novel sphincter-saving procedure for complex disease. Colorectal Disease. 2014;**16**(2):110-115

[116] Tümer H, Bulbuloglu GC. A comparison of laser and fistulotomy techniques in the treatment of fistula-in-ano. Cureus. 2023;**15**(4):e37053

[117] Schurr MO, Arezzo A, Ho CN, Anhoeck G, Buess G, Di Lorenzo N. The OTSC clip for endoscopic organ closure in NOTES: Device and technique. Minimally Invasive Therapy and Allied Technologies. 2008;**17**(4):262-266

[118] Albert JG, Friedrich-Rust M, Woeste G, Strey C, Bechstein WO, Zeuzem S, et al. Benefit of a clipping device in use in intestinal bleeding and intestinal leakage. Gastrointestinal Endoscopy. 2011;**74**(2):389-397

[119] Prosst RL, Joos AK. Short-term outcomes of a novel endoscopic clipping device for closure of the internal opening in 100 anorectal fistulas. Techniques in Coloproctology. 2016;**20**(11):753-758

[120] Prosst R. Minimally invasive surgical clip closure of anorectal fistulas: Current status of OTSC proctology. Minimally Invasive Therapy and Allied Technologies. 2019;**28**(5):261-267

[121] Mennigen R, Laukötter M, Senninger N, Rijcken E. The OTSC® proctology clip system for the closure of refractory anal fistulas. Techniques in Coloproctology. 2015;**19**(4):241-246

Chapter 14

Oral Catechins and Epicatechins as a Treatment Modality for Hemorrhoids

Bhupesh Dewan, Siddheshwar Shinde and Shweta Kondekar

Abstract

Hemorrhoids, a prevalent medical condition impacting millions globally, frequently necessitate effective yet minimally invasive treatment methods. This review delves into the prospects of utilizing oral catechins and epicatechins, naturally occurring polyphenolic compounds present in diverse dietary sources, as an innovative avenue for addressing hemorrhoids. These compounds have antioxidant and anti-inflammatory attributes, which may help alleviate hemorrhoid symptoms. An understanding of the anatomy and pathophysiology of hemorrhoids, emphasizing the need for accessible and versatile treatment options. Subsequently, the focus turns to a detailed exploration of catechin and epicatechin, encompassing their chemical composition, natural origins, and mechanism of action. The core of this review presents a comprehensive analysis of the existing literature, including randomized controlled trials that examine the efficacy of oral catechin and epicatechin supplementation in alleviating hemorrhoidal symptoms. To conclude, this article highlights the potential of oral catechin and epicatechin supplementation as a non-invasive and natural approach to managing hemorrhoids. While promising findings have emerged, further research is essential to solidify their role in hemorrhoid treatment. The comprehensive assessment of existing literature and critical evaluation of these compounds' mechanism of action provides valuable insights into their viability as a treatment modality for this common and often distressing medical concern.

Keywords: hemorrhoids, polyphenolic compounds, catechins, epicatechins, antioxidant, anti-inflammatory

1. Introduction

Anorectal disorders constitute a diverse group of medical conditions that affect the complex anatomical and physiological structures of the anorectal region. These disorders encompass a wide range of conditions, including hemorrhoids, perianal pruritus, anal fissures, functional rectal pain, perianal abscess, condyloma, rectal prolapse, and fecal incontinence among others [1]. Collectively, it can lead to significant discomfort, impaired quality of life, and even life-threatening complications if not promptly and effectively managed.

Despite their prevalence and clinical significance, anorectal disorders remain an under-discussed and often stigmatized area of medical research.

The anorectal region serves critical functions in the human body, including fecal continence, waste elimination, and gas control. Dysfunction in this region can result from various factors, including genetic predisposition, lifestyle choices, and underlying medical conditions. While some anorectal disorders are acute and self-limiting, others can develop into chronic conditions that require complex and multidisciplinary approaches to treatment.

The exploration of anorectal disorders presents a unique challenge due to the intricate interplay between biological, psychological, and sociocultural factors. As such, comprehensive research is essential to unravel the underlying causes, mechanisms, and effective management strategies for these disorders. This review article aims to delve into the intricacies of anorectal disorders, shedding light on their etiology, clinical presentation, diagnostic approaches, and a spectrum of treatment options. By synthesizing existing knowledge, this paper seeks to contribute to a deeper understanding of anorectal disorders and to stimulate further research in this important yet often overlooked field.

In the subsequent sections, we will discuss the prevalence of anorectal disorders, elucidate the anatomical and physiological basis of these disorders, examine the intricate web of contributing factors, and explore therapeutic interventions. By addressing these aspects, we hope to provide clinicians, researchers, and healthcare professionals with a comprehensive resource to enhance their ability to diagnose, treat, and manage anorectal disorders effectively. Moreover, this research aims to foster greater awareness and destigmatization of anorectal disorders, encouraging individuals to seek timely medical attention and ultimately improve their overall well-being.

2. Pathophysiology of hemorrhoids

The pathophysiology of hemorrhoids involves a complex interplay of vascular, mechanical, and anatomical factors that contribute to the enlargement and swelling

Pathophysiological theories of hemorrhoids	Description
Vascular theory	Weakening of connective tissue supporting anal cushions leads to blood vessel engorgement.
Increased venous pressure	Elevated intra-abdominal pressure from straining or constipation causes vein dilation.
Congenital weakness	Genetic predisposition to weak blood vessel walls and connective tissue in the anal area.
Dysfunction of smooth muscle	Abnormalities in smooth muscle function result in blood vessel dilation and pooling.
Inflammation and microtrauma	Chronic inflammation or repeated microtrauma from bowel movements leads to vascular congestion.
Genetic and hereditary factors	Family history suggests a genetic susceptibility to weakened blood vessels and tissue.

Table 1.
Key mechanisms in pathophysiological theories.

of blood vessels within the anal canal and rectum. Hemorrhoids are thought to originate primarily from the vascular cushions present within the anal canal, which play a crucial role in maintaining anal continence and preventing leakage of stool and gas. Several risk factors, including pregnancy, elderly age, constipation, chronic diarrhea, and internal rectal prolapse, have been reported to be associated with the formation of hemorrhoids [2]. While the exact etiology remains multifactorial and not fully elucidated, several key mechanisms have been proposed in **Table 1**.

3. Current management of hemorrhoids

The management of hemorrhoids spans from making adjustments to one's diet and lifestyle to undergoing extensive surgery, with the chosen approach contingent upon the extent and seriousness of the symptoms. Treatments can be grouped into three categories namely conservative, office-based, and surgical [3].

3.1 Lifestyle modification

Lifestyle modifications and dietary factors should be advised as primary and preventive measures for patients with any degree of hemorrhoids. They are as follows: [2, 4, 5]

- Increase in the dietary fiber consumption
- Ensure adequate water and fluid intake
- Reduce the consumption of fat
- Warm sitz bath is recommended
- Daily physical exercise for 20–30 minutes
- Maintain proper anal hygiene
- Sit on the toilet with resting feet six-inch high from surface
- Abstain straining and reading on the toilet
- Avoid medicines that cause constipation or diarrhea

3.2 Fiber supplement

The recommended intake of dietary fiber for adults is 25 g/day (women) to 30 g/day (men) [6]. Fiber helps in maintaining stool consistency, preventing it from becoming overly hard or loose [7]. Fiber supplementation has shown an effective beneficial effect in the treatment of symptomatic hemorrhoids. In studies with multiple intervals of follow-up, results indicated positive outcomes associated with fiber supplementation concerning issues like prolapse, pain, and itching [8].

3.3 Non-operative treatment

3.3.1 Sclerotherapy

Sclerotherapy, using agents like phenol in oil, vegetable oil, quinine, or hypertonic salt solution, is a recommended treatment for first and second-degree hemorrhoids. The precise injection into the submucosa at the hemorrhoidal tissue aims to induce fibrosis, fixing the mucosa to the underlying muscle [2].

3.3.2 Rubber band ligation

Rubber band ligation is an effective treatment for first- and second-degree hemorrhoids as well as a few cases of third-degree hemorrhoids. Reduced blood supply causes ischemic necrosis and subsequent scarring of the hemorrhoidal tissue, ending in fixation to the rectal wall. Multiple anal locations can be treated at once. Severe pain can be avoided by carefully placing the band, particularly near the dentate line. Sitz baths and analgesics may help in alleviating the pain [2].

4. Need for a natural alternative

The need for an oral dietary supplement for the treatment of hemorrhoids arises from several key factors and considerations in the management of this common and often uncomfortable medical condition:

Prevalence and impact: hemorrhoids are highly distressing and frequently observed an anorectal condition, involving half of the population at some stage in their lives [9]. This high prevalence underscores the need for accessible and effective treatment options.

Variability in severity: hemorrhoids can range from mild discomfort to severe pain and bleeding. Most common complications vary from heavy bleeding, chronic unremitting prolapse of mucosal tissue, and ulceration, to thrombosis [10]. Despite centuries of treating this condition, its precise etiology is unclear and thus, a definitive treatment has yet to be established [11]. The severity of symptoms varies among individuals, and treatment should be tailored to the specific needs of each patient. An oral dietary supplement can provide a non-invasive and potentially versatile option for a wide range of patients.

Minimizing invasiveness: many treatment options are proposed for the management of hemorrhoids. Dietary interventions, lifestyle modification and medication treatment are adopted but surgical procedures or office-based interventions such as rubber band ligation are normally utilized [11]. These can be painful and associated with potential complications. Many patients thus prefer less invasive treatment options that can be administered orally.

Managing chronic symptoms: hemorrhoids can become a chronic condition for some individuals, requiring long-term management. An oral supplement may offer the advantage of sustained and convenient treatment over extended periods, potentially reducing the recurrence of symptoms.

Holistic approach: many times, patients are interested in holistic and natural approaches to healthcare. Dietary supplements made from natural compounds like catechin, epicatechin, etc. align with this preference for non-pharmaceutical, plant-based interventions.

Potential health benefits beyond hemorrhoids: these dietary supplements often contain bioactive compounds with broader health benefits. Catechin and epicatechin, for example, are known for their antioxidant and anti-inflammatory properties and may provide additional health advantages, making them attractive options for individuals looking to enhance overall well-being.

Patient preferences: patient preferences and adherence to treatment regimens are crucial for successful outcomes. An oral dietary supplement is typically more convenient and easier to incorporate into daily life than other treatment modalities.

In conclusion, the need for an oral dietary supplement for the treatment of hemorrhoids is driven by the desire to provide patients with effective, non-invasive, and versatile options for managing this prevalent and sometimes chronic condition. Such supplements have the potential to address underlying causes, reduce the invasiveness of treatment, and align with patients' preferences for holistic and natural approaches to healthcare.

5. Naturally available phytochemicals

Hemorrhoids involve the initiation of physiological and pathological changes by free radicals. Antioxidants play a key role in managing hemorrhoids by neutralizing these free radicals, contributing to their eradication. A vital but often overlooked aspect of therapy for hemorrhoids is the use of botanical and nutritional approaches. Herbal medicines have shown efficacy in enhancing vascular tone, microcirculation in the perivascular amorphous substrate, strengthening connective tissue, and improving capillary flow [12].

Moreover, herbal extracts containing phyto-antioxidants such as polyphenols, flavonoids, tannins, and related compounds are recognized for their favorable impact on health, leading to a decreased occurrence of diseases. Consequently, there is a considerable emphasis on exploring natural antioxidants, aiming to deliver substantial health advantages with minimal associated toxicities [13].

5.1 Phytochemicals used in the treatment of hemorrhoids

Based on different chemical structural groups, phytochemicals are categorized into phenolics, flavonoids, alkaloids, plant steroids, terpenes, lignans, saponins and glycosides.

Flavonoids, known for their antioxidant, anti-inflammatory, anti-mutagenic, and anti-carcinogenic properties, are associated with a diverse range of health-enhancing effects. They serve as essential components in various applications, including nutraceuticals, pharmaceuticals, medicinal products, and cosmetics.

5.1.1 Flavonoids

Flavonoids, naturally occurring compounds with different phenolic contents, are present in bark, roots, stems, flowers, and fruits. The different flavonoids like flavones, isoflavones, neoflavonoids flavonols, flavanones, flavanonols, flavanols or catechins, and anthocyanins, are categorized based on their ring position. The antioxidant activity of the flavonoids is related to the degree of unsaturation, and oxidation of the rings [14].

Flavonoids like proanthocyanidins comprising catechins and epicatechins have Flavanols, a subgroup of flavonoids, present as stereoisomers in cis or trans configuration [(−)-epicatechin (cis) and (+)-catechin], have been reported with free radical scavenging, antioxidant, anti-inflammatory and anti-allergic activity [15]. A meta-analysis of flavonoids for hemorrhoidal treatment suggested that flavonoids decreased the risk of bleeding, persistent pain and itching, and also reduced the recurrence rate [16].

5.1.2 Catechin and epicatechin

Proanthocyanidins are a type of flavonoids that include procyanidins [17]. They are oligomeric flavonoids and polymers of flavan-3-ols, mainly catechin and epicatechin [18].

Catechins, diverse isoforms of polyphenol compounds within the flavonoid family, consist of two steric forms: (+)-catechin and its enantiomer. These include compounds like epigallocatechin gallate, epigallocatechin, and epicatechin gallate [19].

Currently, catechin and epicatechin have garnered significant interest due to their status as non-toxic, plant-derived natural antioxidants that effectively neutralize free radicals within the human body [20].

5.2 How do they act?

Flavonoids are a group of plant compounds known for their antioxidant properties. Research suggests that various types of flavonoids, including flavones and catechins, exhibit strong antioxidant activity, and protect the body against reactive oxygen species [14]. Proanthocyanidins (catechins and epicatechins) may act via the following mechanisms:

- Proanthocyanidins crosslink the collagen fibers in the vessel basement membranes which makes them stronger and less permeable.

- The proanthocyanidins or monomeric catechins increase plasma antioxidant activity and also show beneficial effects on capillary fragility and permeability.

- Inhibition of enzymes such as hyaluronidase, elastase and collagenase which degrade the connective tissue leads to increased capillary permeability.

- Proanthocyanidins prevent the release and synthesis of compounds associated with inflammation and allergies such as histamine, serine proteases, prostaglandins and leukotrienes.

- They carry vitamin C to the basement membranes which leads to increased production of collagen making vessels (veins) strong.

5.3 Published literature

Throughout history, the community has relied on traditional remedies derived from plants and herbs to address hemorrhoids. The World Health Organization promotes the exploration of herbal medicines rooted in traditional wisdom [21]. Nevertheless, for these herbal treatments to gain acceptance within modern medicine, they must be substantiated by scientific evidence. The comprehensive details of natural sources and their phytochemical activity in hemorrhoids are given in **Table 2**.

Sr. no.	Plant name	Phytoconstituents	Pharmacological activity
1	*Achillea biebersteinii Afan* [22]	Flavonoids, tannins	Antioxidant
2	*Achillea millefolium L.* [23]	Flavonoids, tannins	Antispasmodic, anti-inflammatory, anti-hemorrhoidal
3	*Achillea wilhelmsii K.Koch* [3]	Flavonoids, tannins	Antioxidant, anti-inflammatory
4	*Anthemis austriaca Jacq* [5]	Flavonoids	Antioxidant
5	*Anthemis pseudocotula Boiss* [8]	Tannins, Flavonoids	Antioxidant and Anti-inflammatory
6	*Arum balansanum R.R. Mill* [24]	Alkaloids, polyphenols, glycosides (flavonoids, saponin and cyanogenic groups), monoterpenes, sesquiterpenes, lectin	Anti-hemorrhoidal
7	*Arum elongatum steven ssp.* [24]	Alkaloids, polyphenols, glycosides (flavonoids, saponin and cyanogenic groups), monoterpenes, sesquiterpenes, lectin	Anti-hemorrhoidal
8	*Arum maculatum L.* [25]	Alkaloids, polyphenols, glycosides (flavonoids, saponin and cyanogenic groups), monoterpenes, sesquiterpenes, lectin	Anti-hemorrhoidal
9	*Commiphora molmol* [26]	Flavonoids	Anti-inflammatory, anti-hemorrhoidal
10	*Commiphora mukul* [27]	Flavonoids, terpenes, phytosterols	Anti-hemorrhoidal, astringent antiseptic, anti-inflammatory, demulcent
11	*Dracunculus vulgaris Schott* [28]	Saponins, tannins, Flavonoids	Treatment of hemorrhoids
12	*Eryngium campestre L.* [29]	Flavonoid	Anti-hemorrhoidal
13	*Gardenia gummifera* [30]	Flavonoids	Antioxidant, anti-inflammatory
14	*Mesua ferrea* [31]	Flavonoids	Anti-inflammatory, anti-ulcer, and anti-microbial
15	*Opopanax hispidus Friv. Gris* [32]	Flavonoids	Antioxidant, anti-hemorrhoidal
16	*Petroselinum crispum Miller* [33]	Flavonoids	Antioxidant, anti-inflammatory
17	*Sambucus ebulus L* [34, 35]	Flavonoids, Tannins	Antioxidant, anti-inflammatory, anti-hemorrhoidal
18	*Sambucus nigra L.* [36]	Flavonoids	Anti-hemorrhoidal
19	*Tagetes erecta* [37]	Flavonoids	Wound healing, antioxidant, analgesic

Table 2.
Natural sources and their phytochemical activity in hemorrhoids.

6. Conclusion

Anorectal disorders, including hemorrhoids, pose a significant medical challenge due to their impact on quality of life and the complex interplay of biological, psychological, and sociocultural factors. Hemorrhoids, a common condition affecting the anal canal's blood vessels, are associated with oxidative stress, making natural antioxidants like flavonoids, catechins, and epicatechins an appealing treatment option.

This review emphasizes the need for a natural alternative in hemorrhoid treatment, focusing on the potential of phytochemicals to combat oxidative stress. In summary, these natural antioxidants show promise in alleviating hemorrhoidal symptoms and improving anal canal health, offering a valuable addition to treatment options for this common condition.

Conflict of interest

The authors declare no conflict of interest.

Author details

Bhupesh Dewan*, Siddheshwar Shinde and Shweta Kondekar
Zuventus Healthcare Limited, Mumbai, Maharashtra, India

*Address all correspondence to: bhupesh.dewan@zuventus.com

IntechOpen

© 2024 The Author(s). Licensee IntechOpen. This chapter is distributed under the terms of the Creative Commons Attribution License (http://creativecommons.org/licenses/by/3.0), which permits unrestricted use, distribution, and reproduction in any medium, provided the original work is properly cited.

References

[1] Cohee MW, Hurff A, Gazewood JD. Benign anorectal conditions: Evaluation and management. American Family Physician. 2020;**101**(1):24-33

[2] Lohsiriwat V. Anatomy, physiology, and pathophysiology of hemorrhoids. In: Ratto C, Parello A, Litta F, editors. Hemorrhoids. Coloproctology. Vol. 2. Cham: Springer; 2018. pp. 9-17. DOI: 10.1007/978-3-319-53357-5_2

[3] Altundag E, Ozturk M. Ethnomedicinal studies on the plant resources of East Anatolia, Turkey. Procedia Social and Behavioral Sciences. 2011;**19**:756-777. DOI: 10.1016/j.sbspro.2011.05.195

[4] De Marco S, Tiso D. Lifestyle and risk factors in hemorrhoidal disease. Frontier in Surgery. 2021;**8**:729166. Published 2021 Aug 18. DOI: 10.3389/fsurg.2021.729166

[5] Simsek I, Aytekin F, Yesilada E, et al. An ethnobotanical survey of the beypazari, ayas, and Güdül district towns of Ankara Province (Turkey). Economic Botany. 2004;**58**:705-720. DOI: 10.1663/0013-0001(2004)058[0705:AESOTB]2.0.CO;2

[6] ICMR NIN-Nutrient requirements for Indians. Available from: https://www.nin.res.in/RDA_short_Report_2020.html

[7] Davids JS, Ridolfi TJ. Hemorrhoids. In: Steele SR, Hull TL, Hyman N, Maykel JA, Read TE, Whitlow CB, editors. The ASCRS Textbook of Colon and Rectal Surgery. Cham: Springer; 2022. DOI: 10.1007/978-3-030-66049-9_11

[8] Boukhary R, Aboul-Ela M, El-Lakany A. Review on chemical constituents and biological activities of genus *Anthemis*. Pharmacognosy Journal. 2019, 2019;**11**(5):1155-1166. DOI: 10.5530/pj.2019.11.180

[9] Sheikh P, Mital K, Maheshwari U, Prabakaran J, Sharda P, Dumbre R. Clinical presentation of hemorrhoids and its correlation with chronic venous disease in India: A subgroup analysis of the international CHORUS survey. The Indian Journal of Surgery. 2021;**83**:513-521. DOI: 10.1007/s12262-020-02426-1

[10] Jacobs D. Clinical practice. Hemorrhoids: New England Journal of Medicine. 2014;**371**(10):944-951. DOI: 10.1056/NEJMcp1204188

[11] Hardy A, Chan CL, Cohen CR. The surgical management of haemorrhoids – A review. Digestive Surgery. 2005;**22** (1-2):26-33. DOI: 10.1159/000085343

[12] Chen M, Tang TC, He TH, Du YJ, Qin D, Zheng H. Management of haemorrhoids: Protocol of an umbrella review of systematic reviews and meta-analyses. BMJ Open. 2020;**10**(3):e035287. DOI: 10.1136/bmjopen-2019-035287

[13] Chiaretti M, Fegatelli DA, Pappalardo G, Venti MDS, Chiaretti AI. Comparison of Centella with flavonoids for treatment of symptoms in hemorrhoidal disease and after surgical intervention: A randomized clinical trial. Scientific Reports. 2020;**10**(1):8009. DOI: 10.1038/s41598-020-64772-0

[14] Panche AN, Diwan AD, Chandra SR. Flavonoids: An overview. Journal of Nutritional Science. 2016;**5**:e47. DOI: 10.1017/jns.2016.41

[15] Safe S, Jayaraman A, Chapkin RS, Howard M, Mohankumar K, Shrestha R. Flavonoids: Structure-function and

mechanisms of action and opportunities for drug development. Toxicology Research. 2021;**37**(2):147-162. DOI: 10.1007/s43188-020-00080-z

[16] Alonso-Coello P, Zhou Q, Martinez-Zapata MJ, et al. Meta-analysis of flavonoids for the treatment of haemorrhoids. The British Journal of Surgery. 2006;**93**(8):909-920. DOI: 10.1002/bjs.5378

[17] Sambasivam A, Sangameswaran K, Senthilkumar K, Sasirekha V. Theoretical investigation on the structure and antioxidant activity of (+) catechin and (−) epicatechin – A comparative study. Molecular Physics. 2020;**118**(17):1-12. DOI: 10.1080/00268976.2020.1745917

[18] Yu K, Dixon RA, Duan C. A role for ascorbate conjugates of (+)-catechin in proanthocyanidin polymerization. Nature Communications. 2022;**13**(3425):1-17. DOI: 10.1038/s41467-022-31153-2

[19] Kim JM, Heo HJ. The roles of catechins in regulation of systemic inflammation. Food Science and Biotechnology. 2022;**31**(8):957-970. DOI: 10.1007/s10068-022-01069-0

[20] Nie F, Liu L, Cui J, Zhao Y, Zhang D, Zhou D, et al. Oligomeric proanthocyanidins: An updated review of their natural sources, synthesis, and potentials. Antioxidants. 2023;**12**(5):1004. DOI: 10.3390/antiox12051004

[21] WHO. WHO Traditional Medicine Strategy: 2014-2023 [Internet]. 2023. Available from: https://www.who.int/publications/i/item/9789241506096 [Accessed: August 16, 2023]

[22] Özgen U, Kaya Y, Houghton P. Folk medicines in the villages of Ilıca District (Erzurum, Turkey). Turkish Journal of Biology. 2012;**36**:93-106. DOI: 10.3906/biy-1009-124

[23] Mahmoudi A, Seyedsadeghi M, Miran M, Ahari S, Layegh H, Mostafalou S. Therapeutic effect of Achillea millefolium on the hemorrhoids: A randomized double-blind placebo-controlled clinical trial. Journal of Herbal Medicine. 2023;**39**:100657. DOI: 10.1016/j.hermed.2023.100657

[24] Kozuharova E, Naychov Z, Kochmarov V, et al. The potential of Arum spp. as a cure for hemorrhoids: Chemistry, bioactivities, and application. Advance in Traditional MedICINE (ADTM). 2020;**20**:133-141. DOI: 10.1007/s13596-020-00425-x

[25] Serafeim Z, Giannakou K, Lavranos G, Lamnisos D. Alternative herbal medicine for hemorrhoids. Effect of *Arum maculatum* on the quality of life of patients: A randomized controlled trial. Journal of Applied Pharmaceutical Science. 2019;**9**(S1):40-45. DOI: 10.7324/JAPS.2019.S105

[26] Haffor AS. Effect of Commiphora Mukul; on leukocytes proliferation in relation to histological alterations before and during healing from injury. Saudi Journal of Biological Sciences. 2010;**17**(2):139-146. DOI: 10.1016/j.sjbs.2010.02.007

[27] Yousefi M, Mahdavi MR, Hosseini SM, et al. Clinical evaluation of Commiphora Mukul, a botanical resin, in the Management of Hemorrhoids: A randomized controlled trial. Pharmacognosy Magazine. 2013;**9**(36):350-356. DOI: 10.4103/0973-1296.117832

[28] Tuzlaci E, Aymaz PE. Turkish folk medicinal plants, Part IV: Gönen (Balikesir). Fitoterapia. 2001;**72**(4):323-343. DOI: 10.1016/s0367-326x(00)00277-x

[29] Soumia B. Chapter 7 - *Eryngium campestre* L.: Polyphenolic and flavonoid compounds; applications to health and disease. In: Watson RR, Preedy VR, Zibadi S, editors. Polyphenols: Mechanisms of Action in Human Health and Disease. 2nd ed. USA: Academic Press; 2018. pp. 69-79. DOI: 10.1016/B978-0-12-813006-3.00007-6

[30] Kekuda PT, Raghavendra HL, Shilpa M, Pushpavathi D, Petkar T, Siddiqha A. Antimicrobial, antiradical and insecticidal activity of Gardenia gummifera Lf (Rubiaceae). International Journal of Pharmacy and Pharmaceutical Sciences. 2017;**9**(10):265-272

[31] Tripathi RK, Bolegave SS, Shetty PA, et al. Efficacy and safety of a polyherbal formulation in hemorrhoids. Journal of Ayurveda Integrated Medicine. 2015;**6**(4):225-232. DOI: 10.4103/0975-9476.172382

[32] Tuzlacı E, Erol MK. Turkish folk medicinal plants. Part II: Eğirdir (Isparta). Fitoterapia. 1999;**70**(6):593-610

[33] Chauhan ES, Aishwarya J. Nutraceuticals potential of Petroselinum Crispum: A review. Journal of Complementary Medicine and Alternative Healthcare. 2018;**7**(2):1-6. DOI: 10.19080/JCMAH.2018.07.555707

[34] Shokrzade M, Saravi SSS. The chemistry, pharmacology and clinical properties of *Sambucus ebulus*: A review. Journal of Medicinal Plants Research. 2010;**4**(2):95-103. DOI: 10.5897/JMPR09.026

[35] Jabbari M, Daneshfard B, Emtiazy M, Khiveh A, Hashempur MH. Biological effects and clinical applications of Dwarf Elder (*Sambucus ebulus* L): A review. Journal of Evidence Based Complementary and Alternative Medicine. 2017;**22**(4):996-1001. DOI: 10.1177/2156587217701322

[36] Sargin SA, Selvi S, López V. Ethnomedicinal plants of Sarigöl district (Manisa), Turkey. Journal of Ethnopharmacology. 2015;**171**:64-84. DOI: 10.1016/j.jep.2015.05.031

[37] Priyanka D, Shalini T, Navneet VK. A brief study on marigold (Tagetes species): A review. International Research Journal of Pharmacy. 2013;**4**:43-48